Positive Prevention

Reducing HIV Transmission among People Living with HIV/AIDS

Positive Prevention
Reducing HIV Transmission among
People Living with HIV/AIDS

Edited by

Seth C. Kalichman

University of Connecticut
Storrs, CT

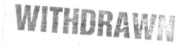

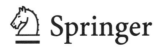 Springer

ISBN 0-306-48699-7

Springer Science+Business Media, Inc.
233 Spring Street, New York, New York 10013

Springeronline.com

10 9 8 7 6 5 4 3 2

A C.I.P. record for this book is available from the Library of Congress.

Permissions for books published in Europe: permissions @ wkap.nl
Permissions for books published in the United States of America: permissions @ wkap.com

Printed in the United States of America

This book is dedicated to Sydney, Rita, Moira, and Hannah Fay Kalichman, my sources of inspiration.

Contributors

Shalini Bharat, Tata Institute of Social Sciences, Mumbai

Heiner C. Bucher, University Hospital Basel, Switzerland

Nicole Crepaz, Centers for Disease Control and Prevention

Maria Ekstrand, University of California San Francisco

Jonathan Elford, City University, London

Amy Elkavich, Center for HIV Identification, Prevention, and Treatment Services, Department of Psychiatry University of California, Los Angeles

Jeffrey D. Fisher, Center for Health/HIV Intervention and Prevention, University of Connecticut

William A. Fisher, University of Western Ontario and Center for Health/HIV Intervention and Prevention

Diane Flannery, Center for HIV Identification, Prevention, and Treatment Services, Department of Psychiatry University of California, Los Angeles

Andrea Fogarty, University of New South Wales, Australia

Rise Goldstein, Center for HIV Identification, Prevention, and Treatment Services, Department of Psychiatry University of California, Los Angeles

Lauren K. Gooden, University of Miami School of Medicine

Christopher Gordon, National Institute of Mental Health

Robert S. Janssen, Centers for Disease Control and Prevention

Ida M. Onorato, Centers for Disease Control and Prevention

Patricia Jones, Center for HIV Identification, Prevention, and Treatment Services, Department of Psychiatry University of California, Los Angeles

Susan M. Kiene, Center for Health/HIV Intervention and Prevention, University of Connecticut

Susan Kippax, University of New South Wales, Australia

Lisa R. Metsch, University of Miami School of Medicine

David W. Pantalone, University of Washington

Jeffrey T. Parsons, Hunter College and the Graduate Center of the City University of New York

Thomas L. Patterson, Department of Psychiatry, University of California, San Diego

David W. Purcell, Centers for Disease Control and Prevention

Jayashree Ramakrishna, National Institute of Mental Health and Neurosciences in Bangalore

Patrick Rawstorne, University of New South Wales, Australia

Mary Jane Rotheram-Borus, Center for HIV Identification, Prevention, and Treatment Services, Department of Psychiatry University of California, Los Angeles

Leckness C. Simbayi, Human Sciences Research Council, Cape Town South Africa

Jane M. Simoni, University of Washington

Steffanie A. Strathdee, Division of International Health and Cross Cultural Medicine, Department of Family and Preventive Medicine, University of California, San Diego

Paul Van de Ven, University of New South Wales, Australia

Lance S. Weinhardt, Center for AIDS Intervention Research, Medical College of Wisconsin

Richard J. Wolitski, Centers for Disease Control and Prevention

Foreword

Acknowledgments: This foreword was aided by a meeting sponsored by the NIMH and CDC to overview state-of-the-science interventions, which was held in conjunction with the 2003 National HIV Prevention Conference in Atlanta.
Note: The views expressed in this foreword do not necessarily represent those of the National Institute of Mental Health nor any other agency of the federal government.

It is rare for edited scientific texts to be as timely as this one. Each section addresses pivotal issues in HIV prevention with positive persons, new data are presented, and innovative recommendations are offered. The chapters cover the prevention priority areas outlined by the CDC (Janssen et al., 2001; Wolitski et al. in this volume), which are supported by the relevant divisions and centers of the National Institutes of Health (NIH) and the Health Resources and Services Administration. In addition to detailed interpretation of available data, the chapter authors are adept at framing important research directions, which aids my task. I will identify the most critical "positive prevention" issues. When possible, I offer my comments with reference to the categories of the domestic prevention initiative; namely, reduction of barriers to early HIV diagnosis and increased access to, utilization of, and adherence to quality medical care, HIV treatment, and prevention services. In my position as a program officer for HIV prevention and treatment adherence at the National Institute of Mental Health, I am privileged to work with many careful thinkers, so I thank them in advance for stimulating these ideas, both informally and formally.

The need for targeted interventions for persons living with HIV is becoming acute due both to our fiscal environment and to the shift in federal prevention strategy described in the first Chapter. There is a finite pool of resources for research and implementation that is competing with an expanding set of recommendations for how these monies should be allocated. Ideally, all of the questions identified in this book could be answered. In reality, research initiatives need to be triaged, and efforts to prioritize are often inextricably linked with cost-effectiveness concerns. Funders, researchers and providers must grapple with the complexities of sexual behavior, relationships, and HIV risk-reduction, and balance this understanding with practical realities that call for feasible models for change—that is, for interventions to be cheaper and briefer to implement. This challenge can be daunting when multiple factors and levels of influence may be associated with risk behavior (e.g., drug use, poverty, stigma, racism, unstable housing, disparate access to prevention and treatment systems).

In terms of early HIV diagnosis, Weinhardt in this book and others (e.g., Crepaz and Marks, 2002) have underscored the importance of HIV serostatus knowledge for risk reduction. We know that the majority of persons who learn their HIV-positive serostatus take measures to reduce risk for themselves and others. However, the field has yet to fully capitalize on this process through theory and intervention development to understand and sustain these changes. Data presented by Weinhardt preliminarily suggests that initial risk-reduction may be followed by a subsequent rebound to pre-testing risk levels for some individuals. Moreover, although there have been numerous studies of factors associated with a decision to get tested for HIV, there are relatively fewer studies of interventions to increase HIV-testing rates. The paucity of studies in this area is particularly troubling because the huge problem of ethnic health disparities for HIV testing (and treatment access) remains poorly understood. It is imperative that our research, policy and interventions begin to close the gaps that are responsible for delay in testing and access to treatment among minority populations, especially women of color. Individual, structural, and social factors likely contribute to these disparities, and interventions to reduce HIV stigma as a barrier to HIV-testing are rare. Parsons highlights the need for more creative approaches to testing and prevention that target relatively untapped risk venues for gay and bisexual HIV-positive and HIV-negative men. The CDC has also recommended to routinize HIV testing in some settings, and early model programs suggest that these programs can be cost-effective and lead to follow-up HIV care (Walensky et al., in press).

These approaches may reduce some barriers to HIV testing, but we also lack critical information about how individuals navigate through the public and private health care system in order to get tested for HIV, access medical care and HIV treatment (if necessary), access HIV prevention services (regardless of test results), and connect to other services that might accompany HIV treatment (e.g., mental health care, substance use treatment, and other supportive services). In communities that lack integrated systems of care, successful outcomes often rely on "referrals" that may require sophisticated knowledge and persistence on the part of patients and providers. Yet, we only have the most rudimentary notions about whether and how these linkages occur, what to do to increase their likelihood, and there is no overarching framework to guide HIV/AIDS service integration.

Once people living with HIV/AIDS are connected to a prevention or treatment setting, research can be enhanced throughout the intervention continuum—from development to dissemination, adaptation, and community/clinic adoption. As echoed by several chapter authors in this book, theoretical models tested for prevention interventions with HIV-positive persons have been largely limited to variants of social-cognitive theory. Although some trials incorporate contextual factors in conceptualizing interventions, most completed trials have utilized cognitive-behavioral skill-building interventions to target behavior change of individuals and small groups. This pattern of intervention development mirrors early generations of primary HIV prevention interventions for high-risk HIV-negative persons, and it suggests areas to further expand future interventions for HIV-positive persons—i.e., to focus more efforts on structural factors, community-level interventions, media, and multiple systems simultaneously. Several ongoing studies to reduce HIV-infections through other levels of influence have been launched, including modification of social/structural influences to reduce risk behavior, family- and couples-based prevention, coping, and adherence approaches, internet-based interventions, and mass media campaign evaluation.

To be clear, behavior change interventions for individuals still have an important place in the national HIV prevention plan. As Holtgrave (2004) has pointed out, perhaps only a minority of HIV-positive men and women actually may need more intensive services, but for these persons the individual level of attention may be critical. Individuals who are struggling with such problems as substance use, severe and persistent mental illness, relationship abuse, childhood sexual abuse, poverty, or transient housing may need to be referred to prevention case management or one of the efficacious interventions detailed in this volume. The efficacy and effectiveness of such programs for individuals struggling with multiple health and social problems continues to need careful study (Stall, et al., 2003). Although only a few efficacious interventions are currently in the literature, methodological descriptions and outcome data for several trials are pending publication (e.g., Wingood et al., in press; Purcell et al., in press; Rotheram-Borus et al., in press; Fisher et al., in press).

However, future prevention outcomes still depend on a fuller appreciation that HIV is transmitted in inherently relationship-driven contexts (Auerbach, in press). Very little research has investigated relational dynamics, condom use decision-making for both HIV transmission *and* acquisition when one partner is HIV-positive, intimacy, the ways that partnerships are affected by culture and more proximal social contexts, and the translation of these findings into effective interventions. In this volume, Simoni and Pantalone and Parsons speak to the importance of these questions, and to the relative dearth of studies in these areas.

The sustainability of intervention effects is also understudied. Successful prevention involves not only the initiation of behavior change but also maintenance over long periods of time. This is especially important for prevention with HIV-positive persons, given the long survival periods after initial HIV infection now achievable in the antiretroviral era. The simplest solution may be to recommend that the length of trials and the assessment intervals be extended, and there may be settings where this is appropriate, such as when a brief, one-time intervention may be all that is possible (e.g., during an emergency room visit). However, perhaps the conventional randomized controlled trial (RCT) design limits the range of questions that can be answered. Typically, a RCT entails an intervention period of specific frequency, duration, and intensity (usually with a closely prescribed intervention manual), followed by an assessment period to evaluate intervention efficacy. Alternative models have been proposed (e.g., Glasgow, et al., 2003) that may better capture factors that affect implementation. A more flexible design could allow for intervention features to be tailored to the needs of the individual or family, structure, or other target, and also permit the intervention to adapt and evolve based on changing needs. Process evaluation and outcome assessment would be ongoing. A useful example may be drawn from the integration of prevention messages with HIV medical care as described in this book, where routine brief risk assessments could cue a level of intervention that meets individual needs.

Finally, diffusion, translation, effectiveness and operational research should be high priorities in order to bridge research and practice. Metsch and colleagues present a novel overview of how community agencies and state HIV prevention planners (i.e., National Alliance of State and Territorial AIDS Directors) are responding to the challenge of HIV prevention with positive persons. They identify useful insights from those who attempt to deliver interventions that demonstrate efficacy in rigorous RCTs. It is clear that it is no longer sufficient to view the final stage of technology transfer as one of end-users waiting for an intervention package when a trial is completed. For prevention to stay ahead of an evolving epidemic, multi-agency and multi-sectoral cooperation is essential in all research phases. Contextual influences that are experienced by individuals in their organizations, cities, and clinics should be routinely communicated to researchers and funders to improve intervention effectiveness and inform future research. Although it is becoming more common for researchers to solicit input and conduct formative research with consumer/community members in intervention development, the degree and quality of this process varies widely.

Elkavich and her co-authors highlight the salience of this issue for interventions designed for young people living with HIV. As a field, we have not benefited from and applied principles of market research in the design and packaging of HIV prevention interventions.

Many other understudied issues for intervention effectiveness are likely to determine whether an intervention works outside of a RCT. What is the minimal and optimal assistance needed to help providers deliver interventions? In most cases, for the interventions that have demonstrated efficacy, skilled interventionists are a key component. Resource-intensiveness for intervention implementation appears to be a critical issue, yet rarely discussed in trial outcome reports. Some other research questions might include: What organizational factors are related to adoption and implementation of interventions and ongoing outcomes assessment? How much can interventions be tailored or adapted to suit local needs before intervention fidelity and/or effectiveness is lost?

Finally, in international settings, nearly all of the aforementioned priorities, and the calls for research described in this book, will be critical. Globally, it is imperative that we learn from lessons that accompanied improved treatments in the U.S., and develop and test proactive and systematic approaches to ensure that prevention and adherence messages are routinely provided to HIV-infected persons.

Christopher M. Gordon
National Institute of Mental Health
Center for Mental Health Research on AIDS

REFERENCES

Auerbach, J. D. (in press). Principles of positive prevention. *JAIDS*.

Crepaz, N., and Marks, G. (2002). Towards an understanding of sexual risk behavior in people living with HIV: a review of social, psychological, and medical findings. *AIDS:25*; 135–149.

Fisher, J. D., Cornman, D. H., Osbom, C. Y., Amico, K. R., Fisher, W. A., and Friedland, G. H. (in press). Clinician-initiated HIV-risk reduction intervention for HIV-positive persons: Formative research, acceptability, and fidelity of the Options project. *JAIDS*.

Glasgow, R. E., Lichtenstein, E., and Marcus, A. C. (2003). Why don't we see more translation of health promotion research to practice? Rethinking the efficacy-to-effectiveness transition. *Am J Pub Health: 93*; 1261–1267.

Holtgrave, D. R. (2004). Estimation of annual HIV transmission rates in the United States, 1978–2000. *JAIDS:35*; 89–92.

Janssen, R. S., Holtgrave, D. R., Valdiserri, R. O., Shepherd, M., Gayle, H. D., and De Cock, K. M. (2001). The Serostatus Approach to Fighting the HIV Epidemic: prevention strategies for infected individuals. *Am J Pub Health: 91*; 1019–1024.

Purcell, D., Metsch, L., Latka, M., Santibanez, S., Gomez, C., Eldred, L., Latkin, C., and the INSPIRE Team. (in press). INSPIRE: An integrated behavioral intervention with HIV-positive drug users to address medical care, adherence, and risk reduction. *JAIDS*.

Rotheram-Borus, M. J., Swendenmen, D., Comulada, W. S., Weiss, R., and Lightfoot, M. (in press). Prevention for substance using HIV positive young people: telephone and in-person delivery. *JAIDS*.

Stall, R., Mills, T. C., Williamson, J., Hart, T., Greenwood, G., Paul, J., Pollack, L., Binson, D., Osmond, D., and Catania, J. A. (2003). Association of co-occurring psychosocial health problems and increased vulnerability to HIV/AIDS among urban men who have sex with men. *Am J Pub Health: 93*; 939–942.

Walensky, R. P., Losina, E., Skolnik, P. R., Hall, J. M., Malatesta, L., Barton, G. E., O'Connor, C. A., McGuire, J. F., and Freedberg, K. A. (in press). Voluntary HIV testing as part of routine medical care—Massachusetts, 2002. *MMWR*.

Wingood, G. M., DiClemente, R. J., Mikhail, I., Lang, D. L., and Hardin, J. W. (in press). A Randomized controlled trial to reduce HIV transmission risk behaviors and STDs among women living with HIV: The *WiLLOW* program. *JAIDS*.

Preface

This book is meant to fill a gap in the HIV prevention literature. With few exceptions, behavioral scientists have conducted empirical studies on the sexual relationships of people living with HIV infection since 1996. Before then, such research was considered by some of the leading behavioral researchers as 'a political minefield'. Concerns that I recall hearing ranged from entering the unknown, straying from the traditional paths taken in HIV prevention, and potentially 'blaming the victim'. But so much changes in HIV/AIDS so too have views of HIV as a chronic illness and henceforth the legitimacy of asking people living with HIV about their sexual lives and behavior. This book aims to bring together this relatively young body of literature, with an emphasis on what is central to HIV transmission risk reduction interventions for people living with HIV/AIDS.

There are other books available on this topic and more are coming. Books that are based on the results of qualitative research, political discourse, and policy analysis offer those unique perspectives. This book, however, is meant to be empirically grounded. The question that I hoped could be answered here is "what do we know about the sexual and drug using risks for HIV transmission among people living with HIV/AIDS and what are the most promising avenues of interventions for addressing the risk reduction needs of people who know that are HIV positive?"

After some consideration, I came to the conclusion that this book would be better edited than written. All of the authors included in this volume have considerable expertise in their respective areas. The essential topics for this book are much better served by this array of authors than I could accomplish alone. The authors have been working extensively with HIV positive populations for years, in most cases long before it was popular to do so. I feel quite fortunate to have collaborated with such a remarkable group of scholars in formulating this book. For me, the authors of this volume represent the 'A' team; I called all of my first choices for authors for this book and they all said yes and they all delivered chapters. My hope was that the chapters could accomplish two things. First, the authors were asked to provide current thinking on aspects of HIV risk and risk reduction for people living with HIV in their respective areas of expertise. Second,

I asked the authors to focus on what they thought most important, most compelling, most exciting about their area. I decided against a uniform structure for the chapters and instead asked the authors to be innovative and creative. My hope was that the authors could convey their enthusiasm, resulting in interesting and exciting chapters. I believe that this goal was achieved.

I also asked the authors to include international aspects of HIV risk and risk reduction for people living with HIV/AIDS in their chapters. In some cases this was easier to achieve than others. In addition to including material that is internationally relevant within chapters, there is also a chapter dedicated to international perspectives. The International Perspectives chapter was a wonderful experience to edit. This chapter includes authors from Europe, Australia, India, and South Africa. It helps to place HIV prevention for people living with HIV/AIDS in a global context. Another unique feature of this book is its emphasis on risk reduction interventions for people living with HIV/AIDS. Every chapter includes information relevant to behavioral interventions to reduce risks among people living with HIV/AIDS. Because there have been fewer published risk reduction intervention studies for people living with HIV than there are chapters, some of the chapters foreshadow intervention trials that are in progress and even interventions that are in the pipeline. I believe that the goal of providing useful and practical information regarding interventions to assist people living with HIV/AIDS manage HIV transmission risks has also been achieved.

In addition to acknowledging my debt to the chapter authors for their contributions to this book, there are many others to whom I owe thanks. Bill Tucker at Kluwer approached me to consider editing this book, despite my inexperience as a book editor. I especially owe Bill thanks for giving me creative license, which allowed me to give the authors creative license. I also thank Tom Patterson for his early support in putting this book together as well as suggesting the importance of including an international perspective in the book. Tom's contributions to this book therefore extend well beyond his and Steffanie's own Chapter. I also thank Chris Gordon at NIMH for agreeing to write the Foreword to this book as well as his contributions to shaping this field. I am also indebted to Lisa Eaton for all of her hard work in assisting me with early copyediting and conforming the manuscript to Kluwer style. The final production of this book occurred in half the usual time because of Lisa's careful work. I also thank the V&A Waterfront and Frieda's Coffee shop in Cape Town South Africa for allowing me the space to do my final edits on the manuscript. I owe special thanks to Jeff Graham and the entire AIDS Survival Project in Atlanta for providing a home for our AIDS behavioral research and the more than

2500 people living with HIV/AIDS who have participated in our studies. Chauncey Cherry, Demteria Cain, Moira Kalichman, Howard Pope and the rest of the SHARE Project research team are also thanked for their countless contributions to this field. Finally, I should thank Hannah Kalichman for her inspiration. I dedicated my first book on AIDS to the hope that Hannah would grow up in a world without AIDS, a dream not realized but a hope not diminished.

SCK
Storrs, CT

Contents

Chapter One   An Overview of Prevention with People
Living with HIV 1
*Richard J. Wolitski, Robert S. Janssen, Ida
M. Onorato, David W. Purcell, and
Nicole Crepaz*
Introduction 1
Rationale for Prevention with People Living
with HIV/AIDS 2
Historical Overview 4
Elements of Prevention for People Living
with HIV/AIDS 6
Conclusions 17
References 20

Chapter Two   **HIV Diagnosis and Risk Behavior** 29
Lance S. Weinhardt
Introduction 29
"How Long Do Reductions in Risk Behavior
Persist Following an HIV Positive
Diagnosis?" 51
"What Needs to Be Done, in Practice and
Research, to Maximize the Beneficiam
Effects of an HIV Diagnosis on
Transmission Risk Behavior?" 54
Recommendations for Future Research 56
Conclusions 59
References 60

Chapter Three   **HIV Disclosure and Safer Sex** 65
Jane M. Simoni and David W. Pantalone
Introduction 65
Theoretical Considerations 69
Review of the Literature 71

Interpretation and Integration of Research
Findings 84
Implications for Research 85
Implications for Practice 89
Implications for Policy 92
Conclusions 93
References 94

Chapter Four   **HIV-Positive Gay and Bisexual Men** 99
Jeffrey T. Parsons
Introduction 99
Sexual Risk Behaviors of Gay and Bisexual
Men in the Third Decade of HIV/AIDS 100
Sexually Charged Environments 102
The Internet 108
Barebacking 114
Club Drugs 120
Conclusions 127
References 129

Chapter Five   **HIV-Positive and HCV-Positive Drug Users** 135
Steffanie A. Strathdee and Thomas L. Patterson
Introduction 135
The Epidemiology of HIV/AIDS among IDU
Populations 137
Behavioral Interventions for Injection Drug
Users 138
Applications to HCV-Seropositive IDUs 147
The Epidemiology of MSM Who Use Drugs 149
Conclusions 152
References 155

Chapter Six   **Young People Living with HIV** 163
*Amy Elkavich, Mary Jane Rotheram-Borus, Rise
Goldstein, Diane Flannery, and Patricia Jones*
Introduction 163
Epidemiology of HIV/AIDS among Young
People 164
Current Interventions Designed and
Evaluated 167
Organization of Care for YPLH 171
Goals 172

Theoretical Frameworks for Preventive
Interventions 173
Ethnographic Study of HIV Positive Youth 175
Teens Linked TRO Care—TLC 177
Intervention Delivery Formats 182
Adaptation of Evidence-Based Interventions 184
Conclusions 187
References 188

Chapter Seven   **Interventions in Community Settings** 193
Lisa R. Metsch, Lauren K. Gooden, and David W.
Purcell
Introduction 193
Tested Interventions Addressing Prevention
for People Living with HIV/AIDS 195
Current Practices Regarding Prevention with
HIV-Positive Persons in Community
Settings 200
Barriers to Implementing Prevention with
People Living with HIV/AIDS 203
Facilitators to Implementing Prevention with
People Living with HIV/AIDS 207
The Voices of People Living with HIV/AIDS 209
Resources for HIV/AIDS Prevention
Technology Transfer and Capacity
Building 210
Conclusions 213
References 214

Chapter Eight   **Interventions in Clinical Settings** 219
Susan M. Kiene, Jeffrey D. Fisher, and William A.
Fisher
Introduction 219
HIV Risk Behavior among People Living
with HIV/AIDS in Clinical Care 220
Priority to Develop Interventions for HIV
Positive Adults 221
Barriers to HIV Prevention in Clinical Settings ... 222
Effectiveness of Prevention Interventions in
Clinical Settings 225
Conclusions 237
References 238

Chapter Nine   **International Perspectives** 245
                Jonathan Elford, Heiner C. Bucher, Patrick
                Rawstorne, Andrea Fogarty, Paul Van de Ven,
                Susan Kippax, Maria Ekstrand, Shalini Bharat,
                Jayashree Ramakrishna, Leckness C. Simbayi,
                and Seth C. Kalichman
                Introduction 245
                United Kingdom: Jonathan Elford, City
                  University, London 246
                Switzerland: Heiner C. Bucher, University
                  Hospital Basel, Switzerland 253
                Australia: Patrick Rawstorne, Andrea
                  Fogarty, Paul Van de Ven, and Susan
                  Kippax, University of New South Wales,
                  Australia 256
                India: Maria Ekstrand, University of
                  California San Francisco, Shalini Bharat,
                  Tata Institute of Social Sciences, Mumbai,
                  Jayashree Ramakrishna, National Institute
                  of Mental Health and Neurosciences in
                  Bangalore 263
                South Africa: Leckness C. Simbayi, Human
                  Sciences Research Council, Cape Town
                  South Africa and Seth C. Kalichman,
                  University of Connecticut 268
                Conclusions 273
                References 274

Index 279

CHAPTER ONE

An Overview of Prevention with People Living with HIV

Richard J. Wolitski, Robert S. Janssen,
Ida M. Onorato, David W. Purcell, and
Nicole Crepaz

INTRODUCTION

Extraordinary progress has been made since the first few cases of acquired immune deficiency syndrome (AIDS) were identified in the United States in 1981. More than 20 years of intense research has yielded invaluable information about human immunodeficiency virus (HIV), the virus that causes AIDS, how it is transmitted, how infection can be prevented, and how at-risk persons can be motivated to protect themselves from HIV (Wolitski et al., 2004). Remarkable advances in the detection and treatment of HIV have significantly improved the quality of life for persons living with HIV and have reduced AIDS-related deaths (Karon et al., 2001). These successes have ushered in a new era in the AIDS epidemic. In this era, HIV infection that is detected early can be successfully managed with proper medical care, allowing the majority of HIV-seropositive persons to lead active and productive lives that may extend for decades (Egger et al., 2002; Porter et al., 2003).

Working effectively with people living with HIV to reduce the risk of HIV transmission has become even more important in this new era. As a result of treatment advances, the number of people living with HIV has grown considerably. It is estimated that there are now 850,000 to 950,000 persons living with HIV in the US (Fleming et al., 2002). This number is

1

likely to increase in coming years due to decreases in AIDS-related deaths and a stable rate of new HIV infections. Given that each person living with HIV has the ability to prevent new cases of HIV infection or to contribute to the spread of the virus, it is important to carefully consider the potential role of people living with HIV in changing the course of the epidemic. This chapter provides a rationale for prevention with people living with HIV/AIDS and reviews the emergence of this issue as a public health priority. It summarizes a comprehensive framework for HIV prevention that was developed by the Centers for Disease Control and Prevention (CDC) that aims to improve the health of HIV-seropositive persons and to prevent new cases of HIV infection. Effective interventions and strategies that fit within this framework are discussed. Issues and challenges in the development and implementation of prevention programs for people living with HIV are presented, and areas for future research are identified.

RATIONALE FOR PREVENTION WITH PEOPLE LIVING WITH HIV/AIDS

An estimated 40,000 people contract HIV each year in the US (Fleming et al., 2002), and recent evidence indicates that the number of new HIV diagnoses has increased in some communities (CDC, 2003d, 2004a). The major factors associated with these infections, and most other HIV infections in the US, are sexual contact and the sharing of contaminated needles, syringes, and other injection paraphernalia with a person living with HIV (CDC, 2004b). Approximately one-quarter of people living with HIV in the US do not know that they carry the virus (Fleming et al., 2002). It is not known with certainty how many new infections result from unsafe encounters with people who know that they are infected. One analysis suggests that a disproportionate percentage of new sexually transmitted HIV infections may be attributable to HIV-seropositive persons who are not aware of their serostatus (Marks et al., 2004). If true, this conclusion would be consistent with earlier estimates suggesting that the majority of HIV transmissions may take place during the first stages of infection when newly infected persons are highly viremic (Koopman et al., 1997).

Many people who test positive for HIV reduce or eliminate behaviors that can transmit HIV to others (Higgins et al., 1991; Weinhardt et al., 1999; Wolitski et al., 1997). This reduction is not absolute, however, and persons who initially adopt reduced risk practices may not sustain these changes for a lifetime (McGowan et al., 2004). Numerous studies have documented unprotected sex and syringe sharing among people who know that they are HIV seropositive (Ciccarone, et al., 2003; Crepaz and Marks, 2002; Kalichman, 2000; Kok, 1999; Marks et al., 1999; McGowan et al., 2004; Metsch et al., 1998; Schiltz and Sandfort, 2000). One review indicates that about one-third of persons with diagnosed HIV infection may engage in sexual practices that place others at risk for HIV (Kalichman, 2000), but the rates of unprotected sex reported in these studies vary widely due to differences in research methods, the specific behaviors and recall periods assessed, and whether the serostatus of sex partners was taken into account. Despite these differences, the conclusion from these studies is the same—the number of HIV-diagnosed men and women who report risky sex or injection practices is too large for public health to ignore.

The benefits of prevention with HIV-seropositive persons go beyond the potential of public health programs to prevent new cases of HIV infection. The reduction of unprotected sex and nonsterile drug injection protects people living with HIV from sexually transmitted infections (STIs), blood borne infections, and the possibility of HIV reinfection, all of which may adversely affect their health (Blackard et al., 2002; Filippini et al., 2001; O'Brien et al., 1999; Wiley et al., 2000). Programs for people living with HIV also may reduce the incidence of HIV-related disease and mortality by facilitating access to quality medical care and improving adherence to HIV treatment (Janssen et al., 2001). Timely and appropriate medical care can reduce HIV to levels that cannot be detected with current technology, prevent the development of opportunistic infections, and improve patients' quality of life (Sabin, 2002; Volberding, 2003). Mental health and social service programs improve the health and well-being of HIV-seropositive people by helping them cope with stresses of living with HIV, providing access to tangible resources (such as housing, meals, transportation, substance treatment, medications, and financial assistance) and facilitating entry and maintenance in medical care (Conviser and Pounds, 2002).

Communities also benefit from prevention programs that improve the health and well-being of HIV-seropositive people. Improving the health of people living with HIV benefits communities by helping families remain intact, reducing the needs of people living with HIV for acute medical care, and making it possible for HIV-seropositive men and women to remain productive and contributing members of society. Promoting access to care and adherence to antiretroviral therapy may also reduce HIV transmission rates by lowering viral load or affecting the transmission fitness of the virus (Brown et al., 2003; Janssen et al., 2001; Quinn et al., 2000). Thus, improved access and adherence to antiretroviral treatments among HIV-seropositive people may benefit the community as a whole by slowing the spread of HIV.

HISTORICAL OVERVIEW

Despite the strong rationale for prevention programs with HIV-seropositive persons, most HIV prevention efforts historically have focused on the general population or members of at-risk subgroups. With few exceptions, prevention services for HIV-seropositive persons were limited to the single session of post test counseling that was provided when they received their test results and assistance with notifying persons with whom they had sex or had shared injection equipment (partner counseling and referral services or PCRS). Although there were many support groups and social service programs for people living with HIV, few resources existed for those who struggled with maintaining safer sex and injection practices. A paper published in the *Journal of the American Medical Association* in 1989 promoted the integration of prevention messages with medical services for people living with HIV (Francis et al., 1989). Some programs did integrate prevention with medical and other services early in the epidemic, including interventions provided by California's Early Intervention Programs, the Plus Seminar sponsored by Los Angeles Shanti, and AIDS Survival Project's weekend retreats in Atlanta (AIDS Survival Project, 2004; California Department of Health Services, 2002; Francis et al.,1992; Los Angeles Shanti, n.d.).

It was not until highly active antiretroviral therapies (HAART) became available that the need for targeted prevention programs for HIV-seropositive persons began to be widely recognized. This recognition was precipitated by a number of influential events that foreshadowed the coming paradigm shift in HIV prevention. In 1995, two prominent AIDS activists wrote editorials that called into question community norms and prevention approaches that failed to address the responsibility of HIV-seropositive people to protect others (Rotello, 1995; Signorile, 1995). This debate was introduced in the professional literature in 1996 when a commentary was published in the *New England Journal of Medicine* that posed a series of pointed questions about the responsibility of HIV-seropositive people to prevent HIV transmission (Bayer, 1996). The lack of interventions for HIV-seropositive persons was recognized by the CDC, which made funds available for research leading to the development of risk reduction interventions for HIV-seropositive men who have sex with men (MSM) in 1996 (Wolitski et al., in press). The most important endorsement of the need for interventions for people living with HIV came in 1997 from a National

Institutes of Health consensus panel ("Interventions to Prevent HIV Risk Behaviors," 1997) that concluded:

"Programs must be developed to help individuals already infected with HIV to avoid risky sexual and substance behavior. This National priority will become more pressing as new biological treatments prolong life. Thus, prevention programs for HIV-positive people must have outcomes that can be maintained over long periods of time, in order to slow the spread of infection." (p. 28)

Another influential review addressed the need for prevention with HIV-seropositive persons, and specifically called for additional efforts to integrate prevention into medical care (Institute of Medicine, 2000). By 2000 a consensus had begun to emerge in the professional literature regarding the importance of prevention with people living with HIV/AIDS (e.g., Kok, 1999; Marks et al., 1999; Schiltz and Sandfort, 2000). What had not yet emerged was a clearly articulated plan for developing and implementing programs for people living with HIV.

In 2001, CDC announced a comprehensive strategy to prevention with HIV-seropositive persons (Janssen et al., 2001). The Serostatus Approach to Fighting the Epidemic (SAFE) defined a framework for prevention programs with people living with HIV that focused on 5 basic goals (see Table 1.1). These goals recognize the need to identify persons with undiagnosed HIV infection, ensure that persons diagnosed with HIV have access to high-quality medical and social services, and to motivate the adoption and maintenance of behaviors that reduce transmission of HIV and other STIs.

Two years later, CDC introduced the Advancing HIV Prevention (AHP) initiative, which included a significant allocation of public health resources to identify undiagnosed cases of HIV infection and further limit HIV transmission by persons living with HIV (CDC, 2003b). As shown in Figure 1.1, AHP introduced a new model for HIV prevention that includes prevention with persons living with HIV as one of three core elements of CDC's HIV prevention activities. In this model, efforts to reduce HIV

Table 1.1. Primary Goals of the CDC's Serostatus Approach to Fighting the Epidemic (SAFE)

1. Increase the number of HIV-infected persons who know their serostatus.
2. Increase the use of health care and preventive services among people diagnosed with HIV.
3. Increase high-quality care and treatment for people diagnosed with HIV.
4. Increase adherence to HIV therapy among persons diagnosed with HIV.
5. Increase the number of persons diagnosed with HIV who adopt and maintain behaviors that reduce the risk of HIV and STI transmission.

Source: Janssen, RS et al. (2001).

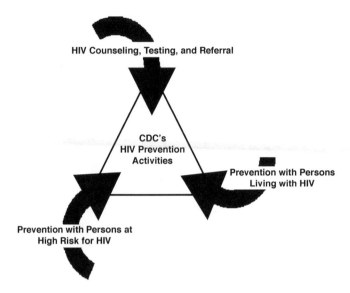

Figure 1.1. HIV prevention activities of the Centers for Disease Control and Prevention

infection is the US are based on: (1) HIV counseling, testing, and referral services, (2) prevention programs with uninfected persons who are at high risk for HIV, and (3) prevention programs with persons living with HIV.

AHP represented a fundamental paradigm shift that elevated the relatively new concept of prevention with HIV positive individuals to a level of importance equal to that of prevention with persons at-risk for HIV infection. More importantly, AHP was backed up by financial resources to implement large-scale demonstration projects and to support community-based prevention programs that were designed to implement four specific strategies: (1) make HIV testing a routine part of medical care, (2) implement new models for diagnosing HIV infections outside medical settings, (3) prevent new infections by working with persons diagnosed with HIV and their partners, and (4) further decrease perinatal HIV transmission.

ELEMENTS OF PREVENTION WITH PEOPLE LIVING WITH HIV/AIDS

Prevention with people living with HIV encompasses the five public health activities shown in Table 1.1. These activities begin with efforts to provide HIV testing to those who are infected and continue after

HIV diagnosis by addressing the medical, psychosocial, and prevention needs of people who know they are HIV-positive. In the following sections we discuss the potential contribution of each activity to decreasing the spread of HIV and improving the health and well-being of people living with HIV.

Early Diagnosis of HIV Infection

All efforts to directly affect the behavior of people living with HIV start with HIV-seropositive persons' knowledge of their serostatus. HIV testing has been available to the public since 1985, but, as stated previously, about one-fourth of people with HIV do not know that they are infected (Fleming et al., 2002). These persons are at considerable risk of transmitting the virus to others and may miss important opportunities to initiate HIV treatment before the virus does significant damage to the immune system (Janssen et al., 2001; Valdiserri, Holtgrave, and West, 1999). HIV/AIDS surveillance data from 33 states indicate that 37% of persons newly diagnosed with HIV either had AIDS at the time of HIV diagnosis or progressed to AIDS within a year, suggesting that most had been infected with HIV years before they were diagnosed (Kamimoto and McKenna, 2004).

Improving the early detection of HIV infection depends on being better able to reduce personal and structural barriers to HIV testing, make HIV testing routinely available to at-risk persons, and increase the proportion of tested persons who learn their test results. New strategies are needed to encourage at-risk persons to seek HIV testing and to accept it when it is offered to them. The most significant individual barriers to HIV testing are thinking that one is not at risk for HIV infection and fearing an HIV-positive test result (Exner et al., 2002; Kellerman et al., 2002). Although persons from different groups often give similar reasons for not having been tested, reasons for not testing can vary from group to group. For example, a 2001 survey of high-risk persons found that MSM (67%) and heterosexual STI clinic patients (63%) were more likely than injection drug users (32%) to indicate that they had not been tested because they thought that they were HIV-negative (CDC, 2004b). Among injection drug users, the most frequently given reason for not testing (endorsed by 59%) was that they did not want to think about being HIV-seropositive. The stigma of having an STI is also a barrier to HIV testing. Community members who perceive that a high level of stigma is associated with STIs are less likely to be tested for HIV than are persons who perceive less stigma (Fortenberry et al., 2002).

A number of strategies have been implemented to overcome these barriers to testing (Valdiserri et al., 1999). These have included efforts to make testing available in non-clinic settings by using mobile testing vehicles or providing testing in alternative venues that are frequented by persons at greatest risk for HIV infection (Keenan and Keenan, 2001; O'Connor, Patsdaughter et al., 1998; Spielberg et al., 2003). Other strategies have included social marketing campaigns for at-risk adolescents and other at-risk populations that were specifically designed to motivate test seeking behavior (Davis et al., 2003; Futterman et al., 2001; Zahn et al., 2003).

Making HIV testing more readily available in settings where patients receive routine and emergency health care is a strategy for normalizing HIV testing that may reduce stigma and direct testing resources to those at considerable risk of HIV infection. A health care providers' recommendation that an individual be tested for HIV is an important motivator of testing behavior (Fernandez et al., 2003; Kellerman et al., 2002). Other strategies for normalizing HIV testing include routine testing for pregnant women and making testing available to all persons entering settings with a high proportion of at-risk persons (e.g., drug treatment, jails, and prisons). Because some people with HIV do not recognize that they are at-risk or do not seek out testing, the CDC has recommended that screening for HIV infection be incorporated into medical care in settings with an HIV prevalence of $\geq 1\%$ or other facility-level indicators of increased HIV risk (CDC, 2003a).

Increasing early detection of HIV infection will require regular testing in high-risk populations. Regular testing may be especially important among MSM and other subpopulations with a high prevalence of HIV infection. For example, a study of nearly six thousand young MSM found that 77% of those who tested HIV-positive incorrectly believed that they were uninfected (MacKellar et al., 2002). Most of these men had previously tested negative for HIV infection (82%), and 59% believed that they were at low or very low risk. These data indicate that, in populations with a high prevalence of HIV, many persons with HIV may incorrectly believe that they are uninfected. To address the risks associated with unrecognized seroconversion, the CDC recommends annual HIV testing among sexually active MSM (CDC, 2002c).

Even when at-risk persons are tested for HIV, the time between sample collection and reporting of test results is a barrier to people learning their serostatus. Standard HIV antibody tests need to be conducted in a lab and, although they take relatively little time to perform, are usually done in batches to reduce costs (Kassler, 1997). Sending tests out to a lab makes it necessary to give results at a follow-up visit. These visits are typically scheduled 1 to 2 weeks after the initial visit so that the confirmatory testing of positive samples can be completed. Depending on the setting and population, 10% to more than 50% of people who take the test may not come back to receive their results (CDC, 2001; Molitor et al., 1999; Sullivan et al., 2004; Tao et al., 1999).

The most promising strategy for increasing the percentage of persons who know their test results is the use of rapid HIV-antibody tests that make it easier to provide test results in a single visit. As of January 2004, the Food and Drug Administration had approved 4 rapid HIV tests (Food and Drug Administration, 2004). Only one of these, OraQuick®, is currently approved for use outside of a laboratory setting. This test provides results in as little as 20 minutes, and can be conducted by existing counseling staff in clinical and non-clinical settings (CDC, 2002a). Evaluations of rapid testing have found it to be accurate, preferred by clients over standard testing, and able to increase the percentage of persons who receive their test results to almost 100% in some settings (Kassler et al., 1997; Keenan and Keenan, 2001; Marmor et al., 1999). Despite these advantages, structural barriers have slowed the implementation of rapid testing in some publicly funded test sites. CDC's experience indicates that barriers to the implementation of rapid testing include the increased cost of the test kit, the need to adapt existing counseling protocols to rapid testing, the need for quality assurance programs and training, the resources needed to train staff, test site certification requirements, and state regulations or laws. Many of these barriers are being overcome and rapid testing is becoming increasingly available across the US.

Improve Access to Care and Utilization of Care

Although it may be reasonable to assume that most people with HIV seek medical care and supportive services shortly after receiving their test results, many do not. Upon learning their serostatus, some HIV seropositive persons may adopt passive or avoidant coping strategies, including denial, that may adversely affect health-promoting behavior or delay access to medical and supportive services (Chesney and Folkman, 1994; Knight et al., in press). An 8-state study of people living with HIV/AIDS reported that 17% of respondents had not received HIV-related medical care one year after diagnosis (Osmond et al., 1999). Similarly, a 3-state study reported that 16% of participants who were interviewed a median of 6 months following diagnosis had not received medical care for HIV (CDC, 2000). Among patients who initially access care, some are not maintained in care and, as a result, are at risk of negative health outcomes. These patients may miss regular medical appointments or drop out of care entirely (Catz, McClure, Jones, and Brantley, 1999; Israelski et al., 2001). One study found that 20% of patients had discontinued care within six months of initial treatment for HIV infection (Samet et al., 2003).

Efforts to help HIV-seropositive persons overcome barriers to HIV care have shown some success. Preliminary results from the Antiretroviral Treatment Access Study (ARTAS) demonstrate that case management improves access to medical care among persons recently diagnosed with HIV infection (Gardner et al., 2003). Participants in this randomized trial who received case management were more likely to enter HIV care than were those who received passive referrals to care (78% vs. 60%, respectively). Other evaluations of case management have shown decreases over time in perceived barriers to care, increases in access to care, and improved health status among persons receiving case management (Brown et al., 2000; Conviser and Pounds, 2002; Katz et al., 2001; Rollison et al., 2002) Integration of care into nontraditional settings and other strategies for improving patient access to care have received less study, but some of these approaches also show promise (Altice et al., 2003; Andersen et al., 2003).

Other factors that exist outside of the individual (e.g., cost of health care, HIV-related stigma, insensitive/culturally inappropriate care, historical events) may also affect health-care seeking and utilization, and patient-level interventions cannot directly affect these influences. At best, patient-level interventions can only change individuals' perceptions of these external influences, link them to advocacy services, or enhance their ability to overcome these barriers. An inability to access affordable health care is more likely to be affected by influences that individuals have little or no control over such as lack of insurance or the presence of other competing financial needs. Affecting these barriers requires structural and policy interventions to make HIV-related care more readily available to those who need it.

Improve the Quality of Care

The quality of care that HIV-seropositive persons receive varies widely and does not always meet standards established by Department of Health and Human Services guidelines for opportunistic infection prophylaxis and antiretroviral therapy (Marx et al., 1995; Shapiro et al., 1999). The quality of care that HIV-positive patients receive greatly affects their health status and the potential spread of the epidemic. Individuals who do not receive indicated prophylaxis against opportunistic infections are at risk for developing life-threatening illnesses. Persons who do not receive appropriate antiretroviral therapy are at greater risk of disease progression and, if their viral load increases, may be more infectious. In addition, failure to screen patients for high-risk sexual and drug-use practices and to test for STIs may represent missed opportunities to reduce the risk of preventable disease among patients or their partners (CDC, 2003c).

Quality of care is affected by the timely prescription of prophylaxis for the prevention of opportunistic infections and the prescription of HAART. The Adult/Adolescent Spectrum of HIV Disease (ASD) Project, which is conducted at more than 100 facilities in 10 US cities, found that 20% of patients for whom *Pneumocystis carinii pneumonia* (PCP) prophylaxis was indicated had not received PCP prophylaxis (Wolfe et al., 2004). Women, Latinos, drug injectors, new patients, and those who were seen less frequently by their health care provider were among those patients participating in the ASD Project who were least likely to receive PCP prophylaxis.

The ASD Project also found that among patients for whom HAART is indicated, some are more likely to be prescribed HAART than are others (McNaghten et al., 2003). Women and those who were diagnosed as alcoholics were less likely to have been prescribed HAART than were men and non-alcoholics. Hispanics, those who contracted HIV through heterosexual contact, and those who received care in a private facility were more likely to have been prescribed HAART. Other studies have shown that improved access to HAART is associated with being male, being white, being older, having insurance, living in an urban area, missing fewer physician appointments, and not having a history of drug injection (Cohn et al., 2001; Cunningham et al., 2000; Giordano et al., 2003; Keruly et al., 2002; Palacio et al., 2002).

Individuals who receive care from physicians who specialize in HIV or have more experience treating HIV-seropositive patients are more likely to receive quality care that includes (when indicated) prophylaxis against PCP, regular monitoring of CD4 and viral load levels, receipt of HAART, earlier access to new HIV treatments, and more frequent primary care visits and referrals to specialists (Gardner et al., 2002; Kitahata et al., 1996, 2003; Kitahata et al., 2000; Landon et al., 2003). The most important benefit of better care by physicians with more experience treating HIV-seropositive patients is reduced mortality—patients who receive better care live longer (Kitahata et al., 1996, 2003). Because of the possible association between viral load and HIV transmission, another potential benefit of high-quality care is that patients who achieve undetectable or very low viral loads may be less infectious than patients with high viral loads.

Specific efforts to improve the quality of care received by HIV-seropositive patients have included the training of medical students and continuing medical education for practicing physicians and other health care providers (Lalonde et al., 2002; Lewis et al., 1993; Madan et al., 1998; Neff et al., 998). The use of computer-based systems to improve the quality of care is also being explored. For example, an electronic clinical reminder system that prompts providers to initiate regular and specifically indicated care has shown promise in improving the quality of medical services received by HIV-seropositive patients (Kitahata et al., 2003).

Improve Adherence to Treatment

The successful treatment of HIV infection is heavily dependent upon medication adherence. Poor adherence contributes to the development of drug-resistant HIV, and high levels of medication adherence are associated with sustained reductions in viral load, decreased risk of developing AIDS, and enhanced survival (Natasha et al., 2002). For example, a study of homeless persons with HIV found that all of those who had taken 98–100% of medication doses had an undetectable viral load, compared to 25% of those who had taken 73–97% of prescribed doses, 22% of those who had taken 48–73% of doses, and none of those who had taken 47% or fewer doses (Bangsberg et al., 2000). Poor adherence also has been associated with persistent shedding of HIV in semen, which is likely to increase the risk of HIV transmission during unprotected sexual intercourse (Barroso et al., 2003).

There is not yet a clear consensus as to what constitutes "good" adherence to HIV treatment, but recent studies have shown that very high levels of adherence (at least 90–95% of doses) may be needed to realize superior treatment outcomes (Gifford et al., 2000). Such high levels of adherence are not achieved by many patients. Pill counts and other objective measures indicate that the average patient with HIV takes about 60–80% of the pills that he or she is prescribed (Bangsberg et al., 2000; Golin et al., 2002; Miller et al., 2002). Unfortunately, even those who achieve near-perfect adherence may experience treatment failure. One study found that 23% of HIV-drug resistance occurred among persons who took 92–100% of prescribed pills (Bangsberg et al., 2003). Drug-resistant virus not only has negative consequences for the health of the HIV-seropositive patient, but it can be transmitted to uninfected partners (Wensing and Boucher, 2003).

Improvements in HIV medications have made it easier for some patients to adhere to their prescribed regimen by reducing the number of pills that have to be taken or easing dosing restrictions. Despite these improvements, some people living with HIV still face large pill burdens and complex dosing restrictions (e.g., some medications are taken with food, others are taken on an empty stomach, some are taken once a day, others twice a day, and others three times a day). Barriers to achieving good adherence to HIV medications have been reviewed extensively in the literature (Chesney, 2003; Ickovics and Meade, 2002; Turner, 2002). A review of 20 studies identified five factors that were most often associated with nonadherence to HAART: (1) symptoms and medication side effects, (2) negative life events or stressors, (3) lack of family or social support, (4) treatment regimen complexity, and (5) low self-efficacy for medication taking (Ammassari et al., 2002).

These reviewers and others have identified a number of other factors that are associated with adherence in some, but not all, studies. These include influences such as age, race, income, treatment beliefs, homelessness, substance use, and mental health (Chesney, 2000; Ickovics and Meade, 2002; Turner, 2002). Even though adverse situations and events may interfere with adherence, it is important to recognize that some injection drug users, homeless men and women, and others experiencing difficult life circumstances are able to achieve high levels of adherence (Bangsberg et al., 2000; Evan et al., 2003). In recognition of this finding, public health guidelines recommend that "no patient should automatically be excluded from antiretroviral therapy simply because he or she exhibits a behavior or characteristic judged by the clinician to indicate a likelihood of nonadherence" (CDC, 2002b; p. 7).

Instead, all patients should be considered at-risk for poor adherence, and physicians should take steps to encourage high levels of adherence to HIV treatment. Overcoming various barriers to adherence requires interventions that address characteristics of the treatment regimen, provider behavior, and patient behavior. Developing new treatments or formulations of existing drugs that simplify dosing, ease dietary requirements, and reduce pill burdens continues to be an important strategy that should be pursued.

Numerous efforts to modify patient adherence behavior have been reported—a recent review identified 21 published pilot studies or intervention trials that evaluated strategies to improve HIV treatment adherence (Simoni et al., 2003). Some strategies focus on improving patients' motivation to take medications as prescribed through individual or group counseling that is provided by a physician, pharmacist, or peer. Other strategies sought to improve patients' ability to plan and monitor their own pill taking behavior (e.g., by using pill boxes), involve others in helping remind patients to take pills, or provide electronic reminders when pills should be taken. Directly observed therapy, a strategy that has a long history in the treatment of tuberculosis, also has been evaluated. This strategy involves staff going to patients or patients coming to a clinic to be administered all or some of their scheduled medication doses. The ability of most of these strategies to bring about long-term behavior change is not yet known, and much remains to be learned about how to determine which approach is likely to work best (and be most cost effective) for a given patient.

Implement Interventions to Reduce Risk Behavior

In order to have the greatest impact on the course of the epidemic it will be necessary to bring about behavior change among people living with HIV whose behavior places others at risk. At present, there are few rigorously evaluated interventions for people who have been tested for HIV and know that they have the virus. The results of these studies show the ability of behavioral interventions to reduce transmission risk behavior, but also provide evidence that it may be difficult to bring about sustainable change in some circumstances.

Two early interventions that were designed to reduce depression and increase the ability of HIV-seropositive persons to cope with HIV-related stress demonstrated that behavioral interventions can reduce risk behavior among people living with HIV (Coates et al., 1989; Kelly et al., 1993). Since that time, a number of other studies have been initiated, but only a small number of published intervention trials have provided compelling data showing significant reductions in transmission risk behavior among HIV-seropositive persons (Kalichman et al., 2001; Margolin et al., 2003; Rotheram-Borus et al., 2001). In most cases, these studies evaluated group-level interventions to reduce HIV risk behaviors among people living with HIV. They found that participants receiving these interventions reported a greater reduction in risk behavior relative to those who were assigned to a comparison group. Each of the interventions was designed for a different population and setting, and each used different intervention messages and strategies to bring about behavior change.

Kalichman and colleagues randomized participants to either a 5-session risk reduction intervention based on social-cognitive theory or a 5-session health-maintenance intervention (Kalichman et al., 2001). The health maintenance intervention used a support group format, contained information related to the health of people living with HIV, and served as an attention control. The risk reduction intervention, named Healthy Relationships, addressed issues related to serostatus disclosure and the prevention of HIV transmission, which were framed in terms of benefiting participants by reducing their own level of stress. The intervention included activities to enhance motivation through self reflection, development of HIV disclosure decision making skills, active listening, assertiveness, and problem solving for disclosure. The intervention also included condom use and communication skills training, individual feedback about participants' own level of risk, and development of a personal risk reduction plan. Interviews at 6 months following intervention showed that participants in the Healthy Relationships intervention significantly reduced unprotected sex and increased condom use with negative or unknown status partners compared to participants in the health maintenance intervention.

An intervention for HIV-seropositive youth receiving medical care in four US cities was tested by Rotheram-Borus and colleagues (Rotheram-Borus, Lee et al., 2001). The intervention took place over six months and included two modules: (1) Stay Healthy, which consisted of 12 sessions and focused on improving health, coping with HIV, disclosure of HIV status and (2) Act Safe, which consisted of 11 sessions that addressed sexual practices and substance use. A third module, Being Together, also was delivered and consisted of eight additional sessions that focused on improved quality of life (Rotheram-Borus, Murphy et al., 2001). Participation in the Act Safe module was limited—only 80 out of 180 eligible youth in the intervention group attended at least one Act Safe session and returned for follow up assessment. Analyses comparing these 80 participants with 30 HIV-seropositive youth who received a standard level of clinic services found that at the 3-month follow up, intervention participants reported fewer unprotected sex acts and were more likely to report no sexual risk behavior than were those assigned to the standard-of-care group.

The third group intervention was tested by Margolin and colleagues with HIV-seropositive drug injectors entering a methadone maintenance program (Margolin et al., 2003). Participants were randomized to one of two interventions that were conducted over a six-month period of time: (1) a comparison intervention, which included daily methadone maintenance, weekly individual substance abuse counseling, case management, and a 6-session risk-reduction intervention, or (2) a harm reduction intervention, which included everything in the comparison condition plus manual-guided group psychotherapy sessions two times a week. Three months following intervention, participants assigned to the harm-reduction intervention obtained lower addiction severity scores and were less likely to engage in high-risk sex and drug-use behaviors, compared to those assigned to the comparison intervention.

Providers are important sources of health information (Neumann et al., 2003). Messages provided to HIV-seropositive patients in medical care are another important strategy for reducing unsafe sexual and injection practices. Unfortunately, a substantial number of people living with HIV do not receive STI or HIV prevention messages from their health care providers (Duffus et al., 2003; Margolis et al., 2001; Marks et al., 2002). In one study, one-in-four HIV-seropositive MSM reported that their current provider had never spoken with them about safer sex (Margolis et al., 2001). In order to address this issue, evidence-based recommendations for incorporating HIV prevention into the medical care of people living with HIV recently have been issued by CDC, HRSA, the NIH, and the HIV Medicine Association of the Infectious Diseases Society of America (CDC, 2003c). These recommendations cover a wide range of structural and individual approaches that health care providers can implement in order to reduce HIV/STI risk among HIV-seropositive patients.

The ability of clinic-based messages to motivate behavior change among persons receiving medical care has been demonstrated by a study of HIV-seropositive patients receiving care at HIV clinics in California (Richardson et al., 2004). This study examined the efficacy of gain- and loss-framed messages in the context of a brief intervention for HIV-seropositive persons in care. Gain-framed messages, used in two clinics, emphasized the positive consequences or benefits of safer sex, whereas the loss-framed messages, used in two other clinics, emphasized the negative consequences or risks of unsafe sex. Messages were presented to patients in written form (brochures, posters) and reinforced by providers during the patient's medical examination and at subsequent clinic visits. In the clinics that implemented the loss-framed messages, there was a 38% reduction in the prevalence of unprotected anal or vaginal intercourse in patients with risky profiles (those with two or more sex partners) at baseline. There were no intervention effects in patients who reported only one sex partner at baseline or in patients who received the gain-framed messages.

A number of other intervention strategies show promise, but have not yet been subjected to rigorous evaluation in a randomized intervention trial. These include interventions for HIV-seropositive men who are being released from prison and those with hemophilia (Butler et al., 2003; Grinstead et al., 2001; Parsons et al., 2000). Other interventions are currently being evaluated and include prevention case management (PCM). PCM is an intensive intervention that combines individual HIV risk-reduction counseling with case management to provide on-going support to clients who face challenging life circumstances that create barriers to initiating or maintaining reduced-risk practices (Purcell et al., 1998). Given that some interventions with people living with HIV have not been successful (Cleary et al., 1995; Patterson et al., 2003; Sorensen et al., 2003), it is important that

Exhibit 1.1. Key questions related to prevention with people living with
HIV/AIDS.

- What are the most efficient strategies for making HIV testing more readily available to those who are at greatest risk of seroconversion?
- How can barriers to the use of rapid testing in private and public settings be overcome?
- As the number of people who know that they are HIV-seropositive grows, will funding for HIV treatment and care keep up with demand?
- What theoretical models best guide the development of behavioral interventions for persons diagnosed with HIV?
- How does risk behavior change over time following HIV diagnosis? When are persons at greatest risk of transmitting HIV? Do persons who have recently learned their HIV status need different interventions than those who have been living with HIV for years?
- What role should disclosure of HIV status play in HIV prevention efforts? Who should do partner notification? What role should providers and public health play? Why does disclosure not consistently lead to risk reduction with uninfected partners?
- What role should knowledge of serostatus play and partner selection based on this knowledge play in prevention programs? Will risk reduction strategies based on partner selection reduce risk at the population level?
- What strategies are needed to bring about life-long adherence to HIV treatment and safer sex recommendations?

these and other interventions for this population be subjected to rigorous trials to determine their efficacy so that limited prevention resources can be used wisely.

CONCLUSIONS

The prioritization of prevention efforts with people living with HIV represents a significant change in HIV prevention efforts. Like any major change, it has raised new concerns and questions about the future. In addition, it has brought to light existing gaps in our knowledge about how to best meet the prevention needs of people living with HIV and support their adoption and maintenance of reduced risk practices. Many more questions will be raised and will need to be answered in order to ensure the success of these programs. Some of the questions that have already emerged are listed in Exhibit 1.1.

The expansion of public health efforts to diagnose undetected HIV infection raises practical and ethical issues. There is an ethical responsibility and a clear public health need to make medical and mental health services available to those who learn that they are HIV seropositive. Unfortunately, some people with HIV in the US are not able to afford HAART or gain access to it in a timely manner. AIDS drug assistance programs in some states have not been able to meet the demand for their services and as a result have capped enrollment, made eligibility criteria more stringent, or have limited the drugs that are covered (Davis et al., 2003). As the number of persons who learn that they are HIV seropositive grows, it is essential that HIV treatment and other services also expand to meet the needs of these individuals. The availability of these services represents an important incentive for people to know their serostatus. Furthermore, good medical care plays a critical role in reducing HIV-related deaths and the further spread of the virus. Investing in the medical care of people living with HIV has the potential to pay substantial benefits by preventing new infections that would otherwise tax an already overburdened health care system.

It is important to recognize that people living with HIV share some common experiences, but they are not a homogeneous population. There is a pressing need to better understand and meet the needs of individuals and subgroups of individuals within this population. For example, many of the challenges faced by HIV-seropositive women are different than those faced by men. Among women and men, needs and challenges may vary according to income, employment and insurance status, age, race/ethnicity, sexual orientation, care-giving responsibilities, and the nature of relationships with partners, children, and other family members. Other life circumstances (e.g., pregnancy, drug addiction, homelessness, mental illness) affect the type of services needed and the ways that these services can best be provided. Influences that exist outside of individuals also affect the services that are needed and their availability. The level of HIV-related stigma, amount of public funding for health care, and whether one lives in a large urban area or in a rural community all affect the accessibility and quality of care received by people living with HIV in the US.

Existing interventions may not be appropriate for all settings and may not meet the needs of some populations. Some of these interventions may be able to be adapted to other settings and populations. It is also possible that some interventions that have been found to be effective for at-risk populations can be successfully modified to be relevant and appropriate for people living with HIV. The process of adapting existing interventions or developing new ones is not necessarily straightforward and may not always be successful.

Facilitating the development of effective interventions depends on answering some very basic questions about the content of intervention messages for people living with HIV. For example, how much emphasis should these messages place on protecting oneself from the consequences of unprotected sex versus protecting others from HIV? Placing greater emphasis on messages that encourage self protection may fail to motivate behavior change among HIV-seropositive persons who believe that the risks they face are acceptable and inconsequential compared to the risks associated with having HIV. On the other hand, messages that place too great an emphasis on protecting others have the potential to contribute to stigma, trigger negative reactions, and be counterproductive to prevention goals. It is likely that messages that place an equal emphasis on personal risks and risks to others may ultimately prove to be most successful, but this has not yet been empirically tested. HIV-related stigma and discrimination not only affect the mental health of people living with HIV, they may also perpetuate the epidemic by causing some people to delay HIV testing and entry into medical care and by decreasing their willingness to disclose their HIV status to sex partners and others (Chesney and Smith, 1999).

We believe that a comprehensive approach to prevention with HIV-seropositive people is needed. There will be no "silver bullet." Rather a wide range of intervention programs and public health activities are needed that vary in terms of when they engage people living with HIV, where they reach people, and how they seek to bring about behavior change. The duration and intensity of the programs will also need to vary. Many people living with HIV already receive regular medical care and maintain safer sex practices. These individuals may only need minimal support from health care providers to maintain their existing health-promoting behaviors. For persons with very high viral loads, access to HAART may impact their ability to transmit HIV. For other individuals, access to substance abuse treatment, mental health services, or a multi-session behavioral intervention may have the most impact. Greater attention should be paid to assessing the individual needs of persons served by prevention programs and providing services that are best suited to meeting these needs (O'Leary et al., 2002).

The public health argument for the expansion of prevention programs targeting persons living with HIV is compelling. As health departments, community-based organizations, and other groups work toward implementing these programs it is essential that they are based on strong science and that they are sensitive to the needs and perspectives of HIV-seropositive persons. These programs have the potential to contribute to the stigma and discrimination experienced by persons with HIV. This is sure to be the case if prevention with people living with HIV/AIDS implicitly blames HIV-seropositive persons for the on-going epidemic of HIV infection, does not recognize their concerns, or fails to build upon the preexisting motivation of many people living with HIV to protect their partners from infection.

HIV-seropositive persons have a responsibility to protect others, and many people living with HIV have internalized this responsibility

(Wolitski et al., 2003). It is important to recognize, however, that this responsibility does not exist in a vacuum (Marks et al., 1999). Uninfected persons have a responsibility to discuss HIV with their partners, avoid high-risk behaviors, and protect themselves from contracting HIV. Society has a responsibility to make HIV information available, reduce barriers to adopting risk reduction strategies, and foster norms, values, and mores that promote the health and well-being of its members. Health care providers have a responsibility to assess the risk behavior of their patients, to reinforce healthy practices, and to encourage the reduction of high-risk behaviors. Public health agencies have a responsibility to ensure that prevention programs are available to those who need them and that these programs are based on the best scientific information available, are implemented well, and are cost-effective. Society also has a responsibility to prevent the stigma and discrimination that create barriers to disclosure, contribute to mental health problems that are associated with risky sexual practices, and affect access to quality medical care. As public health priorities shift, it is essential to remember that preventing HIV transmission is not the sole responsibility of any one group. We all share in the responsibility to prevent the further spread of HIV, and it will take all of our efforts in order to have a significant impact on the future course of the epidemic.

REFERENCES

AIDS Survival Project. (2004). *Thrive Weekend.* Retrieved March 15, 2004 from http://www.aidssurvivalproject.org/programs/thrive.html
Altice, F. L., Springer, S., Buitrago, M., Hunt, D. P., and Friedland, G. H. (2003). Pilot study to enhance HIV care using needle exchange-based health services for out-of-treatment injecting drug users. *J Urban Health*, 80, 416–427.
Ammassari, A., Trotta, M. P., Murri, R., Castelli, F., Narciso, P., Noto, P., Vecchiet, J., Monforte, A. D., Wu, A. W., Antinori, A., and AdICoNA Study Group. (2002). Correlates and predictors of adherence to highly active antiretroviral therapy: Overview of the published literature. *JAIDS*, 31 (Suppl 3), S123–S127.
Andersen, M., Paliwoda, J., Kaczynski, R., Schoener, E., Harris, C., Madeja, C., Reid, H., Weber, C., and Trent, C. (2003). Integrating medical and substance abuse treatment for addicts living with HIV/AIDS: Evidence-based nursing practice model. *Am J Drug Alcohol Abuse*, 29, 847–859.
Bangsberg, D. R., Hecht, F., Charlesbois, E., Zolopa, A., Holodniy, M., Sheiner, L., Bamberger, J. C. M., and Moss, A. (2000). Adherence to protease inhibitors, HIV-1 viral load, and development of drug resistance in an indigent population. *AIDS*, 14, 357–366.
Bangsberg, D. R., Charlesbois, E. D., Grant, R. M., Holodniy, M., Deeks, S. G., Perry, S., Conroy, K. N., Clark, R., Guzman, D., Zolopa, A., and Moss, A. (2003). High levels of adherence do not prevent accumulation of HIV drug resistance mutations. *AIDS*, 17, 1925–1932.
Barroso, P., Schlechter, M., Gupta, P., Bressan, C., Bomfim, A., and Harrison, L. (2003). Adherence to antiretroviral therapy and persistence of HIV RNA in semen. *JAIDS*, 32, 435–440.

Bayer, R. (1996). AIDS prevention–sexual ethics and responsibility. *N Engl J Med*, 334, 1540–1542.

Blackard, J., Cohen, D., and Mayer, K. (2002). Human immunodeficiency virus superinfection and recombination: Current state of knowledge and potential clinical consequences. *Clin Infect Dis*, 34, 1108–1114.

Brown, A. J. L., Frost, S. D. W., Mathews, W. C., Dawson, K., Hellmann, N. S., Daar, E. S., Richman, D. D., and Little, S. J. (2003). Transmission fitness of drug-resistant human immunodeficiency virus and the prevalence of resistance in the antiretroviral-treated population. *J Infect Dis*, 187, 683–686.

Brown, V. B., Smereck, G. A., German, V., Hughes, C., Melchior, L. A., and Huba, G. J. (2000). Change in perceived barriers and facilitators to treatment among women with HIV/AIDS as a function of psychosocial service utilization. *AIDS Patient Care STDs*, 14, 381–390.

Butler, R. B., Schultz, J. R., Forsberg, A. D., Brown, L. K., Parsons, J. T., King, G., Kocik, S. M., Jarvis, D., Schultz, S. L., Manco-Johnson, M., and CDC Adolescent HBIEP Study Group. (2003). Promoting safer sex among HIV-positive youth with haemophilia: Theory, intervention, and outcome. *Haemophilia*, 9, 214–222.

California Department of Health Services, Office of AIDS. (2002, December). *California and the HIV/AIDS epidemic: The state of the state report, 2001*. Retrieved April 9, 2004, from http://www.dhs.ca.gov/aids/Reports/sos/Adobe/SOS2001.pdf

Catz, S. L., McClure, J. B., Jones, G. N., and Brantley, P. J. (1999). Predictors of outpatient medical appointment adherence among persons with HIV. *AIDS Care*, 11, 361–373.

Centers for Disease Control and Prevention. (2000). Adoption of protective behaviors among persons with recent HIV infection and diagnosis—Alabama, New Jersey, and Tennessee, 1997–1998. *MMWR*, 49, 512–515.

Centers for Disease Control and Prevention. (2001). *HIV counseling and testing in publicly funded sites annual report, 1997 and 1998*. Atlanta, GA: Author.

Centers for Disease Control and Prevention. (2002a). Approval of a new rapid test for HIV antibody. *MMWR*, 51, 1051–1052.

Centers for Disease Control and Prevention. (2002b). Guidelines for using antiretroviral agents among HIV-infected adults and adolescents: Recommendations of the Panel on clinical practices for treatment of HIV. *MMWR*, 51 (RR-7), 1–64.

Centers for Disease Control and Prevention. (2002c). Sexually transmitted diseases treatment guidelines. *MMWR*, 51 (RR-6), 1–84.

Centers for Disease Control and Prevention. (2003a). *Advancing HIV Prevention: Interim technical guidance for selected interventions*. Atlanta, GA: Author.

Centers for Disease Control and Prevention. (2003b). Advancing HIV prevention: New strategies for a changing epidemic—United States, 2003. *MMWR*, 52(15), 329–332.

Centers for Disease Control and Prevention. (2003c). Incorporating HIV prevention into the medical care of persons living with HIV: Recommendations of CDC, the Health Resources and Services Administration, the National Institutes of Health, and the HIV Medicine Association of the Infectious Diseases Society of America. *MMWR*, 52(RR 12), 1–24.

Centers for Disease Control and Prevention. (2003d). Increases in HIV diagnoses–29 states, 1999–2002. *MMWR*, 14, 1145–1148.

Centers for Disease Control and Prevention. (2004a). Heterosexual transmission of HIV–29 states, 1999–2002. *MMWR*, 53, 125–129.

Centers for Disease Control and Prevention. (2004b). *HIV/AIDS Special Surveillance Report: HIV Testing Survey, 2001*. Atlanta, GA: Author.

Chesney, M. (2000). Factors affecting adherence to antiretroviral therapy. *Clin Infect Dis*, 30 (Suppl 2), S171–S176.

Chesney, M. (2003). Adherence to HAART regimens. *AIDS Patient Care STDs*, 17, 169–177.

Chesney, M. A., and Folkman, S. (1994). Psychological impact of HIV disease and implications for intervention. *Psychiatr Clinics North Am*, 17, 163–182.

Chesney, M. A., and Smith, A. W. (1999). Critical delays in HIV testing and care: The potential role of stigma. *Am Behav Scientist*, 42, 1158–1170.

Cleary, P. D., VanDevanter, N., Steilen, M., Stuart, A., Shipton-Levy, R., McMullen, W., Rogers, T. F., Singer, E., Avorn, J., and Pindyck, J. (1995). A randomized trial of an education and support program for HIV-infected individuals. *AIDS*, 9, 1271–1278.

Coates, T. J., McKusick, L., Kuno, R., and Stites, D. P. (1989). Stress reduction training changed number of sexual partners but not immune function in men with HIV. *Am J Public Health*, 79, 885–887.

Cohn, S. E., Berk, M. L., Berry, S. H., Duan, N. H., Frankel, M. R., Klein, J. D., McKinney, M. M., Rastegar, A., Smith, S., Shapiro, M. F., and Bozzette, S. A. (2001). The care of HIV-infected adults in rural areas of the United States. *JAIDS*, 28, 385–392.

Conviser, R., and Pounds, M. B. (2002). The role of ancillary services in client-centered systems of care. *AIDS Care*, 14 (Suppl 1), S119–S131.

Crepaz, N., and Marks, G. (2002). Towards an understanding of sexual risk behavior in people living with HIV: A review of social, psychological, and medical findings. *AIDS*, 16, 135–149.

Cunningham, W. E., Markson, L. E., Andersen, R. M., Crystal, S. H., Fleishman, J. A., Golin, C., Gifford, A., Liu, H. H., Nakazono, T. T., Morton, S., Bozzette, S. A., Shapiro, M. F., Wenger, N. S., and HCSUS Consortium. (2000). Prevalence and predictors of highly active antiretroviral therapy use in patients with HIV infection in the United States. *JAIDS*, 25, 115–123.

Davis, D. A., Wan, C., and Lam, J. (2003, July). *Using marketing clusters to evaluate KNOW NOW, a social marketing campaign for increasing awareness of HIV status.* Paper presented at the 2003 National HIV Prevention Conference, Atlanta, GA.

Davis, M. D., Aldridge, C., Kates, J., and Chou, L. (2003, April). *National ADAP Monitoring Project: Annual Report.* Retrieved April 14, 2004 from the Henry J. Kaiser Family foundation Web site: http://www.kff.org/hivaids/20030430a-index.cfm

Duffus, W. A., Barragan, M., Metsch, L., Krawczyk, C. S., Loughlin, A. M., Gardner, L. I., Anderson-Mahoney, P., Dickinson, G., del Rio, C., and Antiretroviral Access Studies Study Group. (2003). Effect of physician specialty on counseling practices and medical referral patterns among physicians caring for disadvantaged human immunodeficiency virus-infected populations. *Clin Infect Dis*, 1577–1584.

Egger, M., May, M., Chene, G., Phillips, A., Ledergerber, B., Dabis, F., Costagliola, D., Monforte, A., de Wolf, F., Reiss, P., Lundgren, J., Justice, A., Staszewski, S., Leport, C., Hogg, R., Sabin, C., Gill, M., Salzberger, B., and Sterne, J. (2002). Prognosis of HIV-1 infected patients starting highly active antiretroviral therapy: A collaborative analysis of prospective studies. *Lancet*, 360, 119–129.

Evan, W., Montaner, J. S. G., Yip, B., Tyndall, M. W., Schechter, M. T., O'Shaughnessy, M. V., and Hogg, R. S. (2003). Adherence and plasma HIV RNA responses to highly active antiretroviral therapy among HIV-1 infected injection drug users. *Can Med Assoc J*, 169, 656–661.

Exner, T., Hoffman, S., Parikh, K., Leu, C., and Ehrhardt, A. (2002). HIV counseling and testing: Women's experiences and the perceived role of testing as a prevention strategy. *Perspect Sex Reprod Health*, 34, 76–83.

Fernandez, M. I., Bowen, G. S., Perrino, T., Royal, S., Mattson, T., Arheart, K. L., and Cohn, S. (2003). Promoting HIV testing among never-tested Hispanic men: A doctor's recommendation may suffice. *AIDS Behav*, 7, 253–262.

Filippini, P., Coppola, N., Scolastico, C., Rossi, G., Onofrio, M., Sagnelli, E., and Piccinino, F. (2001). Does HIV infection favor the sexual transmission of hepatitis C? *Sex Transm Dis*, 28, 725–729.

Fleming, P. L., Byers, R. H., Sweeney, P. A., Daniels, D., Karon, J. M., and Janssen, R. S. (2002, February). *HIV prevalence in the United States, 2000*. Paper presented at the 9th Conference on Retroviruses and Opportunistic Infections, Seattle, WA.

Fortenberry, J., McFarlane, M., Bleakley, A., Bull, S., Fishbein, M., and Grimley, D. (2002). Relationship of stigma and shame to gonorrhea and HIV screening. *Am J Public Health*, 92, 378–381.

Francis, D. P., Anderson, R. E., Gorman, M. E., Fenstersheib, M., Padian, N. S., Kizer, K. W., and Conant, M. A. (1989). Targeting AIDS prevention and treatment toward HIV-1-infected persons: The concept of early intervention. *JAMA*, 262, 2572–2576

Francis, D. P., Russell, C., and Roger, S. (1992, July). *Early intervention: Effect on sexual behavior changes*. Paper presented at the VIII International Conference on AIDS, Amsterdam.

Futterman, D. C., Peralta, L., Rudy, B., Wolfson, S., Guttmacher, S., Rogers, A., and Project ACCESS Team of the Adolescent HIV/AIDS Research Network. (2001). The ACCESS (Adolescents Connected to Care, Evaluation, and Special Services) project: Social marketing to promote HIV testing to adolescents, methods and first year results from a six city campaign. *J Adolesc Health*, 29(Suppl 1), 19–29.

Gardner, L. I., Holmberg, S. D., Moore, J., Arnsten, J. H., Mayer, K. H., Rompalo, A., Schuman, P., Smith, D. K., and HIV Epidemiology Research Study Group. (2002). Use of highly active antiretroviral therapy in HIV-infected women: Impact of HIV specialist care. *JAIDS*, 29, 69–75.

Gardner, L. I., Metsch, L., Loughlin, A., Anderson-Mahoney, P., del Rio, C., Strathdee, S., Gaul, Z., Greenberg, A., and Holmberg, S. (2003, July). Initial results of the Antiretroviral Treatment Access Studies (ARTAS): Efficacy of the case management trial. Paper presented at the 2003 National HIV Prevention Conference, Atlanta, GA.

Gifford, A. L., Bormann, J. E., Shively, M. J., Wright, B. C., Richman, D. D., and Bozzette, S. A. (2000). Predictors of self-reported adherence and plasma HIV concentrations in patients on multi-drug antiretroviral regimens. *JAIDS*, 23, 286–295.

Giordano, T. P., White, A. C., Sajja, P., Graviss, E. A., Arduino, R. C., Adu-Oppong, A., Lahart, C. J., and Visnegarwala, F. (2003). Factors associated with the use of highly active antiretroviral therapy in patients newly entering care in an urban clinic. *JAIDS*, 32, 399–405.

Golin, C. E., Liu, H., Hays, R. D., Miller, L. G., Beck, C. K., Ickovics, J., Kaplan, A. H., and Wenger, N. S. (2002). A prospective study of predictors of adherence to combination antiretroviral medication. *J Gen Intern Med*, 17, 756–765.

Grinstead, O., Zack, B., and Faigeles, B. (2001). Reducing postrelease risk behavior among HIV seropositive prison inmates: The health promotion program. *AIDS Educ Prev*, 13, 109–119.

Higgins, D. L., Galavotti, C., O'Reilly, K. R., Schnell, D. J., Moore, M., Rugg, D. L., and Johnson, R. (1991). Evidence for the effects of HIV antibody testing on risk behaviors. *JAMA*, 266, 2419–2429.

Ickovics, J. R., and Meade, C. S. (2002). Adherence to HAART among patients with HIV: Breakthroughs and barriers. *AIDS Care*, 14, 309–318.

Institute of Medicine. (2000). *No time to lose: Getting more from HIV Prevention*. Washington, DC: National Academy Press.

Interventions to Prevent HIV Risk Behaviors. (1997, February 11–13). Retrieved April 14, 2004 from the NIH Consensus Statement Online from http://consensus.nih.gov/cons/104/104_statement.htm.

Israelski, D., Gore-Felton, C., Power, R., Wood, M. J., and Koopman, C. (2001). Sociodemographic characteristics associated with medical appointment adherence among HIV-seropositive patients seeking treatment in a county outpatient facility. *Prev Med*, 33, 470–475.

Janssen, R. S., Holtgrave, D. R., Valdiserri, R. O., Shepherd, M., Gayle, H. D., and DeCock, K. M. (2001). The serostatus approach to fighting the HIV epidemic: Prevention strategies for infected individuals. *Am J Public Health*, 91, 1019–1024.

Kalichman, S. C. (2000). HIV transmission risk behaviors of men and women living with HIV-AIDS: Prevalence, predictors, and emerging clinical interventions. *Clin Psychol-Sci Pract*, 7, 32–47.

Kalichman, S. C., Rompa, D., Cage, M., DiFonzo, K., Simpson, D., Austin, J., Buckles, J., Kyomugisha, F., Benotsch, E., Pinkerton, S., and Graham, J. (2001). Effectiveness of an intervention to reduce HIV transmission risks in HIV-positive people. *Am J Prev Med*, 21, 84–92.

Kamimoto, L., and McKenna, M. (2004, February). *A population-based assessment of CD4 test results in newly diagnosed, HIV-infected persons*. Paper presented at 11th Conference on Retroviruses and Opportunistic Infections, San Francisco, CA.

Karon, J. M., Fleming, P. L., Steketee, R. W., and DeCock, K. M. (2001). HIV in the United States at the turn of the century: An epidemic in transition. *Am J Public Health*, 91, 1060–1068.

Kassler, W. J. (1997). Advances in HIV testing technology and their potential impact on prevention. *AIDS Educ Prev*, 9(Suppl 3), 27–40.

Kassler, W. J., Dillon, B. A., Haley, C., Jones, W. K., and Goldman, A. (1997). On-site, rapid HIV testing with same-day results and counseling. *AIDS*, 11, 1045–1051.

Katz, M. H., Cunningham, W. E., Fleishman, J. A., Andersen, R. M., Kellogg, T., Bozzette, S. A., and Shapiro, M. F. (2001). Effect of case management on unmet needs and utilization of medical care and medications among HIV-infected persons. *Ann Intern Med*, 135, 557–565.

Keenan, P., and Keenan, J. (2001). Rapid HIV testing in urban outreach: A strategy for improving posttest counseling rates. *AIDS Educ Prev*, 13, 541–550.

Kellerman, S., Lehman, J., Lansky, A., Stevens, M., Hecht, F., Bindman, A., and Wortley, P. (2002). HIV testing within at-risk populations in the United States and the reasons for seeking or avoiding HIV testing. *JAIDS*, 31, 202–210.

Kelly, J. A., Murphy, D. A., Bahr, R., Kalichman, S. C., Morgan, M. G., Stevenson, Y., Koob, J. J., Brasfield, T. L., and Bernstein, B. M. (1993). Outcome of cognitive-behavioral and support group brief therapies for depressed, HIV-infected persons. *Am J Psychiatry*, 150, 1679–1686.

Keruly, J. C., Conviser, R., and Moore, R. D. (2002). Association of medical insurance and other factors with receipt of antiretroviral therapy. *Am J Public Health*, 92, 852–857.

Kitahata, M. M., Koepsell, T. D., Deyo, R. A., Maxwell, C. L., Dodge, W. T., and Wagner, E. H. (1996). Physicians' experience with the acquired immunodeficiency syndrome as a factor in patients' survival. *N Engl J Med*, 334, 701–706.

Kitahata, M. M., Van Rompaey, S. E., and Shields, A. W. (2000). Physician experience in the care of HIV-infected persons is associated with earlier adoption of new antiretroviral therapy. *JAIDS*, 24, 106–114.

Kitahata, M. M., Dillingham, P. W., Chaiyakunapruk, N., Buskin, S. E., Jones, J. L., Harrington, R. D., Hooton, T. M., and Holmes, K. K. (2003). Electronic human immunodeficiency virus (HIV) clinical reminder system improves adherence to practice guidelines among University of Washington Study Cohort. *Clin Infect Dis*, 36, 803–811.

Kitahata, M. M., Van Rompaey, S. E., Dillingham, P. W., Koepsell, T. D., Deyo, R. A., Dodge, W., and Wagner, E. H. (2003). Primary care delivery is associated with greater physician experience and improved survival among persons with AIDS. *J Gen Intern Med*, 18, 95–103.

Knight, K. R., Dawson-Rose, C., Gomez, C. A., Purcell, D., Halkitis, P. N., and the SUDIS Team. (in press). Sexual risk taking among HIV-positive injection drug users: contexts, characteristics, and implications for prevention. *AIDS Educ Prev*

Kok, G. (1999). Targeted prevention for people with HIV/AIDS: Feasible and desirable? *Patient Educ Counsel*, 36, 239–246.

Koopman, J., Jacquez, J. A., Welch, G. W., Simon, C. P., Foxman, B., Pollock, S. M., Barth-Jones, D., Adams, A. L., and Lange, K. (1997). The role of early HIV infection in the spread of HIV through populations. *JAIDS*, 14, 249–258.

Lalonde, B., Uldall, K. K., Huba, G. J., Panter, A. T., Zalumas, J., Wolfe, L. R., Rohweder, C., Colgrove, J., Henderson, H., German, V. F., Taylor, D., Anderson, D., and Melchior, L. A. (2002). Impact of HIV/AIDS education on health care provider practice: Results from nine grantees of the Special Projects of National Significance Program. *Eval Health Professions*, 25, 302–320.

Landon, B. E., Wilson, I. B., Cohn, S. E., Fichtenbaum, C. J., Wong, M. D., Wenger, N. S., Bozzette, S. A., Shapiro, M. F., and Cleary, P. D. (2003). Physician specialization and antiretroviral therapy for HIV: Adoption and use in a national probability sample of persons infected with HIV. *J Gen Intern Med*, 18, 233–241.

Lewis, C. E., Bursch, B., Klau, M., Konitsney, D., and Conrow, S. (1993). Continuing medication education for AIDS: An organizational response. *AIDS Educ Prev*, 5, 263–271.

Los Angeles Shanti. (n.d.). *Positive Living for Us Weekend Seminar.* Retrieved March 15, 2004, from the LA Shanti Website: http://www.lashanti.org/plus.html.

MacKellar, D. A., Valleroy, L., Secura, G., Behel, S., Bingham, T., Shehen, D., LaLotta, M., Celentano, D., Theiede, H., Koblin, B., and Torian, L. (2002, July). *Unrecognized HIV infection, risk behavior, and misperceptions of risk among young men who have sex with men—6 US cities, 1994–2000.* Paper presented at the XIV International Conference on AIDS, Barcelona, Spain.

McGowan, J. P., Shah, S. S., Ganea, C. E., Blum, S., Ernst, J. A., Irwin, K. L., Olivo, N., and Weidle, P. J. (2004). Risk behavior for transmission of human immunodeficiency virus (HIV) among HIV-seropositive individuals in an urban setting. *Clin Infect Dis*, 38, 122–127.

Madan, A. K., Caruso, B. A., Lopes, J. E., and Gracely, E. J. (1998). Comparison of simulated patient and didactic methods of teaching HIV risk assessment to medical residents. *Am J Prev Med*, 15, 114–119.

Margolin, A., Avants, S. K., Warburton, L. A., Hawkins, K. A., and Shi, J. (2003). A randomized clinical trial for a manual-guided risk reduction intervention for HIV-positive injection drug users. *Health Psychol*, 22, 223–228.

Margolis, A. D., Wolitski, R. J., Parsons, J. T., and Gómez, C. A. (2001). Are health care providers talking to HIV-seropositive patients about safer sex? *AIDS*, 15, 2335–2337.

Marks, G., Burris, S., and Peterman, T. A. (1999). Reducing sexual transmission of HIV from those who know they are infected: The need for personal and collective responsibility. *AIDS*, 13, 297–306.

Marks G., Crepaz, N., and Senterfitt J, W. (2004). Meta-analysis of high-risk sexual behavior in persons aware and unaware they are infected with HIV: Implications for HIV prevention. Under review.

Marks, G., Richardson, J., Crepaz, N., Stoyanoff, S., Milam, J., Kemper, C., Larsen, R. A., Bolan, R., Weismuller, P., Hollander, H., and McCutchan, A. (2002). Are HIV care providers talking with patients about safer sex and disclosure? A multi-clinic assessment. *AIDS*, 16, 1953–1957.

Marmor, M., Titus, S., Hagerty, R., and Harrison, C. (1999, August). *Rapid versus standard HIV testing of persons at high risk of HIV infection.* Paper presented at the 1999 National HIV Prevention Conference, Atlanta, GA.

Marx, R., Katz, M. H., Barreto, A. I., Park, M., Black, T., and Welch, M. (1995). Receipt of recommended medical care in HIV-infected and at-risk persons. *J Gen Intern Med*, 10, 92–95.

McNaghten, A. D., Hanson, D. L., Dworkin, M. S., Jones, J. L., and Adult/Adolescent Spectrum of Disease Project. (2003). Differences in prescription of antiretroviral therapy in a large cohort of HIV-infected patients. *JAIDS*, 32, 499–505.

Metsch, L. R., McCoy, C. B., Lai, S., and Miles, C. (1998). Continuing risk behaviors among HIV-seropositive chronic drug users in Miami, Florida. *AIDS Behav*, 2, 161–169.

Miller, L. G., Liu, H., Hays, R. D., Golin, C. E., Beck, C. K., Asch, S. M., Ma, Y., Kaplan, A. H., and Wenger, N. S. (2002). How well do clinicians estimate patients' adherence to combination antiretroviral therapy? *J Gen Intern Med*, 17, 1–11.

Molitor, F., Bell, R., Truax, S., Ruiz, J., and Sun, R. (1999). Predictors of failure to return for HIV test result counseling by test site type. *AIDS Educ Prev*, 11, 1–13.

Natasha, P., Tyndall, M. W., Wood, E., Hogg, R. S., and Montaner, J. S. (2002). Virologic and immunologic response, clinical progression, and highly active antiretroviral therapy adherence. *JAIDS*, 31, S112–S117.

Neff, J. A., Gaskill, S. P., Prihoda, T. J., Weiner, R. V., and Rydel, K. B. (1998). Continuing medical education versus clinic-based STD and HIV education interventions for primary care service providers: Replication and extension. *AIDS Educ Prev*, 10, 417–432.

Neumann, M. S., Marks, G., and Purcell, D. W. (2003). Delivering HIV transmission prevention services to HIV-seropositive persons in clinical care. In Erwin, J., Smith, D. K., and Peters B. S. (Eds.), *Ethnicity and HIV: Prevention and Care in Europe and the USA* (pp. 141–164). London: International Medical Press.

O'Brien, T., Kedes, D., Ganem, D., Macrae, D., Rosenberg, P., Molden, J., and Goedert, J. (1999). Evidence of concurrent epidemics of human herpes virus 8 and human immunodeficiency virus type-1 in US homosexual men: Rates, risk factors, and relationship to Kaposi's Sarcoma. *J Infect Dis*, 180, 1010–1017.

O'Connor, C. A., Patsdaughter, C. A., Grindel, C. G., Taveria, P. F., and Steinberg, J. L. (1998). A mobile HIV education and testing program: Bringing services to hard-to-reach populations. *AIDS Patient Care STDs*, 12, 931–937.

O'Leary, A., Peterman, T., and Aral, S. (2002). Prevention triage: Optimizing multiple HIV intervention strategies. In A. O'Leary (Ed.), *Beyond condoms: Alternative approaches to HIV prevention* (pp. 221–231). New York, NY: Klewer Academic/Plenum Publishers.

Osmond, D. H., Bindman, A. B., Vranizan, K., Lehman, S. J., Hecht, F. M., Keane, D., Reingold, A., and for the Multistate Evaluation of Surveillance for HIV Study Group. (1999). Name-based surveillance and public health interventions for people with HIV infection. *Ann Intern Med*, 131, 775–779.

Palacio, H., Kahn, J. G., Richards, T. A., and Morin, S. E. (2002). Effect of race and/or ethnicity in use of antiretrovirals and prophylaxis for opportunistic infection: A review of the literature. *Public Health Rep*, 117, 233–251.

Parsons, J. T., Huszti, H. C., Crudder, S. O., Rich, L., and Mendoza, J. (2000). Maintenance of safer sexual behaviours: Evaluation of a theory-based intervention for HIV seropositive men with haemophilia and their female partners. *Haemophilia*, 6, 181–190.

Patterson, T. L., Shaw, W. S., and Semple, S. J. (2003). Reducing the sexual risk behaviors of HIV+ individuals: Outcome of a randomized controlled trial. *Ann Behav Med*, 25, 137–145.

Porter, K., Babiker, A., Darbyshire, J., Pezzotti, P., Bhaskaran, K., and Walker, A. (2003). Determinants of survival following HIV-1 seroconversion after the introduction of HAART. *Lancet*, 362, 1267–1274.

Purcell, D. W., DeGroff, A. S., and Wolitski, R. J. (1998). HIV prevention case management: Current practice and future directions. *Health Soc Work*, 23, 282–289.

Quinn, T. C., Wawer, M. J., Sewankambo, N., Serwadda, D., Li, C., Wabwire-Mangen, F., Meehan, M. O., Lutalo, T., Gray, R. H., and for the Rakai Project Study Group. (2000). Viral load and heterosexual transmission of human immunodeficiency virus type 1. *N Engl J Med*, 342, 921–929.

Richardson, J. L., Milam, J., McCutchan, A., Stoyanoff, S., Bolan, R., Weiss, J., Kemper, C., Larsen, R. A., Hollander, H., Weissmuller, P., Chou, C. P., and Marks, G. (2004). Effect of brief provider safer-sex counseling of HIV-1 seropositive patients: A multi-clinic assessment. *AIDS*, 18, 1179–1186.

Rollison, M. N., Higginson, R. T., Mercier, B. E., and Weir-Wiggins, C. (2002, July). *HIV prevention case management builds an alliance with healthcare providers.* Paper presented at XIV International Conference on AIDS, Barcelona, Spain.

Rotello, G. (1995, April 17). Letter to the editor. *The Nation*, p. 510.

Rotheram-Borus, M. J., Lee, M. B., Murphy, D. A., Futterman, D., Duan, N., Birnbaum, J. M., and Lightfoot, M. (2001). Efficacy of a preventive intervention for youths living with HIV. *Am J Public Health*, 91, 400–405.

Rotheram-Borus, M. J., Murphy, D. A., Wight, R. G., Lee, M. B., Lightfoot, M., Swendeman, D., Birnbaum, J. M., and Wright, W. (2001). Improving the quality of life among young people living with HIV. *Eval Program Plann*, 24, 227–237.

Sabin, C. A. (2002). The changing clinical epidemiology of AIDS in the highly active antiretroviral therapy era. *AIDS*, 4 (Suppl 4), S61–S68.

Samet, J. H., Freedberg, K. A., Savetsky, J. B., Sullivan, L. M., Padmannabhan, L., and Stein, M. D. (2003). Discontinuation from HIV medical care: Squandering treatment opportunities. *J Health Care Poor Underserved*, 14, 244–255.

Schiltz, M. A., and Sandfort, T. G. (2000). HIV-positive people, risk and sexual behaviour. *Soc Sci Med*, 50, 1571–1588.

Shapiro, M. F., Morton, S. C., McCaffrey, D. F., Senterfitt, J. W., Fleishman, J. A., Perlman, J. F., Athey, L. A., Keesey, J. W., Goldman, D. P., Berry, S. H., and Bozzette, S. A. (1999). Variations in the care of HIV-infected adults in the United States: Results from the HIV Cost and Services Utilization Study. *JAMA*, 281, 2305–2315.

Signorile, M. (1995, February). HIV-positive and careless. *The New York Times*, p. E15.

Simoni, J. M., Frick, P. A., Pantalone, D. W., and Turner, B. J. (2003). Antiretroviral adherence interventions: A review of current literature and ongoing studies. *Topics HIV Med*, 11, 185–198.

Sorensen, J. L., Dilley, J., London, J., Okin, R. L., Delucchi, K. L., and Phibbs, C. S. (2003). Case management for substance users with HIV/AIDS: A randomized clinical trial. *Am J Drug Alcohol Abuse*, 29, 133–150.

Spielberg, F., Branson, B. M., Goldbaum, G. M., Kurth, A., and Wood, R. W. (2003). Designing an HIV counseling and testing program for bathhouses: The Seattle experience with strategies to improve acceptability. *J Homosex*, 44, 203–220.

Sullivan, P. S., Lansky, A., Drake, A., and for the HITS-2000 Investigators. (2004). Failure to return for HIV test results among persons at high risk for HIV infection: Results from a multistate interview project. *JAIDS*, 35, 511–518.

Tao, G., Branson, B., Kassler, W., and Cohen, R. (1999). Rates of receiving HIV test results: Data from the US National Health Interview Survey for 1994 and 1995. *JAIDS*, 22, 395–400.

Turner, B. J. (2002). Adherence to antiretroviral therapy by human immunodeficiency virus-infected patients. *J Infect Dis*, 185(Suppl 2), S143–S151.

US Food and Drug Administration. (2004, March 10). *Licensed/approved HIV, HTLV and hepatitis tests*. Retrieved March 12, 2004 from http://www.fda.gov/cber/products/testkits.htm

Valdiserri, R., Holtgrave, D., and West, G. (1999). Promoting early HIV diagnosis and entry into care. *AIDS*, 13, 2317–2330.

Volberding, P. A. (2003). HIV therapy in 2003: Consensus and controversy. *AIDS*, 17(Suppl 1), S4–S11.

Weinhardt, L. S., Carey, M. P., Johnson, B. T., and Bickman, N. L. (1999). Effects of HIV counseling and testing on sexual risk behavior: A meta-analytic review of published research, 1985–1997. *Am J Public Health*, 89, 1397–1405.

Wensing, A. M., and Boucher, C. A. (2003). Worldwide transmission of drug-resistant HIV. *AIDS Rev*, 5, 140–155.

Wiley, D., Visscher, B., Grosser, S., Hoover, D., Day, R., Gange, S., Chmiel, J., Mitsuyasu, R., and Detels, R. (2000). Evidence that anoreceptive intercourse with ejaculate exposure is associated with rapid CD4 loss. *AIDS*, 14, 707–715.

Wolfe, M. I., Hanson, D. L., Teshale, E. H., Brooks, J. T., Kaplan, J. E., and Sullivan, P. S. (2004, February). *Reasons for lack of appropriate receipt of primary PCP prophylaxis in a large cohort of HIV-infected persons in care in the US, 1993–2002*. Paper presented at the 11th Conference on Retroviruses and Opportunistic Infections, San Francisco, CA.

Wolitski, R. J., MacGowan, R. J., Higgins, D. L., and Jorgensen, C. M. (1997). The effects of HIV counseling and testing on risk-related practices and help-seeking behavior. *AIDS Educ Prev*, 9(Suppl 3), 52–67.

Wolitski, R. J., Bailey, C. J., O'Leary, A., Gómez, C. A., and Parsons, J. T. (2003). Self-perceived responsibility of HIV-seropositive men who have sex with men for preventing HIV transmission. *AIDS Behav*, 7, 363–372.

Wolitski, R. J., Janssen, R. S., Holtgrave, D. R., and Peterson, J. L. (2004). The public health response to the HIV epidemic in the United States. In G. Wormer (Ed.), *AIDS and other manifestations of HIV infection* (4th ed., pp. 997–1012). London: Elsevier/Academic Press.

Wolitski, R. J., Parsons, J. T., and Gómez, C. A. (in press). Prevention with HIV seropositive men who have sex with men: Lessons from the Seropositive Urban Men's Study (SUMS) and the Seropositive Urban Men's Intervention Trial (SUMIT). *JAIDS*.

Zahn, M. A., Evans, T., and Bull, S. (2003, July). *"Test Because You Matter": The role of social determinants to influence HIV testing*. Paper presented at the 2003 National HIV Prevention Conference, Atlanta, GA.

CHAPTER TWO

HIV Diagnosis and Risk Behavior

Lance S. Weinhardt

INTRODUCTION

It is clear that when people learn that they are HIV positive, this knowledge can have profound effects in all areas of their lives and that how one reacts to an HIV diagnosis is affected by many factors. The purpose of this chapter is to review available research on the effects that an HIV diagnosis has on the sexual risk behaviors that may have led to infection. Although many cross-sectional and longitudinal studies have demonstrated that a substantial proportion of HIV infected individuals engage in high-risk sexual practices with HIV-negative or unknown serostatus partners (e.g., Crepaz and Marks, 2002; Kalichman, 2000), relatively little information is available on how notification of an HIV diagnosis affects sexual risk behavior or the extent to which these behaviors are prevalent among those newly infected with HIV.

In 1999, a meta-analysis of the effects of HIV testing and counseling on sexual risk behavior found that persons who tested HIV-negative did not change their risk behavior compared to persons who were not tested (Weinhardt et al., 1999). This result was at odds with two hypotheses being discussed at the time: (a) A negative test result leads to increased risk behavior because it reinforces previous risky behavior; and (b) participating in HIV-counseling and testing, even with a negative test result, results in decreased risk behavior in response to the risk reduction counseling or other characteristics of the testing experience. In contrast, we found that people who tested HIV-positive, either alone or with a partner, significantly reduced their sexual risk behavior compared to HIV-negative and untested individuals. These results implied that HIV counseling and testing was not a particularly effective primary prevention strategy, but that an HIV positive diagnosis, at least when coupled with test counseling, does lead to reductions in sexual risk behavior. However, there have been several significant developments since the publication of this meta-analysis, which included only studies published between 1985 and 1997.

First, a major study of the effects of HIV test counseling (Kamb et al., 1998) demonstrated that brief, theory-based test pre and post-test counseling can have a meaningful impact on sexual risk behavior and associated sexually transmitted infections. Project RESPECT (Kamb et al.) enrolled HIV negative participants only and compared HIV risk reduction counseling models of different length. This study indicated that a brief two-session pre and post test counseling model was as effective as a four session intervention. If the Project RESPECT/CDC model of HIV test counseling were disseminated and adopted by service providers, it is likely that many people testing HIV-negative who received this counseling would likely reduce risk behaviors. Second, in 1996, effective treatments for HIV infection were introduced for the first time. The development of highly active anitiretroviral treatment (HAART) fundamentally changed the nature of what it means to be HIV positive (at least in communities with access to effective treatments). As people with HIV began to live longer and healthier lives, many people aware of their HIV diagnosis regained their health and resumed sexual activity, of course whether or not this sexual activity constitutes an HIV transmission risk depends on whether condoms are used, the HIV status of the sex partner, etc. Thus, data from studies conducted before HAART and before Project RESPECT may not be generalizable to people who test HIV positive or negative today.

Another relevant development is the recent change in HIV testing procedures. Rapid tests, which provide initial results in 20 minutes, have been in wide use in many countries for years and are now becoming standard in the US An even more convenient test that provides rapid results from a saliva sample received FDA approval in March 2004. The shift to a rapid test model necessitates an adapted counseling strategy, and the CDC has responded with a model that de-emphasizes pre-test counseling and risk reduction counseling with people who test negative in order to reduce barriers to providing testing to large numbers of people in routine care.

Counseling resources are instead shifted toward working with those who test positive, which is presumably a more cost-effective and direct way to prevent further infections. Even a short term reduction in HIV transmission risk behavior following HIV infection may have large effects on the course of the epidemic. If risk behaviors with uninfected individuals are high at a time when viral load is high, a substantial proportion of new infections could result. Reduction of risk behavior during this period of high viremia may therefore result in significant reductions in transmission (Jacquez et al., 1994).

Given these recent developments, a more current examination of the effects of HIV diagnosis on sexual risk behavior is warranted. In this chapter, I review and synthesize the empirical evidence regarding the effects of HIV diagnosis on sexual risk behavior, and attempt to answer three primary questions. First, "What is the magnitude of reduction in sexual risk behavior resulting from an HIV diagnosis?" This question is placed in the context of HAART; specifically, I examine whether the magnitude of risk behavior reduction decreased following the introduction of HAART. The second question addressed is "How long do reductions in risk behavior persist?" Third, "What needs to be done, in practice and in research, to maximize the beneficial effects of an HIV diagnosis on transmission risk behavior?"

"What Is the Magnitude of Reduction in Sexual Risk Behavior Resulting from an HIV Diagnosis?"

To provide a current answer to this question, studies of sexual behavior proximal to HIV diagnosis were meta-analyzed, using and updating the subset of studies in Weinhardt et al. (1999) that had an HIV-positive group, and using the following procedures.

Studies were identified through three methods: (1) computer searches of MEDLine and PsycINFO databases from January 1985 (the year that HIV-antibody testing was approved for public use) through November 2003, using combinations of the key words "AIDS," "HIV," "test*," "counseling," "serodiagnosis," "serostatus," "sex*," and "behavior"; (2) manual searches of leading public health journals (i.e., *AIDS, AIDS Care, AIDS Education and Prevention, American Journal of Public Health, Health Psychology, Journal of the American Medical Association, Sexually Transmitted Diseases*) for the years 1985 through 2003; and (3) inspection of the reference lists of all identified articles. The latter method was repeated until all potentially relevant articles from these sources were identified.

Identified studies were included if they provided (a) assessment of when, relative to data collection, at least some participants received an HIV-positive diagnosis or test result; (b) sexual behavior outcome data or a proxy measure (e.g., sexually transmitted disease [STD] incidence); (c) two or more assessments with the same participants, to allow examination of behavior change over time; (d) data from a sample independent from earlier studies included in this review and (e) summary or inferential statistics sufficient for the calculation of within-group effect sizes. With regard to criterion 5, two recent studies (Allen et al., 2003; Chamot et al., 1999) were excluded because they provided neither the significance level for the relevant within-group comparison nor other data needed to make the comparisons. However, these studies and their narrative results are included in Table 2.1.

Computation and Analysis of Effect Sizes

The effect size used was d, the standardized mean difference index (Johnson, 1993), computed using sexual risk behavior data from before and after HIV diagnosis. The effect size d can range from zero to plus or minus any number of standard deviations, depending on the direction and magnitude of the effect. Conventionally speaking, an effect size of ± 0.20 is "small," a value of ± 0.50 is "medium," and values exceeding ± 0.80 are "large" (Cohen, 1977). Effect sizes were expressed such that positive effect sizes indicated reductions in sexual HIV-risk behavior. Effect sizes were calculated using means and standard deviations, or if these were not available, using proportions or other data (e.g., n and F, t, or χ^2 values). If only ns and significance levels were presented, this information was used to estimate effect sizes. I used the pooled standard deviation in cases where only the mean and standard deviation were presented. Use of the pooled standard deviation results in effect sizes that may be biased toward zero compared to the use of paired observations. When authors reported dichotomous outcomes, such as the proportion of participants who engaged in unprotected sex during specified periods before and after diagnosis, I treated the proportions as means and derived the pooled standard deviation by following commonly available equations (Hedges, 1981; Hedges and Olkin, 1985; Johnson, 1993; Snedecor and Cochran, 1980). A correction for bias due to sample size was applied to the calculated effect sizes, resulting in the effect size statistic d used for analysis (Hedges, 1981).

For each study, within-group effect sizes were computed separately for each sexual behavior outcome for each group (HIV-positive, HIV-negative, and untested participants, serodiscordant couples, and mixed samples). Effect sizes for serodiscordant couples and mixed samples were calculated separately because these two groups differ from the other three (i.e., each effect size includes data from both HIV-positive and HIV-negative participants). If a study offered more than one follow-up assessment of intervention effectiveness, data from the first follow-up assessment were used. This strategy resulted in a set of 71 effect sizes. When a study yielded more than one effect size for the same outcome in the same serostatus group, these effect sizes were averaged, reducing the number of effect sizes in

Table 2.1. Characteristics and results of 23 studies examining behavior change proximal to receiving an HIV-positive diagnosis

Study (Year)	Study Description				Results			
	Participants	Study Design[a]/Dates of Data Collection	HIV Serostatus	Outcome variable /Precision	n	d	Additional Comments	
Allen, Meinzen-Derr et.al. (2003)	*Total Sample* N = 963 serodiseordant couples living together *Age range:* women 18–35 *M age:* women 29, men 36 *Gender:* 50% male *Ethnicity:* 100% African *Orientation:* 100% Heterosexual *Source:* VCT center in Lusaka, Zambia.	Couples attending research project's VCT clinic/August 1994–November 1998	Positive Men	Condom Use/ Mean (SD) occasions per 3 month period	204 couples	Within-group data not available for meta-analysis	
			Positive Men	Unprotected Sex/ same	204 couples		
			Positive Women Positive Women	Condom Use/ same Unprotected Sex	280 couples 280 couples		
Allen, Serufilira et al. (1992)	*Total sample* N=1,666 *M (SD) age:* NR *Age range:* 20–40 *Gender:* 100% female *Ethnicity:* 100% African *Orientation:* NR *Source:* consecutive visits to prenatal and pediatric clinics at Kigali, Rwanda hospital	C/1998–1991	Positive	STD infections/ Proportion	310	+0.25	Women whose partner was also tested were less likely to seroconvert than those whose partners were not tested.
			Negative	HIV infections/ rate per 100 person-years	970	+0.09	

(Continued)

Table 2.1. (*Continued*)

Study (Year)	Participants	Study Design[a] /Dates of Data Collection	HIV Serostatus	Outcome variable /Precision	n	d	Additional Comments
	Tested n = 1,458 n(%) HIV+: 460 (32) *Untested Controls* n = 208						
Allen, Tice et.al. (1992)	*Total Sample* N = 53 serodiscordant couples, living together *Age range:* women 18–35 *M age:* women 29, men 36 *Gender:* 50% male *Ethnicity:* 100% African *Orientation:* 100% Heterosexual *Source:* consecutive visits to prenatal and pediatric clinics at Kigali, Rwanda hospital	C/1998–1991	Discordant couples	Condom use/ proportion	60	+1.12	All couples completed follow-up assessment
Casadonte et.al. (1990)	*Total Sample* N = 81 *Age range:* 27–63 *Median age:* 37 *Gender:* 100% male *Ethnicity:* 47% Af. Am., 32% Cauc., 21% Latino *Orientation:* 100% heterosexual	B—Participants self-selected into tested group by requesting results from blood drawn for seroprevalence study. Assessments conducted before test result disclosure, 1–3 week	Positive Negative Untested	Unprotected sex / proportion Unprotected sex / proportion Condom use/ proportion	15 31 24	+0.02 +0.14 −0.18	

	Source: Methadone Maintenace Treatment Program, NYC *Tested* N = 50 *n HIV+(%):* 15 (30%) *Controls* n = 31	follow-up, and 8–14 wek follow-up./ November 1985–November 1986	Pre-post data not suitable for meta-analysis	Among those who received post-test counseling, those who were HIV negative had a higher rate of gonorrhea; those who were HIV positive had a nonsignificantly lower rate of gonorrhea
Charnot et al. (1999)	*Total Sample* N = 4031 *Age range:* 15–25 *Gender:* 69% male *Ethnicity:* 99.6% Af.Am., 0.3% Cauc. *Orientation:* NR *Source:* STD Clinic records *n HIV+(%):* 49 (1.2%) *Controls* n = 31	Historical cohort study examining incidence of gonorrhea reinfection after HIV testing/ June 1989—May 1991 RESULTS: no significant association between HIV-positive testing and any variation in gonorrhea rate. Significantly lower rate after first HIV-negative result, but higher after second or third negative test among cohort members		

(Continued)

Table 2.1. (*Continued*)

Study (Year)	Study Description				Results		Additional Comments
	Participants	Study Design[a] /Dates of Data Collection	HIV Serostatus	Outcome variable /Precision	n	d	
Cleary et al. (1991)	*Total Sample (all HIV+)* N = 271 *Age range:* 18 and over *M (SD) age:* NR *Gender:* 78% male *Ethnicity:* 45% Cauc., 31% Af. Am., 24% Latino/a. *Orientation:* 45% heterosexual, 55% homosexual or bisexual *Source:* Blood donors, notified of HIV+ results at New York City Blood Center	E—Data collected during visit to blood center for test-result disclosure and at a 2-week follow-up: M=23 days./June 1, 1986–February 28, 1988	Positive	Unprotected sex/ proportion	196	+0.54	271 of 708 confirmed HIV+blood donors agreed to enroll in the study. 75 (28%) did not return for follow-up assessment.
VCT Group (2000)	*Total sample* N=3120 individuals 1173 couples *Age range:* 18+ *M(SD) age:* TO BE CALCULATED *Gender:* 50.8% female (individuals) *Ethnicity:* Kenyan, Tanzanian, Trinidad	D—Multisite randomized clinical trial of voluntary counseling and testing (VCT) comparing VCT to health information condition, assessments at baseline and two follow ups (average 7.3 and 13.9 months after baseline)	Positive Individuals	Unprotected sex, primary partners	M: 56 F: 148	+0.22 +0.27	All effect sizes computed from participants who received HIV-CT as opposed to health information
			Positive Individuals	Unprotected sex, non-primary partners	M: 56 F: 144	+0.52 +0.37	

Orientation: NR Source: local media and community recruitment Tested (at baseline) n = 1480 individuals, 557 couples n (%) HIV+: 56 (6.4%) individual men, 145 (19.3%) individual women; 43 (15.3%) men in couples, 55 (18.4%) women in couples Controls n=1557 individuals, 584 couples		Positive Couples	Unprotected sex (enrollment partner)	M:73 F:73	+0.89 +1.24
		Negative Individuals	Unprotected sex, primary partners	M:670 F:606	+0.12 +0.16
		Negative Individuals	Unprotected sex, non-primary partners	M:671 F:608	+0.26 +0.22
		Untested Individuals	Unprotected sex, Primary partners	M:765 F:791	+0.18 +0.13
		Untested Individuals	Unprotected sex non-primary partners	M:766 F:789	+0.07 +0.11
Coates, Morin, McKusick (1987)	A/1984–1986				
Total Sample N=502 Age range: NR M (SD) age: NR Gender: 100% male Ethnicity: 91% Caue. Orientation: 98% homosexual Source: bars, bath houses, and newspaper ads in San Francisco. Tested n=205 n(%) HIV+:99 (48%) Controls n=297		Positive	UAI/Proportion	99	+0.85	Participants from San Francisco cohort study.
		Negative	UAI/Proportion	77	+0.69
		Untested	UAI/Proportion	297	+0.30

(Continued)

Table 2.1. (*Continued*)

Study (Year)	Study Description			Results			
	Participants	Study Design[a]/Dates of Data Collection	HIV Serostatus	Outcome variable /Precision	n	d	Additional Comments
Colfax et.al. (2002)	*Total Sample* $N = 66$ *Age range* = 20–44 *Median age* = 31 years *Gender:* 100% male *Ethnicity:* 64% Cauc., 9% Af. Am., 18% Latino *Orientation:* 100% MSM *Source:* STD clinics, advertisements, and other methods; from HIVNET cohort	HIVNET cohort. Recruited April–November 1995	Positive	UIAI HIV-/U	66	+0.81	Study examined behavior during and in early sero-conversion
			Positive	URAI HIV+	66	+0.22	
			Positive	URAI HIV-/U	66	+0.51	
			Positive	URAI HIV+	66	+0.05	
Deren, Beardsley, Coyle, and Singer (1998)	*Total Sample* N=976 injectors, 729 crack users *M age*=38.1 (injectors), 35.7 (crack users) *Gender:* 75% male (i), 52% male (c0 *Ethnicity:* (i)49% Af. Am., 35% Puerto Rican, 16% White and other; (c) 88% Af. Am., 5% Puerto Rican, 6% White and other *Orientation:* NR *Source:* Outreach recruitment	Data from NIDA Cooperative Agreement for AIDS Community-Based Outreach/ Intervention Research Programs. Compared baseline and follow up data from matched (on site, gender, age, and ethnicity) samples of HIV+/−injectors and crack users	Positive Injectors	Unprotected Sex / Proportion	488	+0.43	
			Negative Injectors	Unprotected Sex / Proportion	488	+0.05	
			Positive Crack Users	Unprotected Sex/ Proportion	364	+0.37	
			Negative Crack Users	Unprotected Sex/ Proportion	364	+0.18	

Study	Sample	Method	HIV status	Measure	N	ES	Results
Fox, Odaka, Brookmeyer, and Polk (1987)	*Tested* N=1001 *Age range:* NR *M(SD) age:* 36 (NR) *Gender:* 100% male *Ethnicity:* 95% Cauc. *Orientation:* 100% MSM *Source:* Participants from Study to Help the AIDS Research Effort (SHARE) Baltimore—Washington area. *N informed:* 670 *N (%) HIV+:* 201(30)	B—Behavior assessed for 6-month reporting period at 6 month intervals at assessment 1, 2, 3, and 4. Serostatus disclosed at visit 3/April 1984–April-86	Positive	Partners/mean	175	+0.20	
			Negative	Partners/mean	436	+0.06	
			Untested	Partners/mean	308	+0.14	
			Positive	URAI partners/mean	167	+0.40	
			Negative	URAI partners/mean	428	+0.01	
			Untested	URAI partners/mean	304	+0.21	
			Positive	UIAI partners/mean	167	+0.30	
			Negative	UIAI partners/mean	427	+0.11	
			Untested	UIAI partners/mean	301	+0.16	
George, Green and Murphy (1998)	*Total Sample* N=228 *n (%) HIV+:* 114 (50%—matched controls) *Age range:* 79% between 21 and 35. *M (SD) age:* 33.5 (9.2) *Gender:* 83% male	Longitudinal retrospective case-note survey, HIV+ cases matched on gender, age, country of origin, and risk category with HIV-patients/1994	Positive	STD rate/infections per year	114	+0.32	Rates of STD infections decreased among HIV+ and HIV- patients
			Negative	STD rate/infections per year	114	+0.14	

(Continued)

Table 2.2. (*Continued*)

Study (Year)	Study Description				Results		Additional Comments
	Participants	Study Design[a]/Dates of Data Collection	HIV Serostatus	Outcome variable /Precision	n	d	
	Ethnicity: 43% EU countries, 22% north Africa, 7% sub-Saharan Africa. *Orientation:* 37% Hetero, 61% MSM, *Source:* inner-London STD clinic						
van Griensven et al. (1989)	*Total Sample* N=307 *Gender:* 100% male *Ethnicity:* NR *Orientation:* 100% MSM *M (SD) age:* 36 (NR) *Tested* N=193 N (%) HIV+: 75 (39) *Source:* subsample of prospective study on risk factors for HIV. Amsterdam. *Controls* N=114. *Source:* Subscribers to a homosexually-oriented newspaper in Amsterdam	A-Interviewed at 3 consecutive 6 month intervals. Knew serostatus an average of 6 months at time of first interview./ October, 1984–December, 1986	Positive	UAI/proportion	75	+0.55	
			Negative	UAI/proportion	108	+0.26	
			Untested	UAI/proportion	114	+0.85	
			Positive	Condom use with nonsteady partners/ proportion	75	+0.85	

Study	Sample	Notes	HIV Status	Measure	n	Effect Size
Huggins et al. (1991)	*Total Sample* N=155 *n (%) HIV+:* 22 (14.2) *Age range:* 79% between 21 and 35. *M(SD) age:* NR *Gender:* 100% male *Ethnicity:* 100% Cauc. *Orientation:* 87% MSM *Source:* Participants in MACS, Pittsburgh, PA	B—22 HIV-negative participants randomly selected as comparison group. 12 participants chose not to learn their results and were also used as a comparison group. Resulting N = 56./NR	Positive	RAI Partners/ Mean	22	+0.81
			Negative	RAI Partners/ Mean	22	+0.54
			Untested	RAI Partners/ Mean	12	+0.22
Kamenga et al. (1991)	*Total Sample* N = 149 married serodiscordant couples *M (SD) age:* men 38.9 (NR), women 31.4 (NR) *Gender:* 53% of wives were HIV+ *Ethnicity:* 100% African *Orientation:* 100% heterosexual *Source:* employee HIV screening at textile factory and large commercial bank in Kinshasa, Zaire.	C—Follow-up: Minimum 6 months/ 1987–1989.	Discordant couples	Consistent condom use/ proportion	149	+1.84
			Discordant couples	Abstinence/ proportion	149	+0.88
Magura et al. (1990)	*Total Sample* N=48 *n (%) HIV+:* 9 (18%) *Gender:* 67% male	C—Each of 8 HIV+ participants were matched with an HIV-participant on gender,	Positive	Condom Use/ proportion changed	7	+0.31

(Continued)

Table 2.1. (*Continued*)

Study (Year)	Study Description			Results			
	Participants	Study Design[a]/Dates of Data Collection	HIV Serostatus	Outcome variable /Precision	n	d	Additional Comments
	M Age (SD): NR (NR). 87% < 40. *Ethnicity*: 89% Cauc. *Orientation*: NR *Source* Methadone maintenance program in New York City	ethnicity, and baseline drug-use behavior. One HIV+ participant did not provide follow-up data, resulting in *N* HIV+ = 7 and HIV− = 7 (100% Cauc.)/NR	Negative	Condom Use/ proportion changed	7	0.00	
Ostrow et al. (1989)	*Total Sample N* = 474 *Age range*: NR *Gender*: 100% male *Orientation*: 100% MSM *Source*: Multicenter AIDS Cohort Study *Tested n*=146 *n (%) HIV+*: 50 (34%) *M (SD)*: age: 35.1 (0.7) *Ethnicity* 92% Cauc. *Controls n*=328 *M (SD)* age: 35.7 (0.5) *Ethnicity*: 94% Cauc.	B—Participants from the MACS Chicago cohort only/1984–1987	Positive	Partners/mean	67	+0.50	
			Negative	Partners/mean	88	+0.18	
			Untested	Partners/mean	398	+0.30	
			Positive	Celibate/ proportion	67	+0.03	
			Negative	Celibate/ proportion	88	+0.00	
			Untested	Celibate/ proportion	398	+0.02	
			Positive	Monogamous/ proportion	67	+0.02	
			Negative	Monogamous/ proportion	88	+0.01	
			Untested	Monogamous/ proportion	398	0.00	

Study	Sample	Notes	HIV status	Outcome	n	Effect size
Otten et al. (1993)	*Total Sample* N=5522 *Age:* 48% between 20–29, 23% between 30–49 *Gender:* 73% male *Ethnicity:* 76% Af. Am. *Orientation:* NR *Source:* STD clinic in Miami, FL *Tested* n=797 n (%) HIV+: 331 (42) *Controls* n=4,525	C—Groups based on chart review of test result, and return for post-test counseling/ Charts of patients who received HIV-CT between January 1988 and February 1989 were included.	Positive	Any new STD infection/proportion	331	+0.03
			Negative	Any STD/proportion	666	−0.19
			Untested	Any STD/proportion	4524	−0.06
			Positive	Any new gonorrhea infection/proportion	331	+0.08
					666	−0.14
			Negative	Gonorrhea/proportion	4524	−0.05
Padian et al. (1993)	*Total Sample* N=144 serodiscordant couples n (%) HIV+: 100% of index participants *Age range:* 19–61 (female partner) *Gender:* 112 men, 32 women *Ethnicity:* 68% Cauc., 12% Af. Am., 14% Latino 5% Other *Orientation:* 28% bisexual *Source:* HIV counseling and testing sites in CA.	Data collection began in 1985.	Serodiscordant couples	Condom Use	120	+0.90
			Serodiscordant couples	Abstinence	144	+0.63

(Continued)

Table 2.1. (*Continued*)

Study (Year)	Study Description			Results			
	Participants	Study Design[a]/Dates of Data Collection	HIV Serostatus	Outcome variable /Precision	n	d	Additional Comments
Pickering et al. (1993)	*Total Sample* N=474 *Age range:* NR *Gender:* 100% female *Ethnicity:* African *Orientation:* 100% MSM *Source:* larger study of HIV infection and prostitution in The Gambia	B/September 1989– 1990	Positive Negative	Condom use/ proportion improved Condom use/ proportion improved	11 18	+0.00 +0.13	
Roth et al. (2001)	*Total Sample* N = 684 couples, 66 serodiscordant, 109 seroconcordant HIV+ *Age range:* 21–38, for women at enrollment in this study phase *M (SD) age:* NR *Gender:* 50% women *Ethnicity:* 100% African *Source:* Women with partners previously screened for HIV and malaria, in prenatal and pediatric clinics in Kigali Rwanda.	1991–1992	Sample from earlier Allen studies. Effect sizes not included in meta analysis.	N/A	N/A	N/A	Rates of condom use in all serodiscordant couples increased; Effect most pronounced in couples where man was positive and had not been tested before.

Study	Total Sample	Design	HIV status	Outcome	n	Effect size	Notes
Schechter et al. (1988)	Total Sample N = 361; n (%) HIV+: 130 (36); Age range: NR; M (SD) age: NR; Gender: 100% male; Ethnicity: NR; Orientation: 100% Homosexual; Source: Vancouver Lymphadenopathy AIDS Cohort Study.	B—All Participants tested and aware of result. Comparison between HIV+ and HIV-Participants, and changes in sexual behavior between 3rd and 7th assessments of study (mean duration 28 months)./April 1984–September 1987	Positive	Partners/mean	130	+0.31	Excluded participants who were diagnosed with AIDS during study period.
			Negative	Partners/mean	231	+0.18	
Zapka et al. (1991)	Total Sample N = 249; n (%) HIV+: 65 (26); M (SD) age: 31.7 (NR); Gender: 100% male; Ethnicity: 96% Cauc; Orientation: 100% MSM; Source: Fenway Community Health Center Cohort Study	Data collection began in May 1985	Positive	Partners	25	+1.10	
			Positive	Unprotected Sex	25	-0.19	
			Negative	Partners	81	+1.14	
			Negative	Unprotected Sex	81	-0.32	
			Untested	Partners	12	+0.34	

Note: a = study design: (a) cohort study comparing behavioral data collected before and after antibody testing was introduced, and assessing whether participants had been tested and the result; (b) cohort study comparing the behavioral responses of participants whose blood was sampled for a study, and chose to be notified of test results and receive counseling, with those of individuals who also had their blood drawn but chose not to receive their results; (c) comparing behavioral data collected before and after testing was conducted among people seeking testing at a testing site or among people in treatment for injection drug use; (d) randomly assigning participants who did not originally plan to be tested to a control group; and (e) comparing pre- notification and post-notification behavioral data among individuals who tested HIV-positive when donating blood and received counseling with their test result; n = number of participants in analysis; d = within-groups pre-test v. post-test effect size; * = significantly greater than an effect size of zero, $p < .05$; tested = participants who received pre- and post-test counseling and received their results; untested = control participants who did not receive counseling or test results; Orientation = sexual orientation; MSM = men who have sex with men; HIV+ = HIV-positive; mixed = sample consisted of HIV-positive and HIV-negative participants; Af. Am. = African American; Cauc. = Caucasian; NR = not reported.

the data set to 62. Thus, each participant was included in only one effect size for each outcome to avoid violating the assumption of independence of effect sizes. Analyses followed fixed-effects procedures (Hedges and Olkin, 1985), which assume that larger sample sizes provide more reliable outcomes and therefore assign greater weight to effect sizes from larger studies. The weighted mean effect size, d_+, is an average of the individual studies' effect sizes weighted by the inverse of their variance (i.e., sample size). Separate analyses were conducted for each of the sexual behavior outcomes that were typically reported (i.e., number of partners, condom use, and unprotected intercourse).

To determine whether models implied by weighted mean effect sizes describe studies' effect sizes correctly, a homogeneity of variance statistic, Q, was computed (Hedges and Olkin, 1981). Q has an approximate χ^2 distribution with degrees of freedom equal to the number of effect sizes (k) minus one. A significant Q indicates that the d_+ may not adequately describe the variability in outcomes in a given set of studies.

Summary of Methodological Features of Studies

A detailed description of the individual study methods appears in Table 2.1 and provides a context from which to interpret the results of the studies. Study sample sizes of HIV-positive participants varied widely across studies. Studies were conducted in North America, Africa, and Europe. Five basic research strategies were used to study behavioral responses to diagnosis: (a) cohort studies that compared behavioral data collected before and after antibody testing was introduced (in 1985), and assessed whether participants had been tested and, if so, the result; (b) cohort studies that compared the behavioral responses of individuals whose blood was sampled for the study, and who chose to be notified of test results and receive counseling, with those of individuals who also had their blood sampled but chose not to receive their results; (c) studies that compared behavioral data collected before and after testing was conducted among people seeking testing at a testing site or among people in treatment for injection drug use; (d) studies that included random assignment of participants who did not originally plan to be tested to testing or to one or more control groups; and (e) one study that compared pre-notification and post-notification behavioral data among individuals who tested HIV-positive when donating blood and received counseling with their test result. Some studies were part of larger cohort studies of sexual behavior and HIV infection, such as the Multicenter AIDS Cohort Study (Ostrow et al., 1989).

Sample Characteristics

Most of the studies involved individual participants, whereas some studies recruited couples for participation. In addition to the participants in community cohort studies, who were primarily recruited through targeted advertising and word-of-mouth, samples were recruited from consecutive visits to HIV-testing centers, patients at STD clinics and treatment programs for IDU, and screening of the blood donation system. Other study and sample characteristics are summarized in Table 2.1.

Characteristics of Counseling

With a few notable exceptions (e.g., VCT, 2000), the characteristics of counseling used in studies were generally not described thoroughly, in terms of the duration or specific procedures used. Only five studies included the average length of pre- or post-test counseling sessions, whereas seven studies provided no details of the counseling. Four studies supplemented basic counseling with other educational efforts including peer-group discussion (Magura et al., 1990), videotaped presentations (Allen, Serufilira et al., 1992; Allen, Tice et al., 1992), and partner counseling (in the case of serodiscordant couples; Allen, Tice et al., 1992; Kamenga et al., 1991). Other studies, such as Coates et al. (1987), conducted assessments of participants before and after public HIV-testing became available in 1985 and asked participants whether they had been tested, whether they knew the result, and whether the result was positive or negative. Participants in these studies may have been tested at many different sites, and may have received different types of counseling. The majority of studies did not indicate whether counseling procedures adhered to any particular counseling guidelines. As a result of the inconsistency and limited amount of specific information reported about counseling procedures, analyses of effect sizes by characteristics of counseling could not be conducted.

Outcome Measures

Sexual behavior outcome measures that were used consistently were number of partners, condom use, and unprotected intercourse. These variables were measured with interviews and self-administered questionnaires, with different levels of specificity (e.g., condom use with non-steady v. any partner) and precision (e.g., mean number of partners v. any partner during the reporting period), and used reporting periods ranging from 10 days to 2 years. Some studies provided data on HIV or STD incidence to supplement self-reported sexual behavior data.

Table 2.2. Weighted mean effect size (d_+) and related statistics by behavior and serostatus in studies of people diagnosed with HIV

Outcome	Group	d^*_+	$Q^{\ddagger}_B$	95% Confidence Interval Lower	95% Confidence Interval Upper	$k^{\P}$	Q^{**}_W
Unprotected	HIV+	$0.44^{\dagger\#}$	$121.83^{\S}$	0.37	0.51	10	$25.02^{\S}$
Intercourse	HIV−	0.18		0.12	0.23	8	$28.70^{\S}$
	Discordant Couples	$0.85^{\dagger\#}$		0.71	0.99	4	8.21
	Untested	0.13		0.07	0.18	4	5.48
Condom Use	HIV+	$0.59^{\#}$	$90.47^{\S}$	0.38	0.81	5	6.30
	HIV−	0.26		0.11	0.41	4	1.70
	Discordant Couples	$1.31^{\dagger\#}$		1.14	1.48	3	$24.83^{\S}$
	Untested	0.49		0.37	0.61	3	$10.06^{\S}$
Sexual Partners	HIV+	$0.34^{\dagger}$	10.91	0.20	0.47	5	9.98
	HIV−	$0.24^{\dagger}$		0.15	0.34	5	$31.15^{\S}$
	Untested	0.07		0.03	0.18	4	0.51

$* d_+$ = Mean effect size weighted by sample size; The direction of the effect size for each behavior is such that a positive value reflects a decrease in risk for HIV infection and a negative value reflects increased risk for HIV infection; † Mean weighted effect sizes greater than the untested group at $P < .05$; † Mean weighted effect sizes greater than the HIV-negative group at $P < .05$; ‡ Q_B = Between-group homogeneity statistic for mean weighted effect sizes for each behavior; § Q_B or Q_W significant at $P < .05$; ¶ k = Number of studies contributing an effect size; ** Q_W = Within-group homogeneity statistic.

Effects of Testing HIV-Positive on Sexual Behavior

Within-group effect sizes were computed separately for each sexual behavioral outcome, for each group in each study (HIV-positive, HIV-negative, and untested participants, serodiscordant couples, and mixed samples). The individual effect sizes computed from the 21 studies included are displayed in Table 2.1.

Unprotected Intercourse

Twenty-six effect sizes were based on unprotected intercourse data. As displayed in Table 2.2, the mean weighted effect sizes for the HIV-positive group ($d_+ = 0.44$; 95% CI, 0.37 to 0.51) and the serodiscordant couple group ($d_+ = 0.85$; 95% CI, 0.71 to 0.99) indicated significant risk reduction, and both were greater than the weighted mean effect size effect for the untested ($d_+ = 0.13$; 95% CI, 0.07 to 0.18) and HIV-negative participants ($d_+ = 0.18$; 95% CI, 0.12 to 0.23; $Ps < .001$). Effect sizes in the untested and HIV-serodiscordant couples groups were homogeneous.

Condom Use

As shown in Table 2.2, fifteen effect sizes were based on condom-use measures. Weighted mean effect sizes for the HIV-positive group (d_+ = 0.59; 95% CI, 0.38 to 0.81) and the serodiscordant couple group (d_+ = 1.31; 95% CI, 1.14 to 1.48) were positive and significant and both were greater than the weighted mean effect size for the HIV-negative participants ($Ps < .005$). However, only the discordant couples had larger increases than untested participants.

Number of Sexual Partners

Fourteen effect sizes were based on number of sexual partners. The weighted mean effect size for the HIV-positive group was significantly positive (d_+ = 0.34; 95% CI, 0.20 to 0.47). The HIV-negative effect size (d_+ = 0.24; 95% CI, 0.15 to 0.34) was also positive and significant. Both groups exhibited greater change than the untested group (d_+ = 0.07; 95% CI, 0.03 to 0.18). There was significant heterogeneity of effect sizes in the HIV-negative group, but the HIV-positive and untested groups were homogenous. There were no data regarding numbers of sexual partners from studies of serodiscordant couples.

HIV and STD Incidence

Six additional effect sizes based on HIV and STD incidence data were available from four studies. These data indicated that the incidence of STD infection decreased among HIV-positive individuals (d_+ = 0.18, 95% CI, 0.08 to 0.28), but increased among HIV-negative participants (d_+ = −0.12, 95% CI, −0.22 to −0.02) and among untested participants (d_+ = −0.05, 95% CI, −0.09 to −0.01). The weighted mean effect size among HIV-positive participants was significantly greater than the HIV-negative and untested participants. Chamot et al. (1999) also examined changes in STD rates, but within-group effect sizes could not be derived from the published data. In a record-based study of a STD clinic in New Orleans, Chamot compared rates of gonorrhea re-infection among 4031 patients who had a first lifetime gonorrhea infection within a two year period at the clinic. Seventy-seven percent of these patients were tested for HIV over the monitoring period, and 49 tested HIV positive. The paper reported no association between HIV-positive testing and any variation in gonorrhea rate, although the low number of HIV-positive individuals included in these analyses may have limited statistical power to find an association.

Effect sizes were also not computed for Allen et al. (2003) because pre-post data points were not reported in sufficient detail. Allen et al. examined the sexual behavior of 963 cohabitating heterosexual couples, recruited from an HIV counseling and testing center in Lusaka, Zambia. Fewer than 3% of couples reported condom use prior to testing, whereas over 80% of intercourse was condom protected following HIV diagnosis. This study also examined STD infections and other biological markers of sexual activity and found that individuals who reported 100% condom use following testing also reported significant reductions in gonorrhea, syphilis, and *Trichomonas vaginalis*.

Effects of HIV Diagnosis before and after HAART

To examine evidence for whether the introduction of HAART changed the magnitude of effects of HIV diagnosis on behavior, each study was also coded for the dates of data collection, pre- or post-1996. At present, only three studies have been published that collected post-HAART behavior change data proximal to HIV diagnosis. All three studies provided data on unprotected intercourse among individual participants (as opposed to couples), and these effect sizes were compared to pre-HAART effect sizes among HIV-positive individuals. The mean weighted effect size pre-HAART was $d_+ = 0.42$ (95% CI, 0.34 to 0.50) and post HAART was $d_+ = 0.50$ (95% CI, 0.33 to 0.68), effect sizes that are statistically equivalent. Interpretation of this analysis is complicated by the fact that the post-HAART data was collected in Africa where knowledge of HAART was likely not salient to participants. Further, the low number of effect sizes, particularly post-HAART renders this analysis preliminary.

Summary of Findings

Taken together, these data indicate that an HIV diagnosis, whether provided to an individual patient or to a couple, significantly reduces the occurrence of unprotected intercourse and reduces the number of sexual partners of individual HIV-positive patients. Couples with at least one partner testing positive significantly increase their condom use, although HIV-positive individuals do not evidence a significant increase in condom use relative to individuals not tested. This pattern of results is consistent with the idea that individuals testing HIV positive initially reduce their overall sexual activity compared to pre-diagnosis, and therefore do not increase the number of times they use condoms in the period immediately after being diagnosed. These results provide a positive outlook in terms of reduced transmission risk behavior following an HIV diagnosis.

However, we know that some individuals aware of their HIV status do resume engaging in behaviors that can transmit HIV (for reviews see Crepaz and Marks, 2002; Kalichman, 2000). Due to the fact that the studies included in this meta-analysis do not indicate how long the decreases persisted with, most providing only one or two follow up assessments, we must turn to other data to examine this question in more detail.

"HOW LONG DO REDUCTIONS IN RISK BEHAVIOR PERSIST FOLLOWING AN HIV-POSITIVE DIAGNOSIS?"

To answer this question using recent, HAART-era information, I drew upon a large dataset collected from HIV-positive individuals during 2000–2002. These data are from interviews that were used as a screening instrument and as the baseline assessment for the NIMH Healthy Living Project, a randomized controlled trial (RCT) of a transmission risk behavior reduction and ealth promotion intervention for HIV-infected persons.

Interviews lasting between two and four hours were conducted in private settings in research offices, community-based organizations, and clinics in Los Angeles, Milwaukee, New York, and San Francisco. Persons were recruited and consented first for the survey only. If eligible based on survey responses, a participant was informed of the opportunity to enroll in the RCT. Sexual behavior segments of the interviews were conducted using Audio Computer Assisted Self Interviewing (ACASI) software. Participants completed detailed 3-month retrospective partner-by-partner assessments of sexual behavior for up to five partners of each gender, and aggregate frequency assessments for additional partners. Participants were also asked when they were first diagnosed with HIV infection. The sample reported in this chapter consists of 3,723 HIV positive persons: 1,918 MSM, 978 women, and 827 heterosexual men. Further details on the characteristics of this sample and on assessments and other procedures are available in Weinhardt et al. (2004).

In a previous analysis of these data (Weinhardt et al., 2004) using mathematical modeling taking into account gender of participant, type of behavior (i.e., insertive vs. receptive anal, vaginal), HIV serostatus of partner, effect of HAART on viral load and HIV transmissibility, and local HIV seroprevalence rates in each city, we found that the sexual behavior reported in this sample likely resulted in 30.4 new infections. Extrapolated over a 10 year period, assuming the reported behaviors were maintained, these behaviors would result in 671 new infections. However, the mathematical model did not take into account length of time since diagnosis as it is related to viral load, and assumed that behaviors would be maintained at the same levels.

To examine transmission risk behavior in relation to HIV diagnosis, the length of time since diagnosis was computed by subtracting self-reported date of diagnosis from the date of the interview. For each participant, this interval was then transformed into "quarters since diagnosis", to be consistent with the 3 month recall period of the interview. For the purpose of this chapter, HIV transmission risk behavior was defined as any unprotected vaginal or anal intercourse with an HIV-negative partner or partner of unknown serostatus, or unprotected intercourse with any partner characterized as a casual or one-time partner (i.e., even if identified as an HIV-positive partner).

Figure 2.1, Panel A displays the proportion of individuals in each quarter since their own HIV diagnosis who reported engaging in any HIV transmission risk behavior in the 3 months prior to the interview, for participants within 6 years of diagnosis. Panel B includes men only, and Panel C includes women only. For most participants within 3 months of diagnosis, shown in the leftmost bar of each panel, their interview assessed some behavior that occurred prior to diagnosis. Thus, the rates of HIV transmission risk behavior observed among those in the first quarter post-diagnosis likely reflect their behavior prior to diagnosis. As can be seen in all panels,

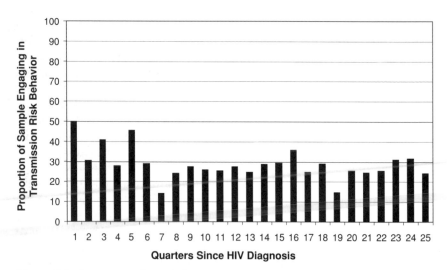

Figure 2.1. Proportion of people living with HIV engaging in HIV transmission risk behavior as a function of quarters since testing HIV positive. Panel A, total sample (among those diagnosed in the past six years). Panel B, men only, Panel C, women only.

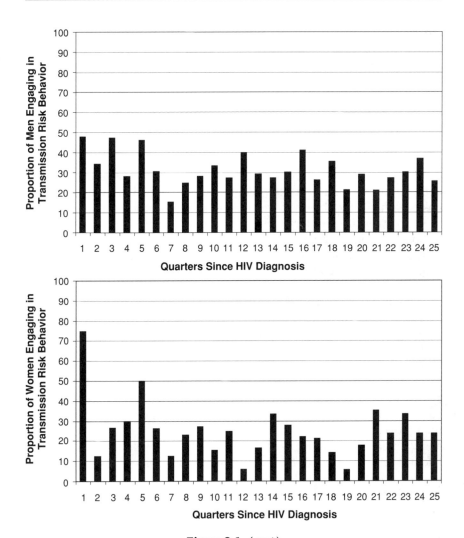

Figure 2.1. (*cont.*)

after the first quarter post-diagnosis, rates of transmission risk behavior decrease considerably.

Three other general patterns can be observed in these data. First, although rates drop off following diagnosis, and again after the first 5 quarters (i.e., behavior that occurred after the first year following diagnosis), there appears to be a relatively stable level (20–30%) of transmission risk behavior occurring among participants in each of these later quarters through the six years charted. Second, within the first year post-diagnosis there appears to be wide fluctuation in rates of risk behavior across quarters. However, there is no evidence here for an increase in transmission risk behavior, or rebound to pre-infection levels, when examining this relatively long post-diagnosis period. This long-term perspective suggests that some individuals newly diagnosed may struggle with reducing sexual risk behavior as they adjust to an HIV diagnosis over the first year. After that period, a relatively stable lower proportion of individuals continue to engage in transmission risk behavior.

Third, according to these data, men and women may respond differently within the first year after diagnosis. The reduction in transmission risk behavior after diagnosis was greater among women than men (75.0% to 12.5% vs. 47.8% to 34.2%). Further, women's rates of transmission risk behavior did not approach pre-diagnosis levels again until the fifth quarter post-diagnosis, whereas men's rates in the third quarter were identical to behavior reported within the first quarter after diagnosis, reflecting pre-testing rates of risk behavior. Finally, rates of transmission risk behavior over the five years after the first year post-diagnosis differ by gender. On average 29% of men in each quarter between their second and sixth year of being HIV-positive engaged in transmission risk behavior compared to 21.7% of women.

Although these cross-sectional data do not allow conclusions as definitive as longitudinal assessments of the same individuals would allow, this analysis is more detailed than previous published studies and includes a larger sample than is available in other existing datasets. It appears that the first year after diagnosis may be a critical period, in which both men and women engage in higher levels of risk behavior than after they have had a chance to adjust to their diagnosis. Strengthening risk behavior reduction interventions that can be implemented during this critical period may help these individuals adjust while engaging in less transmission risk behavior.

"WHAT NEEDS TO BE DONE, IN PRACTICE AND RESEACH, TO MAXIMIZE THE BENEFICIAL EFFECTS OF AN HIV DIAGNOSIS ON TRANSMISSION RISK BEHAVIOR?"

From a behavioral intervention perspective, the above results beg the question of what can be done to increase the likelihood that the newly diagnosed individual will reduce behaviors that can transmit HIV. Currently, there are few studies that address this question directly. The VCT study

(VCT, 2000) in Africa found that providing risk reduction counseling, as opposed to providing simple health education, resulted in larger risk reduction effects. In a retrospective survey, DeRosa and Marks (1998) found in Los Angeles that male HIV-positive patients who had received counseling at post-test and later in their HIV clinic treatment to disclose their serostatus to sexual partners were more likely to disclose to HIV-negative partners, but not to HIV-positive or unknown serostatus partners. Counseling at only one of these times was not associated with higher disclosure rates. The rate of recent condom use was higher with HIV-negative partners to whom participants had disclosed.

Without more relevant intervention outcome data, suggestions for procedures to increase the risk behavior reduction effects of an HIV diagnosis can only be speculations based on studies that focused on risk behavior and intervention among HIV-positive (but not necessarily recently diagnosed) persons. Based on such existing literature, several suggestions can be tested in future research.

Avants et al. (2001) found use of specific coping strategies following an HIV diagnosis was related to transmission risk behavior. Individuals who relied on avoidant coping were more likely to have engaged in recent risk behavior and to have poorer health. Coping Effectiveness Training (CET, Chesney et al., 1996; Chesney et al., 2003) may be a relevant and useful intervention at the time of diagnosis to help the patient develop strategies to actively cope with the new information. CET has been adapted into a 2-session module in the NIMH Healthy Living Project intervention (Rotheram-Borus et al., 2003) that could be implemented in settings where HIV testing and diagnosis is performed

Beyond specific risk reduction counseling approaches that could incorporate disclosure counseling and coping effectiveness-type interventions, encouraging people to seek more intensive transmission risk behavior, mental health (Chesney and Folkman, 1999), and substance use interventions may be effective strategies for improving risk reduction effects of diagnosis. In addition, beginning to discuss sexuality and sexual adjustment (Kalichman, 1998) with the individual may be less threatening than framing messages in terms of risk reduction and protecting others.

Other previous intervention studies such as those conducted by Kalichman et al. (2001) Rotheram-Borus et al. (2001), Parsons et al. (2000), and Patterson et al. (2003) provide strategies for transmission risk behavior reduction among different population segments and are discussed in more detail in other chapters in this volume. The challenge is to adapt these strategies to be practical and effective at the time of HIV diagnosis and immediately thereafter, to realize the full benefits of these programs.

RECOMMENDATIONS FOR FUTURE RESEARCH

The following recommendations are offered to improve future research on the effects of HIV-diagnosis on sexual risk behavior.

Theoretically-Driven Research Is Needed to Further
Understand the Determinants of Behavior Change
Following HIV Diagnosis

For the past decade, other outcome research on HIV-prevention interventions has focused on the psychological determinants of sexual behavior
and of reactions to the interventions. However, the literature reviewed in
this chapter has not been informed by a psychological model of the diagnosis process or of health-related behavior change. Although some parts of the
counseling provided in the reviewed studies are similar to other social cognitive theory-based interventions that have been found to be effective for
risk-behavior reduction, individuals experiencing an HIV diagnosis could
likely benefit from different types of intervention. Thus, new programmatic research is warranted on the psychological determinants of behavior
change associated with HIV diagnosis. Carefully designed and conducted
research such as Project RESPECT (Kamb et al., 1998), which examined
HIV-CT from a transtheoretical model framework, and other studies that
could elucidate the psychological predictors of behavior change in HIV
diagnosis are needed to understand and improve upon the risk-reduction
effects observed in this review and should be adapted and applied to future
studies of HIV positive individuals.

Research is Needed to Enhance Assessment
of Relevant Behaviors and Constructs

Three aspects of the assessments in the reviewed studies warrant discussion. First, there was insufficient distinction between sexual behavior
and sexual risk behavior. To assess accurately whether a participant's behavior has changed toward more risk or less risk for HIV transmission, it is
helpful to know specific information about his or her sexual behavior. For
example, it is important to know whether participants are in a monogamous relationship, and whether they were tested with their monogamous
partner or otherwise know the partner's serostatus. Some of the primary
reasons for being tested are related to starting a new sexual relationship
(Lupton et al., 1995; Leaity et al., 2000); many couples in this situation

are tested together and share their test results. An increase in unprotected intercourse or reduction in condom use between monogamous partners who are both HIV-negative or HIV positive is not necessarily an indication that HIV testing has failed at helping them to reduce their sexual HIV-risk behavior.

A tenable solution to this difficulty would be to assess participants' risk-reduction plans, and to gauge the effects of HIV-CT by their adherence to their plan using behavior frequency data. For example, if a participant is being tested with a partner at the beginning of a monogamous relationship, then his or her subsequent behavior changes in terms of number of partners and the frequency of condom use and unprotected intercourse should be interpreted in terms of this scenario. Using this approach, the participant's relationship status and risk-reduction plan are taken into account, and by using appropriate statistical techniques on frequency data, variability is maintained. Limitations of using this type of partner-specific assessment approach are that there is no guarantee that (a) both partners perceive that they are in a "steady" relationship or will remain monogamous or that (b) both partners will be honest with each other with regard to their HIV-serostatus. Nonetheless, a more fine-grained analysis of sexual behavior is warranted in studies of HIV diagnosis and transmission risk behavior to ensure valid characterization of risk-behavior change, taking into account the context of testing.

A second limitation related to assessment is the reliance on self-reported sexual behavior data. The fidelity of sexual behavior data obtained by self-report has been questioned repeatedly since Kinsey's pioneering surveys of sexuality in the US (Kinsey et al., 1948; Kinsey et al., 1953). In recent years, commentaries have suggested that self-reports of sexual behavior are inherently unreliable and invalid due to multiple sources of bias including under-reports of stigmatized behaviors and over-reports of normative behaviors (Lewontin, 1995). Brody (1995) questioned the validity of self-report data, suggesting that participants in behavioral research are prone to intentional misrepresentation. In the case of the reviewed studies, it is possible that demand characteristics could lead participants, especially HIV-positive participants, to report reduced risk behavior at follow up assessments. The average effect sizes in the HIV-negative and untested groups were small to non-existent and it does not appear likely that there was strong demand effect in these groups. Nevertheless, few of the reviewed studies reported data regarding the psychometric properties of the sexual behavior measures, or referred to other studies containing such data. There has been considerable effort directed at developing self-report measures that are reliable and at gathering evidence supporting their validity (see Catania et al., 1990). In the future, researchers examining effects of HIV diagnosis on risk behavior could bolster more confidence in their self-report outcome data by using measures of risk behavior that have been psychometrically evaluated (e.g., Risk Behavior Assessment; Needle et al., 1995). Further, researchers should ensure that their measures are appropriate for their sample by conducting formative pilot work.

Incidence of HIV or STD infection was reported in four studies included in this review. STD incidence data, although not as sensitive to changes in the frequency of risk-behavior as self-reported data, are arguably more relevant markers of HIV-risk behavior; activity that led to infection with most other STDs could have also resulted in HIV infection. The results indicated that HIV-negative participants in an urban STD clinic had slightly more STD infections after testing negative whereas HIV-positive participants had fewer STD infections after testing. These data, although based on few studies, were generally consistent with the pattern of results emerging from the self-reported sexual behavior data.

Research Is Needed to Determine the Effectiveness of Different Types of Counseling Approaches during Diagnosis of HIV+ Individuals

Few studies reviewed in this chapter allow an examination of the effects of counseling. In Africa, where large numbers of HIV positive participants can be enrolled in studies during routine testing, studies have shown benefits of risk reduction counseling as opposed to health information (e.g., VCT, 2000). This is helpful information and paves the way for similar counseling approaches to be put into widespread practice. However, the next step is to test different models of risk reduction counseling to identify techniques that result in the largest reductions in risk behavior. Research should be conducted to examine the effects of theory-based counseling with different types of content, different modes, and different levels of intensity. This area of research is especially important now that rapid testing is being implemented, which changes the typical structure of test counseling, and more counseling emphasis is placed on individuals who test positive.

It remains to be seen how well the rapid test model works in terms of promoting behavior change among HIV positive individuals. On the one hand, more people who are HIV positive will receive their immediately-available test results; thus we can reasonably expect many of these individuals to reduce their sexual risk behavior and prevent infections among their partners. Of course, these people will also be more likely to receive medical monitoring and treatment which may reduce HIV viral load and transmissibility of the virus. On the other hand, we do not know if receiving an HIV-positive diagnosis without the 'waiting period' required for older tests has the same level of positive effects on behavior as it does with the delayed notification. It is possible that the waiting period provided time for some individuals to seriously reflect on their previous risk behavior and develop a plan for how they would react if they were HIV positive. The emotional uncertainty during this waiting period may have helped some people confront for the first time what it would mean to be HIV positive and to decide for themselves to reduce their risky behavior if they were indeed infected. As Rogers's Protection Motivation model (1975) indicates, it is often a 'fear appeal' that is a cue to action, and perhaps the anxiety associated with the two week waiting period served this function for some people testing HIV positive. Several qualitative studies bear out the intense affective experience of the waiting period, although all were published prior to the advent of HAART. New, well designed studies will be needed to determine the effects of an HIV diagnosis in different testing environments using rapid testing technologies. For example, an important issue is whether there is a difference in behavior change effects between being diagnosed in a doctor's office, where many tests will be routinely conducted in the future under the new CDC guidelines (CDC, 2003) compared to a voluntary HIV testing situation, which is where most previous research has been conducted.

Another important avenue for investigation is the role of detecting acute HIV infection and the role it could have on behavior change. North Carolina has begun statewide testing for acute infection (i.e., prior to development of antibodies), which has resulted in detection of at least one cluster of infections among college students during the early stages of infection characterized by high viremia and transmissibility. Development and evaluation of risk reduction counseling protocols to accompany this type of test are needed.

CONCLUSIONS

The question of the effect of HIV diagnosis on sexual risk behavior is not one that can be answered once and laid to rest. As the context of HIV diagnosis changes, in terms of how HIV tests are conducted, the types of counseling that may be routinely provided with test results, the perceived severity of an HIV infection, and the maturation of cohorts affected by HIV, to name just a few of the relevant factors, it is likely that the magnitude of the impact of an HIV diagnosis also changes for particular segment of those at risk for HIV. In short, effect of the diagnosis is a moving target that depends on the context in which the diagnosis takes place. It remains important, however, to consistently monitor these effects through research and program evaluation and to develop strategies to maximize the amount of risk behavior reduction that results. At the same time, we must respect the rights of newly diagnosed individuals and help them avoid the potential negative social consequences of HIV infection.

ACKNOWLEDGEMENTS Preparation of this chapter was supported by NIH grants R01-AA13567 (Lance S. Weinhardt, Ph.D., PI) and U10-MH57631 (Jeffrey A. Kelly, Ph.D., PI), and NIMH Center grant P30-MH57226 (Jeffrey A. Kelly, Ph.D., PI). Thanks to Allan Hauth, M.S., for bibliographic assistance and Blair T. Johnson, Ph.D., for assistance with meta-analytic techniques. Data from the NIMH Healthy Living Project courtesy of the NIMH Healthy Living Project Team, Principal Investigators Mary Jane Rotheram-Borus, Ph.D., Jeffrey A. Kelly, Ph.D., Anke A. Ehrhardt, Ph.D., Margaret Chesney, Ph.D., and Stephen F. Morin, Ph.D.; NIMH Staff Collaborators: Willo Pequegnat, Ph.D., Christopher M. Gordon, Ph.D.

REFERENCES

Allen, S., Serufilira, A., Bogaerts, J., Van de Perre, P., Nsengumuremyi, F., Lindan, C., Carael, M., Wolf, W., Coates, C., and Hulley, S. (1992a). Confidential HIV testing and condom promotion in Africa: Impact on HIV and gonorrhea rates. *JAMA* 268:3338–3343.

Allen, S., Tice, J., Van de Perre, P., Serufilira, A., Hudes, E., Nsengumuremyi, F., Bogaerts, J., Lindan, C., and Hulley, S. (1992b). Effect of serotesting with counselling on condom use and seroconversion among HIV discordant couples in Africa. *BMJ* 304:1605–1609.

Allen, S., Meinzen-Derr, J., Kautzman, M., Zulu, I., Trask, S., Fideli, U., Musonda, R., Kasolo, F., Gao, F., and Haworth, A. (2003). Sexual behavior of HIV discordant couples after HIV counseling and testing. *AIDS* 17:733–740.

Avants, S. K., Warburton, L. A., and Margolin, A. (2001). How injection drug users coped with testing HIV seropositive: Implications for subsequent health-related behaviors. *AIDS Educ. Prev.* 13:207–218.

Brody, S. (1995). Patients misrepresenting their risk factors for AIDS. *Int. J. STD AIDS* 6:392–398.

Casadonte, P. P., DesJarlais, D. C., Friedman, S. R., and Rotrosen, J. P. (1990). Psychological and behavioral impact among intravenous drug users of learning HIV test results. *Int. J. Addict.* 25:409–426.

Catania, J. A., Kegeles, S., and Coates, T. J. (1990). Towards an understanding of risk behavior: An AIDS-risk reduction model. *Health Educ. Quart.* 17:53–72.

Centers for Disease Control and Prevention. (2003). Advancing HIV prevention: New strategies for a changing epidemic—United States, 2003. *MMWR* 52:329–332.

Chamot, E., Coughlin, S. S., Farley, T. A., and Rice, J. C. (1999). Gonorrhea incidence and HIV testing and counseling among adolescents and young adults seen at a clinic for sexually transmitted diseases. *AIDS* 13:971–979.

Chesney, M. A. and Folkman, S. (1999). The psychosocial management of HIV disease in adults. In: Holmes, K., Sparling, P., Mardh, P., Lemon, S., Stamm, W., Piot, P., Wasserheit, J., (eds.), *Sexually transmitted diseases*, 3rd ed. McGraw Hill, New York, pp. 987–995.

Chesney, M. A., Folkman, S., and Chambers, D. (1996). Coping effectiveness training. *Int. J. STD AIDS* 7(S2):75–82.

Chesney, M. A., Chambers, D. B., Taylor, J. M., Johnson, L. S., and Folkman, S. (2003). Coping effectiveness training for men living with HIV: Results from a randomized clinical trial testing a group-based intervention. *Psychosom. Med.* 65:1038–1046.

Cleary, P. D., Van Devanter, N., Rogers, T. F., Singer, E., Shipton-Levy, R., Steilen, M., Stuart, A., Avorn, J., and Pindyck, J. (1991). Behavior changes after notification of HIV infection. *Am. J. Public Health* 81:1586–1590.

Coates, T. J., Morin, S. F., and McCusick, L. (1987). Behavioral consequences of AIDS antibody testing among gay men. *JAMA* 258:1889.

Cohen, J. (1977). *Statistical power analysis for the behavioral sciences*, 2nd ed. Academic Press, New York.

Colfax, G. N., Buchbinder, S. P., Cornelisse, P. G. A., Vittinghoff, E., Mayer, K., and Celum, C. (2002). Sexual risk behaviors and implications for secondary HIV transmission during and after seroconversion. *AIDS* 16:1529–1535.

Crepaz, N., and Marks, G. (2002). Towards an understanding of sexual risk behavior in people living with HIV: A review of social, psychological, and medical findings. *AIDS* 16:135–149.

Deren, S. Beardsley, M., Coyle, S., and Singer, M. (1998). HIV serostatus and risk behaviors in a multisite sample of drug users. *J. Psychoactive Drugs* 30:239–245.

DeRosa, C. J., and Marks, G. (1998). Preventive counseling of HIV positive men and self-disclosure of serostatus to sex partners: new opportunities for prevention. *Health Psychol.* 17:224–231.

Fox, R., Odaka, N. J., Brookmeyer, R., and Polk, B. F. (1987). Effect of HIV antibody disclosure on subsequent sexual activity in homosexual men. *AIDS* 1:241–246.

George, N., Green, J., and Murphy, S. (1998). Sexually transmitted disease rates before and after HIV testing. *Int. J. STD AIDS* 9:291–293.

Hedges, L. V. (1981). Distribution theory for Glass's estimator of effect size and related estimators. *JSE* 6:107–128.

Hedges, L. V., and Olkin, I. (1985). *Statistical methods for meta-analysis*. Academic Press, Orlando, FL.

Huggins, J., Elman, N., Baker, C., Forrester, R. G., and Lyter, D. (1991). Affective and behavioral responses of gay and bisexual men to HIV antibody testing. *Soc. Work* 36:61–66.

Jacquez, J. A., Koopman, J. S., Simon, C. P., and Longini, I. M. (1994). Role of primary infection in epidemics of HIV infection in gay cohorts. *JAIDS* 7:1169–1184.

Johnson, B. T. (1993). *DSTAT 1.10: Software for the meta-analytic review of research literatures: Upgrade documentation*. Lawrence Erlbaum, Hillsdale, NJ.

Kalichman, S. C. (1998). *Understanding AIDS: Advances in research and treatment*, 2nd ed. American Psychological Association, Washington, DC.

Kalichman, S. C. (2000). HIV transmission risk behaviors of men and women living with HIV-AIDS: Prevalence, predictors, and emerging clinical interventions. *Clin. Psychol. Sci. Pract.* 7:32–47.

Kalichman, S. C., Rompa, D., Cage, M., Di Fonzo, K., Simpson, D., Austin, J., Luke, W., Buckles, J., Kyomugisha, F., Benotsch, E., Pinkerton, S., and Graham, J. (2001). Effectiveness of an intervention to reduce HIV transmission risks in HIV-positive people. *Am. J. Prev. Med.* 21:84–92.

Kamb, M. L., Fishbein, M., Douglas, J. M., Rhodes, F., Rogers, J., Bolan, G., Zenilman, J., Hoxworth, T., Malotte, C. K., Iatesta, M., Kent, C., Lentz, A., Graziano, S., Byers, R. H., Peterman T. A., and Project RESPECT Study Group. (1998). Efficacy of risk-reduction counseling to prevent human immunodeficiency virus and sexually transmitted diseases. *JAMA* 280:1161–1167.

Kamenga, M., Ryder, R. W., Jingu, M., Mbuyi, N., Mbu, L., Behets, F., Brown, C., and Heyward, W. L. (1991). Evidence of marked sexual behavior change associated with low HIV-1 seroconversion in 149 married couples with discordant HIV-1 serostatus: Experience at an HIV counseling center in Zaire. *AIDS*. 5:S61–S67.

Kinsey, A. C., Pomeroy, W. B., Martin, C. E., and Gebhard, P. H. (1953). *Sexual behavior in the human female*. W. B. Saunders, Philadelphia, PA.

Kinsey, A. C., Pomeroy, W. B., and Gebhard, P. H. (1948). *Sexual behavior in the human male*. W. B. Saunders, Philadelphia, PA.

Leaity, S., Sherr, L., Wells, H., Evans, A., Miller, R., Johnson, M., and Elford, J. (2000). Repeat HIV testing: high-risk behavior or risk reduction strategy? *AIDS* 14:547–552.

Lewontin, R. C. (1995). Sex, lies, and social science. *New York Review of Books* 42:24–29.

Lupton, D., McCarthy, S., and Chapman, S. (1995). Doing the right thing: Symbolic meanings and experiences of having an HIV antibody test. *Soc. Sci. Med.* 41:173–180.

Magura, S., Shapiro, J. L., Grossman, J. I., Siddiqi, Q., Lipton, D. S., Amann, K. R., Koger, J., and Gehan, K. (1990). Reactions of methadone patients to HIV antibody testing. *Adv. Alc. Subst. Abuse* 8:97–111.

Needle, R., Fisher, D. G., Weatherbee, N., Chitwood, D., Brown, B., Cesari, H., Booth, R., Williams, M. L., Watters, J., Andersen, M., and Braunstein, M. (1995). Reliability of self-reported HIV risk behaviors of drug users. *Psychol. Addict. Behav.* 9:242–250.

Ostrow, D. G., Joseph, J. G., Kessler, R., Soucy, J., Tal, M., Eller, M., Cmiel, J., and Phair, J. P. (1989). Disclosure of HIV antibody status: Behavioral and mental health correlates. *AIDS Educ. Prev.* 1:1–11.

Otten, M. W., Zaidi, A. A., Wroten, J. E., Witte, J. J., and Peterman, T. A. (1993). Changes in sexually transmitted disease rates after HIV testing and posttest counseling, Miami, 1988 to 1989. *Am. J. Public Health* 83:529–533.

Padian, N. S., O'Brien, T. R., Chang, Y., Glass, S., and Francis, D. P. (1993). Prevention of heterosexual transmission of human immunodeficiency virus through couple counseling. *JAIDS* 6:1043–1048.

Parsons, J. T., Huszti, H. C., Crudder, S. O., Rich, L., and Mendoza, J. (2000). Maintenance of safer sexual behaviours: evaluation of a theory-based intervention for HIV seropositive men with haemophilia and their female partners. *Haemophilia* 6(3):181–190.

Patterson, T. L., Shaw, W. S., and Semple, S. J. (2003). Reducing the sexual risk behaviors of HIV+ individuals: Outcome of a randomized controlled trial. *Ann. Behav. Med.* 25:137–145.

Pickering, H., Quigley, M., Pepin, J., Todd, J., and Wilkins, A. (1993). The effects of post-test counseling on condom use among prostitutes in The Gambia. *AIDS* 7:271–273.

Rogers, R. W. (1975). A protection motivation theory of fear appeals and attitude change. *J. Psychol.* 91:93–114.

Roth, D. L., Stewart, K. E., Clay, O. J., van der Straten, A., Karita, E., and Allen, S. (2001). Sexual practices of HIV discordant couples in Rwanda: Effects of a testing and counseling programme for men. *Int. J. STD AIDS* 12:181–188.

Rotheram-Borus, M. J., Lee, M. B., Murphy, D. A., Futterman, D., Duan, N., Birnbaum, J., and the Teens Linked To Care Consortium. (2001). Efficacy of a preventive intervention for youth living with HIV. *Am. J. Public Health* 91:400–405.

Rotheram-Borus, M., Kelly, J. A., Ehrhardt, A. A., Chesney, M. A., Lightfoot, M., Weinhardt, L. S., Kirshenbaum, S. B., Johnson, M. O., Remien, R. H., Morin, S. F., Kertzner, R. M.,

Pequegnat, W., Gordon, C. M. and the NIMH Healthy Living Project Team. (2003, July). *HIV Transmission Risk Behavior, Medication Adherence, Mental Health, and Substance Use in a Four-City Sample of People Living with HIV: Implications for HIV Prevention—Findings from the NIMH Healthy Living Project.* Paper presented at the 2003 National HIV Prevention Conference, Atlanta, GA.

Schechter, M. T., Craib, K. J. P., Willoughby, B., Douglas, B., McLeod, W. A., Maynard, M., Constance, P., and O'Shaughnessy, M. (1988). Patterns of sexual behavior and condom use in a cohort of homosexual men. *Am. J. Public Health* 78:1535–1538.

Snedecor, G. W., and Cochran, W. G. (1980). *Statistical methods*, 7th ed. Iowa State University Press, Ames, IA.

van Griensven, G. J. P., de Vroome, E. M. M., Tielman, R. A. P., Goudsmit, J., de Wolf, F., van der Noordaa, J., and Coutinho, R. A. (1989). Effect of human immunodeficiency virus (HIV) antibody knowledge on high-risk sexual behavior with steady and nonsteady sexual partners among homosexual men. *Am. J. Epidemiol.* 129:596–603.

Voluntary HIV-1 Counseling and Testing Efficacy Study Group (VCT). (2000). Efficacy of voluntary HIV-1 counseling and testing in Individuals and couples in Kenya, Tanzania, and Trinidad: A randomized trial. *Lancet* 356:103–112.

Weinhardt, L. S., Carey, M. P., Johnson, B. T., and Bickham, N. L. (1999). Effects of HIV counseling and testing on sexual risk behavior: Meta-analysis of published research, 1985–1997. *Am. J. Public Health* 89:1397–1405.

Weinhardt, L. S., Kelly, J. A., Brondino, M. J., Rotheram-Borus, M. J., Kirshenbaum, S., Chesney, M., Remien, R. H., Morin, S. Lightfoot, M., Ehrhardt, A. A., Johnson, M. O., Catz, S. L., Pinkerton, S. D., Benotsch, E. G., Hong, D., Gore-Felton, C., and the NIMH Healthy Living Project Team. (2004). HIV transmission risk behavior among men and women living with HIV in four US cities. *JAIDS, 36*, 1057–1066.

Zapka, J. G., Stoddard, A., Zorn, M., McCusker, J., and Mayer, K. (1991). HIV antibody test result knowledge, risk perceptions among homosexually active men. *Patient Educ. Counsel.* 18:9–17.

CHAPTER THREE

HIV Disclosure and Safer Sex

Jane M. Simoni and David W. Pantalone

INTRODUCTION

"It is difficult to identify a more charged issue in AIDS prevention than that of nondisclosure of positive HIV status to sexual partners." (Ciccarone et al., 2003; p. 949)

Jenenne is a 38-year-old African American woman in Harlem who contracted HIV 10 years ago from her ex-husband, a heroin user. She uses crack cocaine sporadically and is recurrently depressed. Financially, her situation is precarious. Jenenne at first concealed her HIV status from her current boyfriend, Darrell, out of fear he would reject her. Although they began their sexual relationship always using condoms, Darrel later refused. Suspicious of Jenenne's worsening physical condition, Darrell finally confronted her and discovered the truth. Furious, he promptly abandoned her. Eventually, though, he returned and they resumed their relationship, practicing exclusively safer sex. However, Darrell soon began complaining about how condoms were inhibiting his sexual functioning and began pressuring Jenenne to have unprotected intercourse.

Miguel is a 25-year-old Mexican American gay man in Los Angeles who was diagnosed HIV-positive two years ago. He has never used drugs and has stopped drinking since his diagnosis. He works full-time as a waiter. Since his diagnosis, he has had multiple anonymous sexual encounters and a few short relationships. Miguel never revealed his serostatus to any of these partners; however, he scrupulously practiced safer sex, feeling a moral responsibility to protect others. Currently, he is in a committed relationship with another Mexican American man, José, who has never been tested for HIV. Miguel has been very open with José about his

HIV status and his desire to take precautions to prevent transmitting the virus to him. However, José refuses to engage in any discussion of HIV or to practice safer sex. According to José's fatalistic perspective, "If I'm going to get infected, I'm going to get infected, and there's nothing we can do about it." Furthermore, he detests condoms because they disrupt his sexual spontaneity and remind him of Miguel's life-threatening illness. Forced to choose between leaving his boyfriend or having unprotected sex with him, Miguel has chosen to continue the relationship and hope for the best.

The experiences of the (fictitiously named) couples in the preceding case examples illustrate some of the complex internal motivations and external incentives that underlie choices about HIV disclosure and sexual safety. For these couples, as for many individuals living with HIV, the connection between disclosure and safe sex is neither simple nor consistent. Decisions with respect to these issues are further complicated by power differentials between partners, rigid gender roles, community norms, and cultural values. Often, choices about the use of protection cannot be made unilaterally. Cases such as these have sparked questions about the role of disclosure in safer sex. In this chapter, we examine how empirical research can inform the discussion.

To fuel the epidemic, HIV-positive individuals must interact unsafely with HIV-negative individuals. In fact, research indicates that up to one third of individuals diagnosed with HIV continue to have unprotected sex, at times without informing partners, who may be of negative or unknown serostatus (Marks et al., 1994; Wolitski et al., 1998; Kalichman, 2000). Note that nondisclosure in such instances may involve active deception, not merely passive omission (Stein et al., 1998).

In response to reports of increasing numbers of new infections, many public health officials are shifting their HIV prevention efforts from populations at risk for HIV infection to those individuals who are already infected. Notably, CDC in 2000 initiated an innovative Serostatus Approach to Fighting the Epidemic (Project SAFE) and expanded these efforts in 2003 with the initiative Advancing HIV Prevention: New Strategies for a Changing Epidemic (see Chapter 1 and Janssen et al., 2001, 2003). CDC and the public health establishment hope to slow the spread of the epidemic, by, among other approaches, making HIV prevention a part of routine medical care targeting individuals who are already infected, developing interventions to increase rapid testing, facilitating and expediting access to treatment, and decreasing transmission risk behaviors HIV-positive individuals. A major component of preventive efforts directed at HIV-positive individuals involves encouraging them to disclose their HIV serostatus to their sexual partners. Indeed, since the late 1980's the US Public Health

Service has been recommending that all persons with HIV notify their sexual partners of their status and the CDC has been mandating discussions of disclosure to partners in posttest counseling (CDC, 1987). Furthermore, a coalition of public and professional organizations representing a variety of health care providers has come forward to advocate for brief HIV prevention interventions in the context of routine medical care, including discussing safer sex practices with HIV-positive patients and encouraging them to disclose their HIV serostatus to all sex partners (CDC et al., 2004).

Underlying the attempt to encourage HIV-positive individuals to reveal their serostatus to their sex partners is the assumption that disclosure will increase the safety of subsequent sexual activity with informed partners. As Norman et al. (1998) remarked, "... it is reasonable to assume that a couple's diligence in using condoms consistently and correctly would be enhanced by one partner's disclosure of positive serostatus" (p. 341). Miller et al. (1990) concurred that open communication is likely to facilitate safer sex practices. Indeed, disclosure may facilitate the discussion of sexual safe activities or the negotiation of protection. Moreover, it may increase the motivation of the informed partners to use protection to prevent HIV transmission, especially if they are uninfected.

However, significant disincentives and barriers to revealing one's HIV diagnosis persist (Ciccarone et al., 2003). These include fears of rejection and abandonment; discrimination such as in the form of eviction or termination of employment; retribution; violence; and other forms of abuse. Most of these possible outcomes are based on the social stigma that is widely acknowledged to be associated with an HIV diagnosis (Kalichman, 1998). Additionally, divulging that one is HIV-positive may expose other stigmatized behaviors or identities (e.g., that one is gay or an injection drug user; Kalichman and Nachimson, 1999). Disempowered individuals may be particularly reluctant to risk these adverse reactions.

There is another impetus to remain silent regarding one's HIV-positive serostatus. State legislatures and prosecutors emphasized from early in the epidemic that HIV-positive individuals who are sexually active may be liable to prosecution under assault, reckless endangerment, and attempted murder statutes. Case law and statutes now address exposure (whether or not condoms were involved) and not just infection (Stein and Samet, 1999). As of 1999, 31 US states had statutes making sexual contact without disclosure a criminal offense (Shriver et al., 2000). Also, in many states, health professionals are now mandated to report to the appropriate authorities HIV-positive individuals who have unprotected sex without informing their partners of their HIV infection (Lambda Legal Defense Fund, 2002). Civil liberty lawyers contend that these statutes may actually hamper disclosure of HIV status by opening up the possibility of later arrest.

These psychosocial, social, practical, and legal barriers may contribute to the refusal of many individuals with HIV to divulge their serostatus to sexual partners. According to early studies before the advent of antiretroviral therapy, primarily of men who have sex with men (MSM) on the West Coast, nondisclosure to sexual partners ranged from 2% to 52%, with disclosure generally higher for steady than casual partners (O'Brien et al., 2003). In later studies in populations with more diverse samples, nondisclosure to sexual partners ranged from 13% to 41% (O'Brien et al., 2003).

Even when individuals surmount the barriers to disclosure and reveal their HIV serostatus to sexual partners, there is no guarantee of their subsequent sexual safety. As Serovich and Mosach (2003) cautioned, disclosure does not mean individuals will use the information to protect themselves or others; in fact, some will knowingly place themselves at risk for infection. They concluded "Thus, it is erroneous to assume that disclosure would lead to safer behaviors or a lowering of risk" (p. 78). Marks and Crepaz (2001) expressed a similar viewpoint, explaining that some HIV-positive individuals may disclose their status but then eschew protection, what they termed "informed exposure", possibly to attest to their commitment to the relationship or because of the effects of substance use prior to sexual activity. Others engage in informed exposure because their partners made the final decision to forgo protection. In the extreme, a subset of the MSM community seeks out opportunities for "barebacking," or the intentional participation in unprotected anal intercourse (see Chapter 4 and Halkitis et al., 2003).

Similarly, nondisclosure does not necessarily lead to unsafe sex. Some HIV-positive individuals may refrain from divulging their HIV serostatus to protect their privacy and avoid the negative consequences of disclosure such as stigma or rejection. However, they may engage in protected sexual activity, perhaps out of a sense of personal responsibility toward their partners. Marks and Crepaz (2001) labeled this scenario "uninformed protection."

Clearly, disclosure is neither necessary nor sufficient to ensure safer sex. Yet, is the association between disclosure and subsequent sexual safety strong enough to warrant HIV prevention policies that place considerable emphasis on disclosure? To address this important question, we reviewed the available empirical literature on the association between HIV disclosure and safer sex, after first considering theory relevant to the field of HIV disclosure. We end with a discussion of the implications of the findings for future research, practice, and policy.

THEORETICAL CONSIDERATIONS

Self-Disclosure Theory

Most of the early theoretical work on self-disclosure derives from personality and social psychological theory, according to which the sharing of intimate personal information is seen as a stable trait; a unitary construct that can be assessed with a paper-and-pencil inventory. The pioneer in this area was Jourard (1971), who considered self-disclosure to be necessary for intimacy and self-understanding and his research examined how the supposedly unidimensional trait of disclosure was related to the positive, enduring characteristics of an individual associated with psychological well-being and interpersonal success.

However, decades of research attempting to identify individual differences in self-disclosure yielded few consistent or useful findings (Davis and Franzoi, 1987). Researchers therefore switched their focus to asking why individual difference measures of disclosure were sometimes predictive of actual self-disclosure and other times were not. Toward this end, studies examined the methodological limitations of the disclosure scales themselves, the effect of context, the importance of situational factors, the relationship of the target to the discloser, and the role of personality traits of the target (Miller and Read, 1987). These studies tended to be highly descriptive.

In an effort to understand how underlying personality processes might explain variability in self-disclosure, Miller and Read (1987) developed an initial conceptual framework. They proposed that personality traits are stable configurations of four components: (a) an individual's goals, (b) the plans for attaining these goals, (c) the resources required for successfully executing these plans, and (d) the beliefs about the world that would affect the execution of the plans.

Self-Disclosure Theory Applied to HIV Status

Theoretical work on self-disclosure described above has not been highly relevant to disclosure of HIV status. For the most part, disclosure theory does not adequately consider context, including the highly emotionally charged moment when disclosure often takes place, potentially mixed with equal parts sexual desire and substance intoxication; content, which can include the highly stigmatizing nature of an HIV diagnosis; or consequences of HIV disclosure, which are often deleterious and include the potential loss of social support. Indeed, much of the literature on self-disclosure assumes it occurs in the context of a close relationship, involves less socially stigmatized content, and results in the enhancement of intimacy. Hill and Stull (1987) came to similar conclusions in their review of the effect of gender on self-disclosure, citing the need for more consideration of different kinds of disclosures, their varying purposes, and the types of social interactions in which they take place.

An additional limitation of this earlier theoretical work on disclosure is its neglect of cultural values. Traditional communal and collectivist values, in contrast to more individualistic Western norms, may influence an individual's willingness to disclose personal information. For example, the traditional Latino values of *simpatía* and *familismo* may account for the lower rates of HIV disclosure to family, friends, and lovers among less versus more acculturated Mexican American men (Mason et al., 1995) and women (Simoni et al., 1995a).

Finally, although HIV disclosure may be related to certain personality traits, it is likely much more dependent on contextual and situational factors. For example, Zea et al. (2004) found little support for disclosure as a generalized tendency. Instead, they discovered that different factors were influential in disclosure depending on whether the target of disclosure was the individual's mother, father, or closest friend.

HIV Self-Disclosure Theory

Theory specific to the disclosure of HIV is rare. According to Mason et al. (1995), the theory of reasoned action (e.g., Fishbein and Ajzen, 1975) can explain most of the research on disclosure. This theory assumes that people make rational choices based on the information available to them and that behaviors can best be predicted from intentions, which, in turn, are thought to stem at least partially from an individual's relevant attitudes.

Building on work from earlier in the epidemic (e.g., Marks, 1992), Serovich (2001) examined two theories of serostatus disclosure and nondisclosure in one of the few conceptual pieces on the topic. The disease progression theory proposes that individuals disclose their HIV-positive status as their HIV progresses to AIDS because they can no longer hide their illness in the face of hospitalizations and physical deterioration. Numerous prior empirical studies have supported the link between disease progression and disclosure to family and friends; however, the theory has failed to account for disclosure to sexual partners (Mansergh et al., 1995).

The consequence theory of HIV disclosure, based on social exchange theory, presumes that the relationship between disease progression and disclosure is moderated by anticipated consequences of disclosure. According to the consequence theory, persons with HIV will disclose their serostatus to significant others and sexual partners once the anticipated rewards for disclosing (e.g., tangible assistance, medical information, social support and acceptance) outweigh the associated costs (e.g., emotional upset, ostracism, loss of employment or housing). Serovich cited prior empirical support for this theory as well.

Based on structural equation modeling in a sample of HIV-positive gay men, Serovich (2001) found little support for the disease progression theory and good support for the consequence theory. The more important rewards in disclosure decisions were keeping others safe, receiving understanding, and obligation to disclose; main costs were fear of a fight, lecture, or blame. Neither theory was very predictive of disclosure to sexual partners, however. Serovich suggested that a broader measure of consequences might be more informative, perhaps one including relationship variables such as power differentials, need for sex, and strength of partnership.

REVIEW OF THE LITERATURE

Strategy

We searched PsychInfo and Medline for articles published through February 2004 that contained various combinations of the terms HIV/AIDS, infected, infection, positive, seropositive, serostatus, disclosure, self-disclosure, nondisclosure, notification, protected, unprotected, sex, sexual, risk behavior, safer, partner, and prevention. We consulted with experts in the field and inspected the references of the articles we obtained as well.

Findings

Only recently has there been an increase in studies examining disclosure or sexual practices among HIV-positive individuals. Still, very few studies examine and specifically report both of these behaviors for an HIV-positive population, and fewer still collect or report the data in a way that addresses the relationship between disclosure and safer sex. In Table 3.1, we present the 22 studies that even considered both disclosure and sexual safety, whether or not they were explicitly designed to assess the relationship between these two variables.

For each study, when available, we provide information about the sample (i.e., N, basic demographic description, geographic location, and method and date of recruitment,) as well as any descriptive findings related to self-disclosure of HIV and to sexual safety. If any conclusions could be made about the association between disclosure and sexual safety, whether they were explicitly reported in the article or not, these are included as well, along with other noteworthy findings such as correlates of disclosure and sexual safety. In the table, studies are grouped by the gender composition of their samples: only men, only women, or both men and women.

As seen in Table 3.1, we located 10 studies of disclosure and sexual safety with only men in their samples. Two reported no data on the association between disclosure and sexual safety (Norman et al., 1998). Findings among the remaining 8 studies were mixed, with four reporting no significant association (Crepaz and Marks, 2003; Geary et al., 1996; King et al., 1996; Marks and Crepaz, 2001). In both a multi-ethnic sample of men recruited in Los Angeles (De Rosa and Marks, 1998) and a sample of mostly gay or bisexual Hispanic men in Los Angeles (Marks et al., 1991), safer sex was more likely to occur in the context of disclosure with respect to HIV-negative partners but not for partners with a positive or unknown HIV status. Disclosers reported a smaller proportion of partners with whom they had unprotected anal insertive sex than nondisclosers in a multi-ethnic sample of male outpatients from Los Angeles (Marks et al., 1994). Finally, among a US sample of mostly White MSM, no association between disclosure and sexual safety was reported with primary partners, but, among non-primary partners, disclosers were more likely than non-disclosers to report consistent condom use for insertive anal sex (Wolitski et al., 1998).

Four of the articles we located had samples exclusively of women (see Table 3.1). In all four, at least one-third (and up to two-thirds) of the sexually active HIV-positive women and girls reported unprotected sex. Data on disclosure, where reported, indicated most informed their partners. Only Sturdevant et al. (2001) provided data addressing the association between HIV disclosure to sexual partners and safer sex. They concluded that disclosure influenced safer sex among adolescents, based on analyses controlling for perception that partner was also HIV-positive indicating that without disclosure (vs. with disclosure), participants reported less condom use. However, there was no partner-level analysis - condom use was computed for up to three partners for each participant, and the timing of disclosure in relation to safer sex was not considered. Additionally, these results were obtained from a sample of HIV-negative and HIV-positive individuals combined.

In eight studies (shown in Table 3.1), both men and women participated. Two reports did not provide data that would allow us to determine

Table 3.1. Published Studies Examining HIV Disclosure and Sexual Safety

Citation	Sample	Disclosure to sexual partners	Sexual safety	Association between disclosure and sexual safety	Other noteworthy results
MEN ONLY (10)					
Crepaz and Marks (2003)	105 HIV+ male outpatients (64% African American) at HIV clinic in Los Angeles, 1996–1997	53% disclosed their seropositive status to their most recent HIV- or HIV? (i.e., at-risk) partner; 65% talked about using a condom; 48% discussed types of safe activities; 42% agreed very much with their partner about safer sex	28% engaged in unprotected anal or vaginal intercourse with at-risk partner	Disclosure was not related to safer sex; however, disclosers who discussed safer sex (vs. those who disclosed only) had a higher prevalence of protected anal or vaginal intercourse	Disclosure was related to safer sex discussions and was more prevalent with HIV- than HIV? partners and with partners with whom the individual had had sex more than 3 times
Marks and Crepaz (2001)	206 multiethnic HIV+ men whose most recent partner was HIV– or HIV?, recruited at an outpatient clinic in Los Angeles, 1995–1997	52% disclosed to HIV- or HIV? partner; strategies employed were: 40% informed protection; 35% uninformed protection; 12% informed exposure; and 13% uninformed exposure	25% engaged in unprotected anal or vaginal intercourse; unsafe sex was associated with: substance use before sex, having an HIV? partner, less emotional involvement with partner, and more recent HIV diagnosis	Unsafe sex not more prevalent among disclosers than non-disclosers	Disclosure not associated with unsafe sex in any of 25 demographic or partner subgroups

(Continued)

73

Table 3.1. (*Continued*)

Citation	Sample	Disclosure to sexual partners	Sexual safety	Association between disclosure and sexual safety	Other noteworthy results
Prestage, Van De Ven, Grulich, Kippax, Mcinnes, and Hendry (2001)	300 (87% White) gay men who reported casual sex within the last 6 months (20% were HIV+), recruited from the community in Sydney, Australia, 1998	Among HIV+ men, 53% disclosed and 23% asked about any partner's serostatus	Among HIV+ men, 33% engaged in unprotected anal insertive sex (0% with HIV−, 25% with HIV+, and 22% with HIV? partners)	*No relevant data provided*	Overall, 45% were requested to engage in unprotected anal insertive sex
De Rosa and Marks (1998)	255 HIV+ multiethnic men who were sexually active in the last 2 months, recruited at 2 HIV outpatient clinics in Los Angeles, 1992–1993	93% told all their HIV+ partners, 57% told all their HIV− partners, and 23% told all their HIV? partners	Percentage of informed partners with whom all oral, anal, and vaginal sex was protected: 26%; for uninformed partners: 16%	Among HIV− but not HIV+ or HIV? partners: exclusively protected sexual activity occurred with a significantly greater percentage of informed than uninformed partners	Combination of posttest and clinic counseling increased likelihood of informing all partners

(Continued)

Norman, Kennedy, and Parish (1998)	358 mainly White HIV+ heterosexual men with hemophilia in US, 1992	91% of men involved in a close relationship and 50% of uninvolved men had disclosed to most recent partner	84% of involved men reported condom use for vaginal intercourse with main partners, and 100% with other-than-main partners; 82% of uninvolved men consistently used condoms for other-than-main partners	*No relevant data provided*	Involved vs. uninvolved men were more likely to discuss HIV risk reduction; disclosure was negatively correlated with risk reduction discussion barriers
Wolitski, Rietmeijer, Goldbaum, and Wilson (1998)	701 mainly White MSM from 4 US cities who recently received their HIV test result, 1987–1991	89% of HIV+ MSM informed primary sex partner; 34% informed non-primary partner	16% of HIV+ MSM reported inconsistent condom use during anal intercourse with an uninformed non-primary partner within the last 90 days	With primary partners, HIV+ disclosers and non-disclosers did not differ in sexual practices or condom use; with non-primary partners, disclosers more likely than non-disclosers to report consistent condom use for insertive anal intercourse	For HIV+ MSM, likelihood of disclosure not related to number of partners

Table 3.1. (*Continued*)

Citation	Sample	Disclosure to sexual partners	Sexual safety	Association between disclosure and sexual safety	Other noteworthy results
Geary, King, Forsberg, Delaronde, and Parsons (1996)	167 suburban, 77% White HIV+ males (12–25 years old) with hemophilia in US	58% of the 60% who were sexually active did not disclose to their most recent partner	Among disclosers, 64% reported consistent condom use and 81% used a condom during last sexual intercourse; for nondisclosers, 66% and 85%	No significant association found between disclosure and condom use	Most significant predictor of disclosure was perception that peers would disclose; age positively related to disclosure
King, Delaronde, Dinoi, and Forsberg (1996)	306 HIV+ mostly White adolescent males with hemophilia, recruited at 11 hemophilia treatment centers, 1992	HIV status disclosure to all partners was reported by 30% of individuals who used alcohol or other drugs (AOD) as a coping strategy for their diagnosis, and 55% of non-AOD copers	68% reported using condoms every time for sex	No difference in disclosure was found between those who used condoms every time for sex and those who were less consistent	Non-AOD copers associated with disclosure of HIV status, discussion of safer sex, and finding the use of condoms enjoyable
Marks, Ruiz, Richardson, Reed, Mason, Sotelo, and Turner (1994)	609 HIV+ multiethnic men recruited at 2 HIV outpatient clinics in Los Angeles, 1991–1992	86% of HIV+, 46% of HIV–, and 18% of HIV? anal sex partners were informed	9% engaged in unprotected insertive anal intercourse in the past 2 months (3.27 times more likely with HIV+ than HIV- or HIV? partners)	HIV+ respondents had unprotected insertive anal sex with 18% of HIV– partners who were informed and with 23% of HIV– partners who were not informed (26% and 28%, receptive)	

Marks, Richardson, and Maldonado (1991)	138 HIV+ mainly Hispanic sexually active men, mostly gay or bisexual, recruited at a public HIV outpatient clinic in Los Angeles	52% of sexually active men kept their diagnosis secret from at least one partner; disclosure more common to HIV+ than HIV- partners	17% engaged in unprotected insertive anal intercourse with HIV- partners without disclosure (29%, receptive)	Disclosure to HIV+ partners generally occurred in combination with unprotected contact, whereas disclosure to HIV- partners generally occurred in combination with protected contact	Likelihood of disclosure inversely related to number of partners
WOMEN ONLY (4) Sturdevant, Belzer, Weissman, Friedman, Sarr, (2001)	153 HIV+ and 90 HIV- sexually active adolescent girls (73% African American) from 13 US cities	Among HIV+ girls, disclosure related to perception that partner was HIV+	59% of HIV+ and 80% of HIV- girls reported oral, anal, or vaginal sex without condom in past 3 months; among HIV+ girls, non-use of condoms was associated with older partner age, greater partner age difference, partner being HIV+, and longer duration of partnership	Among HIV+ girls, without disclosure (vs. with disclosure) less condom use was reported, after controlling for perception that partner was HIV	HIV+ (vs. HIV-) girls had older and more HIV-positive partners; among HIV+ non-disclosers, non-condom use was associated with perception of partner as HIV-positive and larger partner age difference

(Continued)

Table 3.1. (*Continued*)

Citation	Sample	Disclosure to sexual partners	Sexual safety	Association between disclosure and sexual safety	Other noteworthy results
Simoni, Walters, and Nero (2000)	Multiethnic sample of 105 HIV+ heterosexually-active women in New York City	Disclosure data available for steady partners only: all but one were informed	54% reported unprotected oral, anal, or vaginal sex in last 90 days	*Analyses among steady partners could not examine association between disclosure and unsafe sex because all but one steady partner was informed.*	Unprotected sex associated with having steady (vs. non-steady) partners and current substance use but (among steady partners) not with steady partner's serostatus
Clark, Kissinger, Bedimo, Dunn, and Albertin (1997)	83 HIV+ women (91% African-American) attending an outpatient clinic in New Orleans, LA	77% reported that current sex partner knows their HIV+ status; 91% had ever discussed condom use with current partner and 87% reported that they initiated the conversation; partners were HIV+ (26%), HIV- (46%), or HIV? (28%)	69% reported always using condoms with their primary partner (60% for other partners); 29% said they never used condoms with primary versus (13% for other partners); 65% of the sample with an HIV+ partner did not use a condom the last time they had sex	*No relevant data provided*	23% reported being forced to have sex against their will; 53% sometimes or always were drunk or high on drugs during sex; 74% reported only having 1 sex partner in the last year

Reference	Sample				
Simoni, Mason, Marks, Ruiz, and Richardson (1995)	72 multiethnic HIV+ women recruited at two outpatient clinics in Los Angeles, 1991-1992	81% of the 21 sex partners were informed; all uninformed partners were HIV- or HIV?	68% of those sexually active in the last two months engaged in unprotected oral, anal, or vaginal sex with 14 partners – these were 5 of the 6 HIV+ and 9 of the 15 HIV-/? partners; unprotected sex occurred with 6 informed HIV-/? partners	*No relevant data provided*	71% of sex partners were HIV- or HIV?; 8% of women did not know unprotected sex could transmit virus
BOTH MEN AND WOMEN (8) Ciccarone, Kanouse, Collins, Miu, Chen, Morton, and Stall (2003)	US national probability survey of HIV+ adults in medical care: 606 gay/bisexual men, 287 heterosexual men, and 504 women	1-2% of men and 5% of women reported not disclosing in serodiscordant exclusive partnerships	16% of gay/bisexual men, 5% of heterosexual men, and 7% of women had unprotected anal or vaginal sex without disclosure in last 6 months; for gay/bisexual men only, substantially more sex (both protected and unprotected) without disclosure occurred in nonexclusive partnerships	*No relevant data provided*	Unprotected sex without disclosure occurred equally in seroconcordant and serodiscordant partnerships; most of those reporting sex without disclosure reported only protected sex or oral sex

(Continued)

Table 3.1. (*Continued*)

Citation	Sample	Disclosure to sexual partners	Sexual safety	Association between disclosure and sexual safety	Other noteworthy results
Kalichman, Rompa, Luke, and Austin (2002)	269 HIV-positive men and 114 HIV-positive women (71% African American) from HIV agencies and clinics in Milwaukee, WI	22% of those with a regular partner had not disclosed; 46% for non-regular partner	71% of the 257 who engaged in vaginal or anal intercourse in the last 3 months did so with serodiscordant partners	Percentage of protected intercourse with regular and non-regular serodiscordant partners (68–77%) was similar regardless of whether disclosure had occurred	Frequency of protected and total intercourse (but not percentage protected intercourse) was greater with regular than non-regular serodiscordant partners
D'Angelo, Abdalian, Sarr, Hoffman, and Belzer (2001)	203 HIV+ male and female adolescents who were part of an ongoing national multi-site study	48% of 242 partners were informed; disclosure was more likely to HIV+ (vs. HIV?) and main (vs. casual) partners		Disclosers reported a mean of 14 unprotected sexual encounters (time frame not reported), 41% had HIV-partner(s); Non-disclosers reported a mean of 10 unprotected sexual encounters, 67% had HIV-partner(s)	Disclosure was not related to sociodemographics or substance use

Kalichman (1999)	203 HIV+ men and 129 HIV+ women (67% African American) from HIV agencies and clinics around Atlanta	Nearly half of men and half of women had not disclosed to a sex partner in last 6 months (27% and 28% for last sex partner)	42% of men and 42% of women had unprotected anal or vaginal intercourse (i.e., unsafe sex) in the last six months; 64% of these men and 46% of these women had at least one HIV? partner; 57% of men and 71% of women who had unsafe sex in their last encounter had not disclosed to that partner	*No relevant data provided*	Substance use, emotional distress, maladaptive coping, and relationship status were not predictive of unsafe sex; trading sex and having a higher number of sex partners were associated with unsafe sex
Kalichman and Nachimson (1999)	165 HIV-positive men and 101 HIV-positive women sexually active in last 6 months (67% African American) from HIV agencies and clinics around Atlanta	41% had not disclosed to any sex partners in the last 6 months; 48% of non-disclosers were in exclusive relationships of 6 months or longer; 22% of men and 21% of women had not disclosed to last partner	77% of male and 89% of female non-disclosers had HIV- or HIV? partners in last 6 months	Among men but not women, disclosers reported higher rates of condom-use (especially during anal intercourse) than non-disclosers	Practicing safe sex as a way to avoid disclosure was common; non-disclosers reported more emotional distress than disclosers; substance use was not related to disclosure

(Continued)

Table 3.1. (*Cont.*)

Citation	Sample	Disclosure to sexual partners	Sexual safety	Association between disclosure and sexual safety	Other noteworthy results
Niccolai, Dorst, Myers, and Kissinger (1999)	147 male and female HIV+ outpatients (88% African-American) participating in a risk reduction/partner notification intervention trial in New Orleans, LA, 1994–1998	76% informed (actively or passively) their last partner; African Americans were less likely to disclose, predictors of disclosure include non-African-American race, consistent condom use	76% reported consistent condom use; 85% reported using condoms the last time they had sex; 81% reported having only 1 partner in the previous two months	Those who used condoms consistently were 2.7 times more likely to have disclosed their status than those who reported inconsistent condom use; disclosure also related to condom use at last sex act, and having only 1 sex partner	
Stein, Freedberg, Sullivan, Savetsky, Levenson, Hingson, and Samet (1998)	203 multi-ethnic HIV+ men and women presenting for outpatient care in Boston, MA and Providence, RI, 1994–1996	60% had disclosed to all partners in the past 6 months; among individuals with only 1 partner, 21% had not disclosed; 2+ partners, 58% did not disclose to all (i.e., were inconsistent)	Overall, 43% reported using condoms all the time	Consistent disclosers, inconsistent disclosers, and non-disclosers reported similar rates of condom use; disclosure was related to fewer sexual partners	Disclosure was related to being female, being White/Latino, having high spousal support, and having low friend support

| Sobel, Shine, DiPietro, and Rabinowitz (1996) | 200 HIV-positive male and female outpatients (ethnicity not reported) at a municipal hospital in the South Bronx, NY, 1994 | 77% had disclosed to partners; this proportion did not differ according to partner serostatus | 50% of 119 sexually active in last 4 months reported consistent condom use and 41% reported inconsistent or no condom use; the only difference between these two groups was in proportion of partners who were HIV- or HIV?, which were 65% and 49%, respectively | No difference in proportion of consistent condom users vs. inconsistent/non-users who disclosed |

Note. **HIV+** = HIV-positive. **HIV−** = HIV-negative. **HIV?** = HIV status unknown.

84 - CHAPTER THREE

the relationship between disclosure and safer sex (Ciccarone et al., 2003; Kalichman, 1999). In three of the studies that did provide such data, there was not a significant association. All three of these studies involved men and women who were recruited while seeking outpatient medical care: one researched a sample in the Bronx (Sobel et al., 1996); another sampled a predominantly African-American population in Atlanta (Kalichman et al., 2002); and the third used comparable survey methods in both Providence and Boston (Stein et al., 1998). The three remaining studies did show an association. One outpatient sample in New Orleans demonstrated that consistent condom users were more likely to disclose their status than inconsistent condom users (Niccolai et al., 1999). A study of adolescents indicated an associated between unprotected sexual encounters and disclosure (D'Angelo et al., 2001). The remaining study of predominately African-Americans in Atlanta reported a significant association for men but not women (Kalichman and Nachimson, 1999).

INTERPRETATION AND INTEGRATION
OF RESEARCH FINDINGS

In summary, only 15 of the 22 studies reviewed provided data that allowed us to examine the association between disclosure and safer sex. Fewer still provided a methodologically sound analysis, especially with respect to women. Studies also reported conflicting results, often with a significant effect limited to one subgroup of participants, such as HIV-negative or non-primary partners. Clearly, there is no reason to conclude, as did Chen et al. (2003), that there is an "urgent need" for prevention messages promoting disclosure of HIV serostatus to sex partners (p. 169; note that this conclusion was based on their study that did not assess disclosure).

The failure to demonstrate a consistent association between disclosure and safer sex does not necessarily mean that disclosure is irrelevant to the practice of safer sex. Rather, as Marks and Crepaz (2001) suggested, the inability to empirically demonstrate a statistically significant correlation between disclosure and safer sex may be related in part to the frequency of uninformed protection and informed exposure. Alternatively, Crepaz and Marks (2003) offered that disclosure does not always correlate with safer sex because disclosure is a relatively general communication. It is insufficient to ensure the use of protection because it fails to focus specifically on the target behavior of safer sex. The key to safer sex, they suggested and their data supported, is whether the dyad has explicitly discussed using protection and reached agreement about it.

IMPLICATIONS FOR RESEARCH

Limitations of Research to Date

Our review of the studies in Table 3.1 revealed several methodological limitations of the published literature on disclosure and unsafe sex that future researchers should avoid. The biggest concerns are related: the dearth of partner-level analyses and the failure to assess the timing of HIV disclosure in relation to sexual activity. Researchers need to inquire about specific partners and perhaps even particular sexual events. It does not suffice to know whether an individual has informed partners and then whether protection was used over some specific timeframe. Many studies failed to accurately assess timing, if they considered the issue at all. For example, Ciccarone et al. (2003) acknowledged they did not assess the timing of unprotected sex in relation to disclosure (they assessed only timing of any sex) and that it was possible that some participants had unprotected sex only after disclosing their positive status. They proceeded to label this scenario "unlikely," although that possibility is exactly what studies like theirs are attempting to investigate. Furthermore, it is not sufficient to simply assess the number of partners and whether disclosure (ever) and safer sex (ever) occurred with each, again, because we cannot be sure that disclosure preceded safer sex. Of course, even if we know that disclosure preceded safer sex, the causal association is not assured.

Another major methodological limitation we noted was the failure of most studies to account for confounding variables. Numerous factors have been shown to be associated with disclosure, sexual safety, or both and any of these might account for a demonstrated association or lack of association between disclosure and safer sex. Specifically, type of partnership should always be considered because research has shown it is often related to both disclosure and safer sex. Also, including partnership variables can help researchers avoid the problem of a third variable. As Sturdevant et al. (2001) noted in their study of adolescent girls, "There may be some quality to the relationship, unmeasured in the study, which may not only facilitate disclosure but permits more effective condom negotiation" (p. 68). Research on partnership variables has demonstrated that main/steady/close partnerships are more likely to involve disclosure and more likely to involve unprotected sexual activity than other/casual/unfamiliar partnerships (Misovich et al., 1997). Also, as demonstrated among samples of both gay and bisexual men and heterosexual women, sex without disclosure is more likely in nonexclusive than exclusive partnerships (Ciccarone et al., 2003; Clark et al., 1997). Finally, among HIV-positive women in steady partnerships, Simoni et al. (2000) found that being married, having a longer relationship, and receiving greater partner support were related to safer sex.

Another partner variable that is crucial to include in any analysis of disclosure or safer sex is the HIV status of the sex partner, which has consistently been shown to correlate with both these variables. For example, Marks et al. (1994) reported that HIV-positive MSM disclosed to 90% of their HIV-positive partners, 45% of those who were HIV-negative, and 17% of partners with unknown serostatus. Additionally, Marks et al. (1991) reported that disclosure to HIV positive partners generally occurred in combination with unprotected contact, whereas disclosure to HIV-partners generally occurred in combination with protected contact. HIV positive individuals might be more likely to disclose to a partner whom they know is HIV-positive for many reasons, such as their assessment of lowered risk of rejection. Then, they might be more likely to have unsafe sex with this person because they feel less threatening to his or her health. Indeed, Sheon and Crosby (2004) reported that disclosures of HIV positive status appeared to facilitate unprotected anal intercourse among MSM.

Gender is another important variable with likely effects on disclosure and safer sex that many studies ignored, often collapsing across subgroups of men and women and making it impossible to determine gender's direct effects. Dividing men into self-identified gay/bisexual and heterosexual subgroups, as did Ciccarone et al. (2003), also may be illuminating because behavioral norms may differ in these respective communities. As Ciccarone et al. (2003) pointed out, messages in the gay community encouraging the assumption that every partner is positive may have contributed to norms that consider disclosure optional. Perhaps, alternatively, dividing samples into MSM and others (to capture men living on the "down low," for example; Myers et al., 2003) or separating self-identified gay from bisexual men may be necessary to avoid masking the effects of group differences in the potentially culturally bound behaviors of disclosure and safer sex.

Multiple other factors need to be considered in future research, because they also have been shown to correlate with disclosure, safer sex, or both. Specifically, illness severity and length of time since HIV diagnosis have been shown to positively relate to disclosure (Mansergh et al., 1995). Younger age has been related to less disclosure to a main partner (O'Brien et al., 2003) and greater overall disclosure (Simoni et al., 1995a) as well as more risky sex post-notification (Diamond et al., 2000) and greater risk for transmitting HIV (Kalichman, 1999). Perception of partner's viral load has been associated with unprotected sex among HIV-positive MSM (Kalichman et al., 1998). Race and ethnicity as well as level of acculturation among Latinos have been associated with both disclosure (Mason et al., 1995; Simoni et al., 1995a) and risky behavior (Marks et al., 1998).

Researchers also need to consider the context of the sexual activity, which might affect disclosure. As Serovich and Mosack (2003) explained, there is a difference between making love in one's private residence, where some verbal exchange might be expected, and an anonymous encounter in a public restroom or other public sex venue, where norms of silence may prevail (see Chapter 4). Finally, Marks and Crepaz (2001) found that different patterns of disclosure and sexual risk behavior were related to, among other factors, annual income and the use of alcohol or drugs before sex.

Another limitation of the current research that needs to be addressed in future work is the imprecise and nonstandard operationalization of unprotected sex. Ciccarone et al. (2003) conducted one of the few studies to explicitly define unsafe sex as "unprotected anal insertive sex to ejaculation" (p. 951); in other studies, precise terminology is lacking. Some studies included unprotected oral contact under the category of unsafe sex (e.g., Simoni et al., 1995b, 2000), others limited their definition to unprotected anal or vaginal intercourse (e.g., Crepaz and Marks, 2003), and some studies did not define the term sex at all for their participants (e.g., Stein et al., 1998). In one of the few studies that acknowledged this potential problem, Marks and Crepaz (2001) conducted a secondary analysis of their data, widening their definition of unsafe sex to included unprotected insertive oral sex. The prevalence of unsafe sex in their sample increased from 25% to 40%; however, the association between disclosure and safer sex remained non-significant.

Disclosure itself, though seemingly an uncomplicated behavior, also needs to be more explicitly operationalized and assessed. Some individuals may think they have disclosed their diagnosis when, in fact, their partners remain unaware of their status. For example, some HIV-positive men who encounter HIV-negative men willing to engage in unprotected anal intercourse will assume they must also be HIV-positive; otherwise, they might think to themselves, "why would these men put themselves at risk of infection?" HIV-negative partners, in turn, may be imagining that their partners are also HIV-negative; otherwise, "why would these men be putting others at risk?" As Marks and Crepaz (2001) pointed out, disclosure may be a direct statement of the diagnosis or a more subtle communication such as leaving antiretroviral medications within view. Among MSM in San Francisco inferred preferences for sexual positions such as top or bottom are often construed as tacit disclosures of HIV status (Sheon and Crosby, 2004).

Finally, the effect of socially desirable reporting, which most authors failed to mention, may be a potential limitation in current studies that needs to be addressed in future research. Participants in the studies we reviewed were being asked to acknowledge behaviors that are socially sanctioned and often illegal. Few individuals could be expected to easily admit that they had knowingly exposed loved ones to a life-threatening illness without informing them of their risk. The stigmatizing nature of these assessed behaviors most likely has resulted in underreporting of their prevalence. Most problematic for the interpretation would be participants who might acknowledge one behavior but not the other, perhaps reasoning it is not so incriminating to acknowledge having unprotected sex if they have at least divulged their HIV status, or vice-versa. These observations might partially account for reports of the lack of a demonstrated association between disclosure and safer sex.

The social desirability a participant encounters in a study may be affected by the study's design and procedures. For example, studies that do not assure anonymity or that are conducted by persons affiliated with participants' clinic care may be particularly susceptible to the underreporting of nondisclosure and unsafe sex. Studies conducted in conjunction with behavioral counseling may promote response biases by establishing socially desirable behaviors (e.g., Macalino et al., 2002). Relatedly, longitudinal studies, which exclude patients unwilling to adhere to follow-up visits, are prone to selection bias which may affect reported rates of disclosure or safer sex. In fact, O'Brien et al. (2003) found that nondisclosure to sexual partners was less than 30% in four longitudinal studies that were set in the context of behavioral counseling and greater than 30% in six of eight studies that did not require follow-up or include counseling.

Recommendations for Future Research

It is, of course, easier to critique past studies than to design and conduct improved ones. The host of methodological issues raised here underlies the difficulty of empirically determining whether disclosure of one's HIV-positive status leads in a causal manner to safer sex. Indeed, it is hard to even imagine what the ideal study would involve. For obvious practical and ethical reasons, a researcher could not simply randomly assign HIV-positive people to disclose or not disclose and then assess the safety of their sexual activity with subsequent partners. Furthermore, decisions around sexual safety often cannot be made unilaterally and, even if they are, may vary according to sexual partner. Most problematic is that disclosure, of course, does not actually "cause" safer sex any more than nondisclosure "causes" riskier sex. As suggested by the apt title of Marks and Crepaz (2001), sexual activity takes place "within the context of" disclosure. Finally, no design can possibly control for every possible third variable. For example, a sense of social responsibility might lead an individual to decide always to disclose and always to use condoms. In this case, the disclosure *per se* is not the cause or main reason for the safer sexual practices. A final recommendation for future research in this area is the need for more qualitative studies (e.g., Sobo, 1995; Sheon and Crosby, 2004; Nuss et al., 1995). The complex and multiple emotions and motivations underlying decisions about disclosure and sexual protection might best be illuminated with qualitative methods of inquiry. For example, as Wolitski et al. (1998) uncovered, disincentives to protected sex include the belief that condoms diminish sexual pleasure and intimacy, the desire to avoid facing the risk of HIV infection, the heat of the moment, a shared sense of fatalism, and the desire to conceive among heterosexual couples.

IMPLICATIONS FOR PRACTICE

The partial support we noted in our review for the association between disclosure and safer sex provides some justification for efforts to enhance HIV disclosure to sexual partners. Given the highly stigmatizing nature of HIV and the substantial risks disclosure entails, however, HIV-positive individuals may need help in revealing their HIV diagnosis to others. Moreover, according to some research, such assistance may need to be intensive. For example, even 2.3 years after their initial HIV-positive notification and with repeated counseling about disclosure, 29% of HIV-positive adults had not disclosed to any present partner and 30% had not disclosed to any past partner (Perry et al., 1994). Even with posttest and later clinic counseling, 21% of HIV-positive men in Los Angeles had not informed all their partners (De Rosa and Marks, 1998).

Disclosure efforts might be particularly effective among gay men and their primary partners, because at least some data support the notion that disclosure infrequently leads to negative consequences for this population (e.g., Marks et al., 1994). Wolitski et al. (1998) also cautioned, however, that interventions for HIV-positive individuals should guard against furthering their stigmatization or marginalization by increasing the risk that they will face prejudice or harm; to do otherwise would be a disservice to both HIV-negative and HIV-positive persons.

Crepaz and Marks (2003), based in part on their findings that safer sex may depend on more than just disclosure, suggested going beyond the encouragement of disclosure and including skills-building to bolster individuals' ability to communicate effectively about sexual safety and to negotiate condom use with partners. Norman et al. (1998) similarly stressed the need for communication skills training, with the rationale that improved skills may improve the likelihood of safer sex resulting from HIV disclosure and safer sex discussions.

Research suggests that certain subgroups of individuals living with HIV are more at risk than others of withholding disclosure and of engaging in risky sex and, therefore, should perhaps be especially targeted. Specifically, based on findings from Crepaz and Marks (2003), interventions should target those who have tested HIV-positive recently, are of lower socioeconomic status, and already have experience with at-risk partners. Additionally, we may need to target younger people, given data that, compared to older individuals, they are less likely to disclose to their main partner (O'Brien et al., 2003) and more likely to engage in risky sex postnotification (Diamond et al., 2000). The case of HIV-serodiscordant couples may need special consideration, in light of findings that up to 52% in the US and Europe report continuing to engage in unprotected sex (as cited in van der Straten et al., 1998).

Women with HIV, like their male counterparts, place their HIV-negative partners at risk of HIV infection when they engaged in unprotected sexual intercourse. Especially given the risk of HIV transmission to their child should they become pregnant, women living with HIV have an obligation to have protected sexual activity and should be targeted as well as men in HIV prevention efforts. However, power differentials and gender dynamics complicate the practice of safer sex among women. Although to a large extent an HIV-positive woman can control whether she chooses to disclose, she does not have that same control over condom use. As Sturdevant et al. (2001) pointed out, "Although an empowered woman can supply the condom, place it on the man, and be responsible for knowing it has to stay in place, frequently gender power imbalances and cultural influences put male partners in charge of condom use" (p. 65). This reality is reflected in the finding among adult serodiscordant heterosexual couples that condom use is more likely when the male versus the female partner is uninfected (Kennedy et al., 1993). Interventions targeting women, therefore, need to consider gender roles and power differentials and may need to incorporate male partners (e.g., El-Bassel et al., 2003).

Interventions focused on at-risk populations should be appropriately tailored to these groups. For example, Norman et al. (1998) advised that we might have to design interventions differently for men currently involved in sexual partnerships than for uninvolved men. Based on their findings, they suggested that interventions encouraging disclosure among uninvolved men might appear more credible if they address the commonly perceived negative consequences of disclosing to prospective partners.

Besides targeting certain at-risk groups, interventions might benefit by expanding the range of venues and professionals typically included.

De Rosa and Marks (1998) suggested medical clinic providers should emphasize the importance of disclosure. They found that posttest counseling alone is not as effective as a message reinforced at the patient's clinic, perhaps because the shock of the initial diagnosis diminishes the ability to retain other information. Repetition, according to the authors, is key. Moreover, with the availability of potent antiretroviral regimens, more HIV patients are in care, making HIV providers and public clinics an increasingly valuable setting for HIV prevention interventions such as discussion of HIV status and safer sex with partners. Marks et al. (2002) found that among a random sample of 839 California public HIV clinic attendees, 71% reported a clinic provider had talked with them at least once about safer sex (range across six clinics was 52 to 94%); 50% reported a discussion about disclosing their HIV-positive status to sexual partners. The authors conjectured that structural barriers (e.g., lack of time, procedures for referral) or attitudinal and motivational factors on the part of providers might inhibit discussions. They cited the need to assess and surmount these barriers so that more providers might provide important prevention messages to their patients.

As did the CDC and other agencies (2004), Stein and Samet (1999) promoted the idea that healthcare workers can conduct HIV prevention by encouraging their HIV-positive patients to discuss their serostatus with their sexual partners. They emphasized that motivating a patient to disclose is a process and not a one-time command, wherein motivational interviewing techniques may be helpful. Specifically, they recommended four strategies: (a) express empathy for the difficulty involved in disclosing, (b) have the patient explicitly state the pros and cons of disclosure, (c) avoid persuasion via moral arguments as it is usually ineffective, and (d) describe your own experiences with successful disclosures and their positive outcomes. Of course, they noted that safer sexual precautions still need to be emphasized and that past as well as present partners should be informed, often with the help of voluntary health department contact tracing programs.

Mental health providers also have a great opportunity to assist HIV-positive individuals in the difficult act of divulging their diagnosis to sexual partners. Serovich (2000) advised mental health professionals first to encourage their clients to create a list of all persons they would consider telling and then focus on those to be told first. Disclosure to these individuals should be planned strategically. Clients should pick the time and place, ideally, in a relaxed atmosphere with minimal distractions at a time when the target person is not tired, stressed, or emotionally unavailable. Next, clients should consider before the disclosure just how much they want to share regarding the activities that led to their HIV infections, including the option of not discussing the topic at all. Role-playing likely scenarios can facilitate a successful exchange. Finally, the client should be forewarned that disclosure is not a one-time event but, rather, is an unfolding process involving follow-up conversations regarding the effect of the disclosure.

Understanding the reasons why individuals choose to disclose or not to disclose their serostatus to their sexual partners might facilitate the development of more innovative and effective interventions to increase disclosure. In a study of 78 gay men, Serovich and Mosack (2003) examined reasons for disclosure and nondisclosure to casual sexual partners. A factor analysis of the 15-item disclosure measure they employed revealed a 4-factor solution: Responsibility (e.g., "I felt a sense of duty to tell this person"); Instruction (e.g., "My goal was to teach others about the disease"); Relationship Consequences (e.g., "Wanted to find out if this person would be with me after disclosing"); and Emotional Release (e.g., "Would be able to get information off my chest"). Interestingly, the item "I wanted to emphasize the importance of safer sex" failed to load significantly on any factor. Responsibility was a primary factor according to item means. With respect to the 15 reasons for nondisclosure they assessed, the factor solutions did not fit the data. The authors concluded that prevention messages should focus on others' needs and rights and not merely the personal benefits to the disclosers. Of course, interventionists should remember that motivations for disclosure and safer sex among HIV-positive individuals might not always be altruistic. Therefore, HIV prevention messages directed toward this group might accentuate the benefits of avoiding additional sexually transmitted infections that may compromise their health status, as well as superinfection with a drug-resistant strain of HIV that could (Sagar et al., 2003; Smith et al., 2004) and the potential legal ramifications of not disclosing HIV.

IMPLICATIONS FOR POLICY

Before endorsing interventions to increase disclosure to sexual partners, policy makers need better empirical support for the causal association between disclosure and safer sex that they apparently assume. The research is clear that policy should focus on increasing condom use and other safer sexual techniques more than on disclosure specifically and certainly more than on disclosure exclusively. According to Crepaz and Marks (2003), emphasizing disclosure alone without paying attention to subsequent sex behaviors is not constructive. Similarly, Geary et al. (1996), who found that serostatus disclosure was not related to condom use among adolescents, concluded that their study "raises the question about the effectiveness of focusing primarily or exclusively on disclosing HIV status as a preventive strategy" (p. 422) and suggested it would be more important, at least with adolescents, to focus on safer sex than disclosure.

Most emphatic, Sheon and Crosby (2004) cautioned with respect to their MSM sample in San Francisco: "the men's fundamental unwillingness to ask or disclose suggests that messages focusing on the importance of knowing a partner's serostatus are misguided" (page 2111). More ominously they warned that persons with ambivalent attitudes toward disclosure who are confronted with prevention messages exhorting them to disclosure may be inclined to counter-argue and become more entrenched in their beliefs that they already know their partner's HIV status and this do not need to use condoms.

Public health officials sometimes point with dismay to the high number of HIV-positive individuals who do not disclose. These numbers can be misleading, however, because a large percentage may practice safe sex, as part of what Marks et al. (2001) referred to as uninformed protection. Research suggests that only a small minority of HIV-positive adults do not disclose *and* do not practice safer sex and many of these individuals have HIV-positive partners. Of course, practicing safer sex does not obviate the need for disclosure because of inconsistent safe sex, condom breakage, and the importance of informed consent. As Ciccarone et al. (2003) commented, "Most consider failing to disclose morally indefensible because it precludes the partner's exercising informed choice about the level of risk he or she would like to assume" (p. 949).

Another limitation of the policy of advocating for disclosure on the part of HIV-positive individuals is that it may lead to a false sense of security on the part of HIV-negative individuals. They should not adjust their sexual safety on the basis of a potential partner's disclosure, because an individual claiming to be HIV-negative may be unaware of an actual HIV infection. This may happen even if the individual consistently gets tested because of the delay between exposure and the appearance of detectable antibodies. Additionally, HIV-positive partners can knowingly deceive their partners. In fact, Klitzman and Bayer (2003) reported that over one third of the gay men they interviewed in New York City admitted lying at some point about their serostatus.

CONCLUSIONS

In a review of the published literature, we located 22 empirical studies on disclosure of HIV status and sexual safety, with 15 providing some data on their association. However, methodological limitations in most of these precluded our making interpretations about the association of the two behaviors, let alone determining whether they were causally connected. In most of the studies that did adequately examine the association, the variables were not related. The implicit assumption about HIV status disclosure leading to sexual safety may not be supported empirically because of informed exposure and uninformed protection, as described by Marks and Crepaz (2001). With respect to prevention efforts, the good news is that uninformed exposure is relatively rare; the bad news is that even a small number of such cases can contribute to the HIV epidemic.

Future researchers face the challenge of designing and implementing methodologically rigorous studies that specifically measure disclosure and unprotected sexual behavior, employ a partner-level analysis, and control for potential confounding variables, including partner's HIV status and the type of relationship. Research suggests that practitioners from different disciplines and in multiple venues should not stop at encouraging disclosure of status but, in addition, make the effort to help HIV-positive individuals develop the communication skills necessary to explicitly negotiate safer sex. Policymakers should rely on empirical evidence to guide their decisions in this arena. Based on the findings of this review, although information about a partner's HIV status may play a role in one's choices about safer sex, disclosure alone does not automatically lead to safer sex in the way one might presume.

At this point in the HIV epidemic, given the lack of success in decreasing the number of annual new infections, public health advocates might emphasize more innovative prevention strategies that rely on multiple target areas (e.g., HIV education, availability of barrier protection, communication skills to negotiate safer sex) and multiple messengers (e.g., primary care physician, mental health counselor, public health outreach worker). One lesson we learned from this review of HIV disclosure and sexual behavior may be useful in these endeavors: namely, human relationships and sexual interactions are vastly complex, with myriad motivations, incentives, and risks involved. Deceptively simple HIV prevention interventions such as encouraging disclosure will probably never suffice.

REFERENCES

Chen, S. Y., Gibson, S., Weide, D., and McFarland, W. (2003). Unprotected anal intercourse between potentially HIV-serodiscordant men who have sex with men, San Francisco. *JAIDS* 33:166–170.

Ciccarone, D. H., Kanouse, D. E., Collins, R. L., Miu, A., Chen, J. L., Morton, S. C., and Stall, R. (2003). Sex without disclosure of positive HIV serostatus in a US probability sample of persons receiving medical care for HIV infection. *Am. J. Public Health* 93(6):949–954.

Centers for Disease Control and Prevention. (1987). Public health service guidelines for counseling and antibody testing to prevent HIV infections and AIDS. *MMWR* 36:509–515.

Centers for Disease Control and Prevention. (2003). *HIV/AIDS Surveillance Report 2002, Volume 14.*

Centers for Disease Control and Prevention, Health Resources and Services Administration, National Institutes of Health, HIV Medicine Association of the Infectious Disease Society of America, and the HIV Prevention in Clinical Care Working Group. (2004). Recommendations for Incorporating Human Immunodeficiency Virus (HIV) Prevention into the Medical Care of Persons Living with HIV. *Clin. Infec. Dis.* 38:104–121.

Clark, R. A., Kissinger, P., Bedimo, A. L., Dunn, P., and Albertin, H. (1997). Determination of factors associated with condom use among women infected with human immunodeficiency virus. *Int. J. STD AIDS* 8:229–233.

Crepaz, N., and Marks, G. (2003). Serostatus disclosure, sexual communication and safer sex in HIV-positive men. *AIDS Care* 15(3):379–387.

D'Angelo, L. J., Abdalian, S. E., Sarr, M., Hoffman, N., Belzer, M., and The Adolescent Medicine HIV/AIDS Research Network. (2001). Disclosure of serostatus by HIV infected youth: The experience of the REACH study. *J. Adolesc. Health* 29S:72–79.

Davis, M. H., and Franzoi, S. L. (1987). Private self-consciousness and self-disclosure. In: V. J. Derlega and J. H. Berg (eds.), *Self Disclosure: Theory, research, and therapy*. Plenum Press, New York, pp. 59–80.

De Rosa, C. J., and Marks, G. (1998). Preventive counseling of HIV-positive men and self-disclosure of serostatus to sex partners: New opportunities for prevention. *Health Psychol.* 17(3):224–231.

Diamond, C., and Buskin, S. (2000). Continued risky behavior in HIV-infected youth. *Am. J. Public Health* 90:115–118.

El-Bassel, N., White, S. S., Gilbert, L., Wu, E., Chang, M., Hill, J., and Steinglass, P. (2003). The efficacy of a relationship-based HIV/STD prevention program for heterosexual couples. *Am. J. Public Health.* 93(6):963–969.

Fishbein, M., and Ajzen, I. (1975). *Belief, attitude, intention and behavior: An introduction to theory and research*. Addison-Wesley, Reading, MA.

Geary, M. K., King, G., Forsberg, A. D., Delaronde, S. R., Parsons, J., and the Hemophilia Behavioral Evaluative Intervention Project Staff. (1996). Issues of disclosure and condom use in adolescents with hemophilia and HIV. *Pediatr. AIDS HIV Infect.* 7(6):418–423.

Halkitis, P., Parsons, J. T., and Wilton, L. (2003). Barebacking among gay and bisexual men in New York City: explanations for the emergence of intentional unsafe behavior. *Arch. Sex Behav.* 32(4):351–357.

Hill, C. T., and Stull, D. E. (1987). Gender and self disclosure: Strategies for exploring the issues. In: Derlega, V. J., and Berg, J. H., (eds.), *Self Disclosure: Theory, research, and therapy*. Plenum Press, New York, pp. 81–100.

Janssen, R. S., Holtgrave, D. R., Valdiserri, R. O., Shepherd, M., Gayle, H. D., and De Cock, K. M. (2001). The serostatus approach to fighting the HIV epidemic: Prevention strategies for infected individuals. *Am. J. Public Health* 91(7):1019–1024.

Janssen, R. S., Onorato, I. M., Valdiserri, R. O., Durham, T. M., Nichols, W. P., Seiler, E. M., and Jaffe, H. W. (2003). Advancing HIV Prevention: New Strategies for a Changing Epidemic—US, 2003. *MMWR* 52(15):329–332.

Jourard, S. M. (1971). *The transparent self*. Van Nostrand Reinhold, New York.

Kalichman, S. C. (1998). *Understanding AIDS: Advances in research and treatment*. American Psychological Association, Washington, D.C.

Kalichman, S. C. (1999). Psychological and social correlates or high-risk sexual behaviour among men and women living with HIV/AIDS. *AIDS Care* 11(4):415–428.

Kalichman, S. C. (2000). HIV transmission risk behaviors of men and women living with HIV-AIDS: Prevalence, predictors, and emerging clinical interventions. *Clin. Psych. Science Pract.* 7:32–47.

Kalichman, S. C., and Nachimson, D. (1999). Self-efficacy and disclosure of HIV- positive serostatus to sex partners. *Health Psychol.* 18(3):281–287.

Kalichman, S. C., Nachimson, D., Cherry, C., and Williams, E. (1998). AIDS treatment advances and behavioral prevention setbacks: Preliminary assessment of reduced perceived threat of HIV-AIDS. *Health Psychol.* 17:546–550.

Kalichman, S. C., Rompa, D., Luke, W., and Austin, J. (2002). HIV transmission risk behaviours among HIV-positive persons in serodiscordant relationships. *Int. J. STD AIDS* 13:677–682.

Kennedy, C. A., Skurnick, J., Wan, J. Y., Quattrone, G., Sheffet, A., Quinones, M., Wang, W., and Louria, D. B. (1993). Psychological distress, drug and alcohol use as correlates of condom use in HIV-serodiscordant heterosexual couples. *AIDS* 7(11):1493–1499.

King, G., Delaronde, S. R., Dinoi, R., Forsberg, A. D., and the Hemophilia Behavioral Intervention Evaluative Project Committee. (1996). Substance use, coping, and safer sex practices among adolescents with hemophilia and human immunodeficiency virus. *J. Adolesc. Health* 19:435–441.

Klitzman, R., and Bayer, R. (2003). *Mortal secrets: Truth and lies in the age of AIDS.* The Johns Hopkins University Press, Baltimore, MD.

Lambda Legal Defense Fund. (2002). State criminal statutes on HIV transmission (September 9, 2002). New York, NY.

Macalino, G. E., Celentano, D. D., Latkin, C., Strathdee, S. A., and Vlahov, D. (2002). Risk behaviors by audio computer-assisted self-interviews among HIV-seropositive and HIV-seronegative injection drug users. *AIDS Educ. Prev.* 14(5):367–378.

Mansergh, G., Marks, G., and Simoni, J. M. (1995). Self-disclosure of HIV infection among men who vary in time since seropositive diagnosis and symptomatic status. *AIDS* 9:639–644.

Marks, G., Bundeck, N. I., Richardson, J. L., and Ruiz, M. S. (1992). Self-disclosure of HIV infection: Preliminary results from a sample of Hispanic men. *Health Psychol.* 11(5):300–306.

Marks, G., Cantero, P. J., and Simoni, J. M. (1998). Is acculturation associated with sexual risk behaviors? An investigation of HIV-positive Latino men and women. *AIDS Care* 10:283–295.

Marks, G., and Crepaz, N. (2001). HIV-positive men's sexual practices in the context of self-disclosure of HIV status. *JAIDS* 27:79–85.

Marks, G., Richardson, J., and Maldonado, N. (1991). Self-disclosure of HIV infection to sexual partners. *Am. J. Public Health.* 81(10):1321–1322.

Marks, G., Richardson, J., Crepaz, N., Stoyanoff, S., Milam, J., Kemper, C., Larsen, R. A., Bolan, R., Weismuller, P., Hollander, H., and McCutchan, A. (2002). Are HIV care providers talking with patients about safer sex and disclosure? A multi-clinic assessment. *AIDS* 16(14):1953–1957.

Marks, G., Ruiz, M., Richardson, J. L., Reed, D., Mason, H. R. C., Sotelo, M., and Turner, P. A. (1994). Anal intercourse and disclosure of HIV infection among seropositive gay and bisexual men. *JAIDS* 7:866–869.

Mason, H. R. C., Marks, G., Simoni, J. M., Ruiz, M. S., and Richardson, J. L. (1995). Culturally sanctioned secrets? Latino men's nondisclosure of HIV infection to family, friends, and lovers. *Health Psychol.* 14:6–12.

Miller, A. G., Turner, C. F., and Moses, L. E. (1990). *AIDS: The second decade.* Free Press, Washington, D.C.

Miller, L. C., and Read, S. J. (1987). Why am I telling you this? Self-disclosure in a goal- based model of personality. In: Derlega V.J., and Berg J. H., (eds.), *Self Disclosure: Theory, research, and therapy.* Plenum Press, New York, pp. 35–58.

Misovich, S. J., Fisher, J. D., and Fisher, W. A. (1997). Close relationships and elevated HIV risk behavior: evidence and possible underlying psychological processes. *Rev. Gen. Psychol.* 1(1):72–107.

Myers, H. F., Javanbakht, M., Martinez, M., and Obediah, S. (2003). Psychosocial predictors of risky sexual behaviors in African American men: implications for prevention. *AIDS Educ. Prev.* 15(1SA):66–79.

Niccolai, L. M., Dorst, D., Myers, L., and Kissinger, P. J. (1999). Disclosure of HIV status to sexual partners: Predictors and temporal patterns. *STD* 26(5):281–285.

Norman, L. R., Kennedy, M., and Parish, K. (1998). Close relationships and safer sex among HIV-infected men with haemophilia. *AIDS Care* 10(3):339–354.

Nuss, R., Smith, P. S., Cotton, C., Kisker, T., and the Hemophilia Behavioral Intervention Evaluation Project (HBIEP) Adolescent Education Committee. (1995). Communication about safer sex and serostatus disclosure in HIV-positive adolescents with haemophilia. *Haemophilia* 1:126–130.

O'Brien, M. E., Richardson-Alston, G., Ayoub, M., Magnus, M., Peterman, T. A., and Kissinger, P. J. (2003). Prevalence and correlates of HIV serostatus disclosure. *STD* 30(9): 731–735.

Perry, S. W., Card, C. A. L., Moffatt, M., Ashman, T., Fishman, B., and Jacobsberg, L. B. (1994). Self-disclosure of HIV infection to sexual partners after repeated counseling. *AIDS Educ. Prev.* 6(5):403–411.

Prestage, G., Van de Ven, P., Grulikch, A., Kippax, S., McInnes, D., and Hendry, O. (2001). Gay men's sexual encounters: Discussing HIV and using condoms. *AIDS Care* 13: 277–284.

Sagar, M., Lavreys, L., Baeten, J. M., Richardson, B. A., Mandaliya, K., Chohan, B. H., Kreiss, J. K., and Overbaugh, J. (2003). Infection with multiple human immunodeficiency virus type 1 variants is associated with faster disease progression. *J. Virol.* 77(23):12921–12926.

Serovich, J. M. (2000). Helping HIV-positive persons to negotiate the disclosure process to partners, family members, and friends. *J. Marital Fam. Ther.* 26(3):365–372.

Serovich, J. M. (2001). A test of two HIV disclosure theories. *AIDS Educ. Prev.* 13(4):355–364.

Serovich, J. M., and Mosack, K. E. (2003). Reasons for HIV disclosure or nondisclosure to casual sexual partners. *AIDS Educ. Prev.* 15(1):70–80.

Sheon, N. and Crosby, G.N. (2004). Ambivalent tales of HIV disclosure in San Francisco. *Social Science and Medicine* 58:2105–2118.

Shriver, M. D., Everett, C., and Morin, S. F. (2000). Structural interventions to encourage primary HIV prevention among people living with HIV. *AIDS* 14(S1):S57–S62.

Simoni, J. M., Mason, H. R. C., Marks, G., Ruiz, M. S., Reed, D., and Richardson, J. L. (1995a). Women's self-disclosure of HIV infection: Rates, reasons, and reactions. *J. Cons. Clin. Psychol.* 63:474–478.

Simoni, J. M., Mason, H. R. C., Marks, G., Ruiz, M. S., and Richardson, J. L. (1995b). Women living with HIV: Sexual behaviors and counseling experiences. *Women Health* 23(4):17–26.

Simoni, J. M., Walters, K. L., and Nero, D. K., (2000). Safer sex among HIV-positive women: The role of relationships. *Sex Roles* 42:691–708.

Smith, D., Wong, J., Hightower, G., Kolesch, K., Ignacio, C., Daar, E., Richman, D., and Little, S. (2004). Incidence of HIV superinfection following primary infection. Program and Abstracts of the 11th Conference on Retroviruses and Opportunistic Infections, San Francisco, CA.

Sobel, E., Shine, D., DiPietro, D., and Rabinowitz, M. (1996). Condom use among HIV-infected patients in South Bronx, New York. *AIDS* 10(2):235–236.

Sobo, E. J. (1995). Human immunodeficiency virus seropositivity self-disclosure to sexual partners: A qualitative study. *Holist. Nurs. Pract.* 10(1):18–28.

Stein, M. D., and Samet, J. H. (1999). Disclosure of HIV status. *AIDS Patient Care* 13(5):265–267.

Stein, M. D., Freedberg, K. A., Sullivan, L. M., Savetsky, J., Levenson, S. M., Hingson, R. and Samet, J. H. (1998). Sexual ethics: Disclosure of HIV-positive status to partners. *Arch. Internal Med.* 158:253–257.

Sturdevant, M. S., Belzer, M., Weissman, G., Friedman, L. B., Sarr, M., Muenz, L. R., and the Adolescent Medicine HIV/AIDS Research Network. (2001). The relationship of unsafe sexual behavior and the characteristics of sexual partners of HIV infected and HIV uninfected adolescent females. *J. Adolesc. Health* 29S:64–71.

van der Straten, A., Vernon, K. A., Knight, K. R., Gomez, C. A., and Padian, N. S. (1998). Managing HIV among serodiscordant heterosexual couples: Serostatus, stigma and sex. *AIDS Care* 10:533–548.

Wolitski, R. J., Rietmeijer, C. A. M., Goldbaum, G. M., and Wilson, R. M. (1998). HIV serostatus disclosure among gay and bisexual men in four American cities: General patterns and relation to sexual practices. *AIDS Care* 10(5):599–610.

Zea, M. C., Reisen, C. A., Poppen, P. J., Echeverry, J. J., and Bianchi, F. T. (2004). Disclosure of HIV-positive status to Latino gay men's social networks. *Am. J. Community Psychol.* 33(1–2):107–116.

HIV-Positive Gay and Bisexual Men

Jeffrey T. Parsons

INTRODUCTION

Behavioral research focused on people living with HIV has shown that the minority report sexual practices that would place their partners at high risk of HIV infection. Reviews of the literature have found that about 70% of heterosexual HIV-positive persons remain sexually active after seroconversion, whereas only a third of these individuals report vaginal intercourse without the use of a condom (Crepaz and Marks, 2002; Kalichman, 2000). Similar rates of unprotected anal intercourse have been documented among HIV-positive gay and bisexual men (Kalichman et al., 2002a; Parsons et al., 2003).

Recent studies have reported increases in sexual risk behaviors among gay and bisexual men in the US, Europe, and Australia (Chen et al., 2002; Ekstrand et al., 1999; Kalichman et al., 2002b; Stolte et al., 2001; Van de Ven et al., 2000). In addition, young gay and bisexual men, and particularly men of color, remain at considerable risk of HIV infection as a result of unprotected anal sex (CDC, 2002; Koblin et al., 2000). In New York City, 33% of young African American gay and bisexual men are estimated to be HIV positive and rates among Latinos are also quite high (Valleroy et al., 2000). Other studies have shown increases in HIV incidence (Calzavara et al., 2002) and sexually transmitted infection (STI) rates among young men who have sex with men (Fox et al., 2001). The number of syphilis cases in San Francisco increased from six in 1998 to 115 in 2001, and cases of rectal gonorrhea among gay and bisexual men increased from 162 in

1999 to 237 in 2002 (Chen et al., 2002; Katz et al., 2002). In New York City, cases of primary and secondary syphilis doubled in 2001, predominately among gay and bisexual men (CDC, 2002). Nearly half of these new cases of syphilis were among HIV-positive men. This is of great concern, as syphilis is more likely to facilitate the sexual transmission of HIV than other STIs (Wheater et al., 2003).

These findings underscore the need to more fully understand the safer sexual behaviors of HIV-positive gay and bisexual men. Clearly most men living with HIV neither want to nor intend to transmit HIV (Wolitski et al., 2003). However new infections continue to grow, and in some areas of the US, rates of HIV infection among gay and bisexual men have shown a continued upward trend (Valdisseri, 2003). Gay and bisexual men remain the largest subgroup of persons living with HIV/AIDS in the US; with 14% to 25% of these men living with HIV, a prevalence rate equivalent to that in some sub-Saharan African countries (Catania et al., 2001).

HIV-positive gay and bisexual men can transmit HIV to sexual partners, primarily through unprotected anal sex (Vittinghoff et al., 1999). Placing a partner at risk of HIV infection is particularly dangerous in cases in which HIV-positive men have developed drug resistance, as medication resistant HIV can be transmitted to HIV-negative sexual partners (Hecht et al., 1998). HIV-positive men who engage in unprotected sex, regardless of the HIV status of their sexual partners, risk rapid loss of CD4 cells (Wiley et al., 2000), acquiring pathogens which may lead to opportunistic infections (Renwick et al., 1998), co-infection with Hepatitis C (Spengler and Rockstroth, 1998), and contracting STIs which can lead to further immune system deterioration (Bonnell et al., 2000).

SEXUAL RISK BEHAVIORS OF GAY AND BISEXUAL MEN IN THE THIRD DECADE OF HIV/AIDS

The prevalence of unprotected anal intercourse differs by whether the HIV-positive gay or bisexual man is the insertive or receptive partner (Parsons et al., 2003). Studies have shown that many HIV-positive men intentionally position themselves as the receptive partner for unprotected anal sex, as a method of "strategic positioning" perceived to result in sexual risk reduction (Parsons et al., in press; Van de Ven et al., 2002). It is unclear to what degree such harm reduction efforts actually decrease the likelihood of HIV transmission, although such notions of strategic positioning to reduce the risk of HIV infection are supported somewhat by epidemiological evidence (Vittinghoff et al., 1999).

Other men make efforts to "serosort" their sexual partners, where they limit the risk of HIV transmission by engaging in sexual activity with only men of seroconcordant status (Parsons et al., in press; Suarez and Miller, 2001). Thus, some men who are HIV-positive limit their sexual activity to other HIV-positive men in order to have condomless sex without fear of transmitting HIV to a sexual partner. Inherently problematic in serosorting, however, is the potential for this approach to fail. First, serosorting assumes that HIV status disclosure has occurred. A recent study of HIV-positive gay and bisexual men found that 42% reported sex without disclosing their status, demonstrating considerable inconsistency in disclosure (Ciccarone et al., 2003). Second, serosorting strategies assume that individuals actually know their HIV status in the first place, which is not always the case. Third, the notion of serosorting assumes that gay and bisexual men are fully honest and accurate regarding the disclosure of their status, an assumption that is not fully supported by the literature (Wolitski et al., 1998).

Seropositive and seronegative gay and bisexual men have been shown to make assumptions regarding the HIV status of their sexual partners, typically assuming their partner's HIV status is concordant with theirs when engaging in unprotected sex (Suarez and Miller, 2001). One study of HIV-positive gay and bisexual men in New York City and San Francisco identified comparable rates of HIV sexual risk practices with HIV-positive and HIV status unknown casual sex partners (Parsons, et al., 2003). Qualitative interviews with these same men indicated that in many cases it was assumed that unknown status partners were also HIV-positive (Parsons and Vicioso, in press). However, the strong possibility exists that at least some of these HIV status unknown partners were, in fact, HIV-negative, and thus at risk of HIV infection. As such, serosorting may reduce the risk of HIV transmission in some encounters when seroconcordant sex actually occurs between two HIV-positive men, but questions remain about the effectiveness of this strategy in light of serostatus disclosure, the potential for inaccurate assumptions of serostatus, and accurate knowledge of one's own HIV status.

It is possible that increases in new HIV infections are resulting, in part, from faulty harm reduction techniques utilized by HIV-positive gay and bisexual men, as noted above. It is also important to consider the manner in which HIV treatment advances of the past decade have impacted perceptions regarding the relative risk of unsafe sexual practices. The availability and success of Highly Active Antiretroviral Therapy (HAART) in improving and prolonging the lives of those with HIV has led to increased optimism and reduced concerns, at least in the US, regarding potential HIV infection (Kalichman et al., 1998; Vanable et al., 2002). For some gay and bisexual men, optimism regarding the severity of HIV disease has led to increased complacency in terms of sexual risk behaviors and may be fueling increasing HIV infections among this population (Catania et al., 2001; Wolitski et al., 2001).

It is doubtful, however, that optimism resulting from medical advances in treating HIV is the only reason for continued unprotected sex behaviors among HIV-positive gay and bisexual men and the corresponding increases in new cases of HIV infection. It is more likely that a complex set of interconnected contextual factors is responsible for unsafe sex behaviors among these men. Disentangling these contextual factors, and recognizing the critical importance of the varied social environments in which sexual interactions between men occur, could help to shed light on the current situation of the sexual risk behaviors of HIV-positive gay and bisexual men. To fully understand the sexual lives and sexual risk practices of these men, one must consider the ways in which sexually charged venues and environments that men frequent to look for potential sexual partners may shape their behaviors, the sociological impact of the Internet in facilitating sexual encounters between men, the ways in which the increase in the prevalence and acceptance of "barebacking" (intentional anal sex without condoms) in the gay community may exacerbate sexual risk taking, and the potential for illicit drug use to derail even the most committed intentions to practice safer sex. This chapter examines the ways in which these contextual factors may be hindering the ability of HIV-positive gay and bisexual men to protect their sexual partners from HIV infection. Clearly, the sexual lives of these men and the very nature of their sexual interactions transcend the simplistic messages of "no glove, no love" and other prevention messages of the past two decades that implied the need for consistent condom use in all circumstances.

SEXUALLY CHARGED ENVIRONMENTS

The particular venues in which HIV-positive gay and bisexual men seek and meet their sexual partners directly impact their safer sex decisions. Two such venues that are commonly frequented are commercial and public sex environments. HIV-positive men are more likely than their HIV-negative counterparts to use these venues (Binson et al., 2001). Recent research has shown that nearly half of HIV-positive gay and bisexual men from New York City and San Francisco reported frequenting either commercial or public sex venues, with a substantial number attending both (Parsons and Halkitis, 2003).

Commercial Sex Environments

"A bathhouse is a place—they have like a lot of little rooms that you go in. You pay like twenty dollars and you have your room for like eight hours. It's got a little twin bed. And they also sell booze and drugs in there. And it actually has showers and has a sauna and it has a steam room and it has all that stuff. And it has a work out room and an exercise room and a lounge and a movie room and stuff. So you can walk around there and do what you want. But most people go there for sex." [34-year-old White gay man from New York City]

Commercial sex environments include all business establishments where men go with the intention of finding other men for sex (e.g., bathhouses, saunas, sex clubs, adult movie houses and pornography shops that allow the use of "buddy booths" for previewing movies). Right up to the beginning of the AIDS epidemic, the overt sexuality of these businesses was a source of liberation because here men could publicly display and act on sexual desires that could place them in legal and physical danger in other settings. These venues have served as a place to escape from a hostile society and revel in the very sexuality that made them targets for hostility.

Bathhouses, in particular, came under intense scrutiny early in the first wave of the HIV/AIDS epidemic as sites where gay and bisexual men were engaging in unsafe sex practices (Elwood and Williams, 1998). Mainstream health research began to view bathhouses as sexual venues devoid of any social import and detrimental to the well being of both individual men and the gay community at large because they contributed to unsafe sex, leading to the continued spread of HIV. While these venues may no longer be the target of major government surveillance, their role in the HIV epidemic is still a major topic of scientific investigation and political debate, both outside of and within various gay communities.

Commercial sex venues experienced a major renaissance since 1990 and, as of 2003, there were 4,685 bathhouses and sex clubs known to exist across the US and Canada (Woods et al., 2003). Many HIV-positive gay and bisexual men identify these venues as facilitating escape from thoughts of their HIV status (Elwood and Williams, 1998; Parsons and Vicioso, in press). Since verbal communication is so limited in these venues, discussion of HIV status does not occur, but many men make the assumption that most men frequenting bathhouses and sex clubs are HIV-positive (Haubrich et al., 2004; Parsons and Vicioso, in press). Drug use, particularly club drugs such as methamphetamine, ecstasy, and nitrate inhalants, commonly occurs within these venues, which can substantially impede safer sex decisions (Binson et al., 2001; Haubrich et al., 2004; Parsons and Halkitis, 2002).

Public Sex Environments

"I enjoy group sex. And in a park, if I walk up on a couple of guys who are having sex, and then they notice me, and then they stop having sex but I haven't left the area where they're from, and, in fact, I move closer toward them and provoke some kind of response to my presence from them, to either join them or—or "Back off, you're in my space and don't come any closer." And over the course of whatever, almost three hours, I had sex with one, two, three, four, five, six individuals—six individuals, three of them separately, or respectively, and then three others together." [34-year-old Latino gay man from San Francisco]

Another type of sex venue frequented by HIV-positive men is the public sex environment. Unlike commercial establishments, men can seek sex partners in public venues without having to pay a fee. Public sex venues are not specifically designated sites for sexual interaction; rather they are generally public spaces that men have appropriated for sexual encounters. These areas are open and therefore accessible to the general public (e.g., wooded areas in parks, alleyways in urban areas, bathrooms in department stores, highway rest stops). In most states, sexual activity in public places is illegal and there can be serious consequences for public sex, including arrest and prosecution.

Often, sex in public happens intentionally, with men specifically going to outdoor locations that have a reputation as being a place to have sex with other men. There are directories available on the Internet that provide up-to-date information on thousands of public places for gay and bisexual men to have sex and public places to avoid, organized into a searchable database. Alternatively, sex in these venues can be more spontaneous or unexpected. The spontaneity of a sex encounter can be dictated by the layered structure of public sex environments, in which men can meet one another along the perimeter or deeper within the location, typically where the more intense sexual activities take place (Somlai et al., 2001). Qualitative research has shown that some HIV-positive men report that sex in a public venue "just happens," such as while walking their dog, riding a bike, or trying to clear their head (Parsons and Vicioso, in press). The potential for spontaneous sex, or at least sex that appears to be spontaneous, can be particularly appealing for men who are heterosexually identified, as these men can justify to themselves that they were not seeking out sex with another man. The need to disown such a sexual encounter may be especially important for men who are conflicted about seeking out these experiences due to struggles with one's sexual orientation, internalized homophobia, being in a monogamous relationship, or being HIV-positive.

Commercial and Public Sex Environments
and Unsafe Sex

"HIV, it's like a helicopter hovering around me. And, that doesn't stop me. I just go and do it, you know. I just finish what I went there for because that was the purpose of my visit to [the bathhouse]. And what happens sexually? I don't really care." [41-year-old Latino gay man from New York City]

Both commercial and public sex environments have been described as sites of liberation where gay and bisexual men could seek each other out and freely express their sexuality. On the other hand, they have been described as sources of risk where unsafe sex contributes to HIV transmission. The ecological qualities of these venues, both in terms of physical properties and the social norms that guide behaviors, have been shown to directly impact safer sexual practices (Flowers et al., 1999; Parsons and Vicioso, in press).

Studies have documented a relationship between frequenting commercial sex venues and sexual risk behaviors (Binson, et al., 2001; Haubrich et al., 2004; Parsons and Halkitis, 2002). The desire to escape feelings and thoughts about being HIV-positive, as well as the opportunity to be in a place where most men are assumed to be HIV-positive no doubt has an impact. As such, some men in these venues may feel that they are effectively serosorting, and are willing to engage in unprotected sex with limited concern of infecting partners with HIV. Others may shift their own personal sense of responsibility to that of their sexual partners, by adopting the attitude "everyone here knows what they are getting into." The lack of verbal communication, and the resultant inability to disclose HIV status, however, makes it likely that inaccurate assumptions regarding the serostatus of partners in these venues are common. Even if serosorting were effective, and all unprotected sexual activity in sex clubs and bathhouses occurred between seroconcordant men, concerns regarding reinfection and STI infection and transmission remain.

Like commercial sex establishments, public sex environments may promote sexual risk behaviors, particularly among members of racial and ethnic minority groups (Diaz et al., 1996; Somlai et al., 2001). Such men may lack the financial resources to pay the admission fee to commercial venues, which can often cost $20 to $30, or they may feel that bathhouses and sex clubs are dominated by white men (Parsons and Vicioso, in press). The use of public venues for sexual purposes is a particular concern for young men of color, due in part to rising rates of HIV infection among these men, but also because sex in such venues may constitute their first same-gendered sexual experiences.

Some studies, however, have found that gay and bisexual men, and HIV-positive men in particular, who frequent public sex venues report less unprotected sex than those frequenting commercial venues (Binson et al., 2001; Parsons and Halkitis, 2002). For example, some HIV-positive men who frequent public areas for sexual activity explain that anal intercourse is not possible due to the constant need to be ready at a moment's notice to run from police (Parsons and Vicioso, in press). Similar issues in terms of limited verbal communication, the short-term duration of sexual partnering, and assumptions regarding serostatus that exist in commercial venues exist in public ones, such that it is likely that HIV-positive men who do choose to engage in unprotected sex are not necessarily doing so with HIV concordant partners.

Although quantitative studies have suggested that frequenting commercial and public sex environments is associated with unprotected sexual activity (Diaz et al., 1996; Parsons and Halkitis, 2002), qualitative data reveals a more complicated relationship. Some HIV-positive gay and bisexual men who frequent sexually charged venues are perfectly capable of and committed to safer sex practices in these venues (Parsons and Vicioso, in press). Other men, however, clearly indicate that the spontaneity, anonymity, and lack of verbal communication associated with sex in these sex environments contributes to their engagement in unprotected sexual activity with partners of unknown serostatus. Thus, as is commonly the case, a consistent pattern fails to emerge, and we are left with the understanding that commercial and public sex venues may play an important role in HIV transmission.

Prevention in Commercial and Public
Sex Environments

"I think we should have more sex clubs, and I think that that's a good place to have education. I really think that sex clubs are a good thing. They always have these outreach people there, who are really easy to talk to, and they're funny, and they're informative, and the environment there is really relaxed and safe. I know it influences what I do there." [32-year-old gay man of mixed race/ethnicity from San Francisco]

It's clear that these venues may serve as locations for HIV infections to occur among gay and bisexual men. What is not clear is the full potential to take advantage of commercial and public sex venues for HIV prevention interventions. Two evaluations of HIV prevention interventions delivered in public sex environments have been published (French et al., 2000; Hospers et al., 1999). In one, peer volunteers distributed condoms and safer sex literature to men frequenting a park in the United Kingdom (French et al., 2000). Considerable efforts were made to not intrude by remaining on the periphery of the inner areas in which sexual activity occurred, thereby gaining the trust and acceptance of the men. Evaluation data revealed that condoms were reaching the target population and were being used, and that the intervention was both feasible and acceptable to the participants. A study in the Netherlands compared men who had conversed with HIV prevention volunteers regarding safer sex and those who had not (Hospers et al., 1999). Men who reported interacting with the prevention volunteers reported using condoms more consistently for insertive and receptive anal sex than men who had not. Recognizing the methodological limitations of both studies, including that neither assessed HIV status of respondents, these finding suggest that interventions in public sex venues are feasible and may reduce HIV infections.

No published evaluations of interventions delivered in commercial sex venues could be identified. Although many commercial sex venues display posters related to safer sex and/or provide condoms and lubricant for patrons, few other systematic interventions are offered in these settings. In some cities, efforts have been made to integrate HIV and STI counseling and testing in bathhouses and sex clubs to gay and bisexual men, however these activities exist in only 40% of commercial sex environments (Woods et al., 2001). Rapid HIV testing in these venues may reach men at high risk who fail to access HIV testing in traditional settings. It is important to recognize the ways in which policies may affect the ability to deliver prevention interventions in commercial settings. For example, in San Francisco, closed rooms for purposes of private sex in bathhouses and sex clubs is not permitted, but in New York City, sex is permitted only in closed rooms in these venues.

Intervention efforts need to recognize the unique structural aspects of commercial versus public sex environments. While these venues may set men up for similar HIV risk behavior, there are inherent differences in the venues and the types of men who frequent them. Moreover, the different conditions (public versus private, covertly sexual versus overtly sexual) of these venues provide distinct avenues of arriving at similar risk behaviors. Thus interventions aimed at commercial venues might be built on their overtly sexual nature and it would make the most sense to implement educational campaigns and programs directly in these venues so that you are intervening with men in the heat of the moment. Some have argued that commercial sex venues continue to provide important opportunities for socialization, and as such present outreach workers with a valuable opportunity to provide HIV prevention messages (Binson et al., 2001; Parsons and Vicioso, in press).

Interventions aimed at public sex venues need to take into account the logistics of using condoms in public settings not typically used for sexual activity, as well as the fact that sexual acts often occur in the dark, when the participants are contending with the risk of being caught by police or unsuspecting persons who frequent the venue for non-sexual purposes. Men may benefit from learning how to use condoms more effectively in these settings, as well as how to negotiate safer sex behaviors quickly. The presence of HIV outreach workers in public sex venues may be useful in creating a climate in which safer sex becomes the norm. However, it is likely that the men who frequent these venues due to the anonymity afforded by them will be reluctant to engage in prevention activities. Such efforts need to be persistent in order to become acceptable (French et al., 2000). The limited published work on interventions targeting men who frequent these sexually charged venues represent a missed opportunity, particularly considering the number of HIV-positive men who utilize these venues as well as the potential for the rapid transmission of HIV and STIs resulting from the group sex and multiple partnering common in these environments.

THE INTERNET

"It's hard to remember what we did before the Internet. I guess we actually went to porn shops to get our needs met! I can come home from work, get online, find a streaming video and get off right then and there. You can't browse through porn magazines with your dick in your hand at Border's like you can at home on the net." [40-year-old White bisexual man from Fort Lauderdale]

Utilizing commercial and public sex environments to find other men for sex has been augmented by the opportunity to find sexual partners via the Internet. Most adults in America now have at least some access to the Internet, either through home, work/school, or both. Neilsen/NetRatings, a company that compiles data on Internet usage around the world, estimates that in 2003, 63.2% of Americans were using the Internet, representing an increase of 93.4% from 2000 to 2003. Further data revealed that consumers in the US spent $18.5 billion via online shopping during the 2003 holiday season, an increase of 35% from 2002.

Originally, with regard to sexual activity, the primary use of the Internet was to find pornography and sexually explicit material. Although the Internet is now commonly used for email, trading stocks and mutual funds, purchasing online music, and obtaining the latest news and weather, a significant amount of Internet traffic is aimed at adult content or entertainment. While Amazon.com struggled for years to turn a profit, Internet porn currently generates revenue from $1–2.5 billion annually and is expected to grow into a $5–7 billion business in the next five years. In 2003, the National Research Council estimated that pornographic websites had grown 18-fold in the last six years, with approximately 1.3 million pornographic websites, representing 12% of all websites. Internet Filter Review estimates that 25% of all search engine requests are porn-related. In addition to pornography, one can easily obtain Viagra, sex workers, or sex toys from the privacy of your home computer. It is also important to realize that, in addition to pornography, the Internet has enabled people to purchase condoms, lubricants, and other safer sex products online.

Cooper (1999) proposed that the Internet is used to enhance one's sexual life because of the three A's—access, affordability, and anonymity. The Internet, through the use of gay chat rooms, websites, and listservs, can be easily accessed from individuals with home computers, from computers at work or school, or from Kinko's, Internet cafes, or public libraries. Although some Internet service providers (e.g., America OnLine, Earthlink) and some gay-oriented websites (e.g., M4M4SEX, Gay.com) charge a fee for full membership, others are free to use. The use of email addresses and screen names, as well as the ability to sign-up for certain websites and chat rooms without revealing any contact information, results in a fairly anonymous world with which to initiate sexual contact.

Gay and Bisexual Men Online

"The Internet is like the bathhouse of the millennium! It's like a great big department store online. You can log on and find anything or anybody you want. Tall, short, muscled, thin, hairy, smooth, poz, neg, safe, unsafe, oral, anal—I mean anything you want you can get. And so fast. Sometimes I can go online, go to a chat room, and get a man to come over to my place faster than it takes me to get a pizza delivered." [24-year-old Latino gay man from New York City]

It has been argued that gay and bisexual men comprise one of the largest online communities and these men are significantly more likely to have sex with partners that they meet on the Internet than heterosexual men and women (Bull et al., 2001; Kim et al., 2001; McFarlane et al., 2000). Most studies show no difference between HIV-positive and HIV-negative gay and bisexual men regarding their use of the Internet for finding sexual partners (Benotsch et al., 2002; Elford et al., 2001; Kim et al., 2001; Tikkanen and Ross, 2003). A study of gay and bisexual men in the United Kingdom found that in 2001, two-thirds of gay men reported using the Internet in any given month and over half the men living in London reported use in the past 48 hours (Weatherburn et al., 2003). From 1999 to 2002, use of the Internet to find sex partners among gay and bisexual men in the United Kingdom significantly increased from 28% to 66%. Further analyses of this survey indicated that as the proportion of men using the Internet for sex increased, the proportion of those using public sex venues decreased. In late 2003, a Labour MP in the United Kingdom was exposed for his use of a popular gay Internet dating service. The public, however, was not upset over his sexual orientation, his use of the website, or even his web profile which said how he much enjoyed a "good long fuck." Instead, the public was upset that the photo he posted on the website showed him in briefs rather than boxers, suggesting that public attitudes concerning the use of the Internet to find sexual partners have become quite accepting.

Recent studies have focused on the role that the Internet plays in finding sex partners for gay and bisexual men, as well as the role of this technological advancement in unprotected sex and potential risk of HIV and STIs. Men can utilize the Internet for instant access to identify and eventually meet with a large number of anonymous sexual partners they might not meet otherwise (Ashton et al., 2003; Bull and McFarlane, 2000; Klausner et al., 2000; Tashima et al., 2003). Users can establish member profiles which include information about their sexual likes and dislikes, HIV serostatus, what they are looking for (or not looking for) in a sexual partner, and geographical location. Unlike public and commercial sex venues, where subtle gestures and non-verbal forms are used to communicate information regarding sexual interests and behaviors desired, the Internet permits men to communicate explicitly through written text or even through the use of photos or streaming video.

The relative anonymity afforded by the Internet, as well as the ability to conduct searches of online member profiles, simplifies the process of identifying and interacting with potential sexual partners who meet particular characteristics—in terms of physical characteristics, preferred sexual practices, interest in condom use or non-use, and HIV status and interest in serosorting. Internet terminology and acronyms have developed as a means to convey detailed information regarding interest in combining drug use with sexual activity in more subtle ways. The most common of these, "party and play" (PnP) conveys an interest in combining drug use (typically "party" or "club" drugs, which will be discussed later) with sexual activity. Other commonly used terms include "420 OK" (420 is police code for marijuana), "chem friendly" or "chem sex OK", and "D&D free" or drug and disease free.

The research conducted on gay and bisexual men who seek sex partners using the Internet has some consistent findings. Compared to others, men with online sexual partners or who utilize chat rooms to find sexual partners have been found to be younger (Benotsch et al., 2002; Kim et al., 2001; Tikkanen and Ross, 2003; Weatherburn et al., 2003), more likely to have a previous STI (Elford et al., 2001; McFarlane et al., 2000), to frequent public and commercial sex environments (Mettey et al., 2003; Tikkanen and Ross, 2003), and to identify as non-gay and report also having sex with women (Tikkanen and Ross, 2003; Weatherburn et al., 2003).

Some contradictory findings, however, occur in comparing gay and bisexual men who do and do not use the Internet for finding sex partners. Although some studies have found increased illicit drug use among Internet-using men, specifically poppers, ecstasy, methamphetamine, and Viagra (Benotsch et al., 2002; Mettey et al., 2003), others find no differences in the use of these drugs (Elford et al., 2001). With regard to sociodemographic characteristics, it has been reported that men using the Internet for sex are more likely to be white (Benotsch et al., 2002; Weatherburn et al., 2003) and have less education (Tikkanen and Ross, 2003); however other studies have found no differences in race/ethnicity (Elford et al., 2001) or education (Kim et al., 2001).

Unprotected Sex and the Internet

"I found out about a sex party online one night. So, I went. It was the hottest group of guys I had ever seen, and everyone was going at it. I started in as soon as I walked in the door and could get undressed. I must have had sex with 7 or 8 of them, as a top, as a bottom, oral, anal, three-ways, four-ways— it was amazing. I brought condoms with me, but just sort of got caught up in the whole experience. I didn't really think about it until I got home the next morning. I'm pretty sure most of the guys were poz. Why would someone [who is HIV] negative put themselves at risk like that?" [31-year-old Latino gay man from Los Angeles]

Although HIV-positive gay and bisexual men do report serosorting using the Internet to find other HIV-positive men to have unprotected sex (Elford et al., 2001), other men who use the Internet engage in unprotected sex regardless of HIV status (Halkitis and Parsons, 2003). One study identified two cases of acute HIV infection in men following sexual encounters initiated in gay Internet chat rooms (Tashima et al., 2003). In 1999, a syphilis outbreak among men in San Francisco was traced to users of a gay chat room (Klausner et al., 2000). Similar results have been reported in the United Kingdom, where increasing numbers of men testing positive for syphilis, the majority of whom were co-infected with HIV, reported meeting partners online (Ashton et al., 2003).

The findings regarding sexual risk behaviors among gay and bisexual men who do and do not seek partners via the Internet have revealed contradictory results. Some have found that men using the Internet to find sex partners report a higher number of sexual partners (Benotsch, et al., 2002; McFarlane et al., 2000), are more likely to have had sex with casual partners (Kim et al., 2001; Tikkanen and Ross, 2003), and report more unprotected sex (Benotsch et al., 2002). Other studies, however, have found men using the Internet were more likely to report having used a condom for their most recent sexual encounter (McFarlane et al., 2000), and some have found no differences in the rates of condom use (Kim et al., 2001; Mettey et al., 2003).

A study of men using gay chat rooms in the Netherlands found that the vast majority of these men did engage in sex with men they met through chatting and 30% reported unsafe sex; those reporting a higher number of partners met via the Internet were more likely to report unprotected sex (Hospers et al., 2002). Common reasons for using gay chat rooms in this sample included "to find sex partners," "it turns me on," and "am addicted to it." These researchers also found that the most sexually risky men were those who tended to meet their sexual partners exclusively through the Internet, perhaps indicative of these men receiving less exposure to HIV prevention messages typically disseminated through gay bars, clubs, and other venues. This study, however, did not assess HIV status of respondents, so they were unable to examine potential differences between HIV-positive and HIV-negative men.

When data are analyzed by serostatus, some additional interesting findings emerge. HIV-positive men who report online sexual partners are more likely to have unsafe anal sex with other positive men and report previous gonorrhea (Elford et al., 2001). Among gay and bisexual men in the United Kingdom, HIV-positive men who met partners via the Internet were twice as likely to report unprotected anal sex with a serodiscordant partner, compared to positive men who did not use the Internet to find sex partners (Weatherburn et al., 2003). HIV-negative men with online partners are more likely to report having HIV-positive partners (Kim et al., 2001), more likely to report unsafe anal sex with non-concordant partners (Elford et al., 2001), more likely to report receiving money or drugs for sex (Kim et al., 2001), and report feeling less worry about HIV due to improved HIV treatments (Elford et al., 2001). These findings are particularly a source of concern in terms of increasing the potential for HIV infection among HIV-negative men who utilize the Internet to find sexual partners. Although many commercial sex environments were closed in the 1980s when HIV first affected gay communities, closing virtual venues or shutting down chat rooms or sexually-oriented websites due to the potential for the spread of HIV is not possible (Toomey and Rothenberg, 2000).

HIV Prevention Online

"When I first tested HIV positive a year ago, I didn't know anything. I wasn't really out to many people, and it took me a while to get hooked up with a good doctor. So I did my research using the net. I learned about the meds, the side effects, everything. It took me a few months, but I finally started talking to other positive guys online. They really helped me work through my issues, and even helped me find my doctor. I kind of feel like the Internet kept me sane during all of this hell I was going through." [27-year-old White gay man from Las Vegas]

When the syphilis outbreak occurred in San Francisco in 1999, the Department of Health electronically contacted hundreds of gay chat room users to educate them regarding the outbreak and to provide information on seeking medical evaluation (Klausner et al., 2000). Further, email addresses were used for partner notification purposes regarding possible exposure. Men surveyed after this intervention took place reported that such outreach was helpful and appropriate. The Netherlands study asked men about their preferences for HIV prevention activities on the Internet and found that a safer sex website, an email-based question and answer program, and a safer sex chatroom were the most preferred programs (Hospers et al., 2002). HIV-positive men in London were more likely than other men to have used the Internet to obtain information about HIV and sexual health services and HIV treatments, as well as to get information regarding recreational drugs and Viagra (Elford et al., 2001). Many HIV-positive men utilize the Internet to access health information and such use is associated with more active coping, empowerment, and social support (Kalichman et al., 2003).

It has been argued that men who seek sex on the Internet tend to be well-educated and insured compared to others, and as a result they may be less likely to access prevention messages via traditional methods delivered through the public sector and particularly in need of Internet-based education and prevention (Bull et al., 2001). Further, since many HIV-positive men who use the Internet for sex are engaged in risk practices, delivering HIV prevention messages through this medium targets those most at risk of transmitting HIV to their partners. The Internet could be used to encourage gay and bisexual men to have regular medical check-ups, and to promote HIV and STI testing through the use of emails, banner ads, or other mechanisms, at a cost significantly less than in-person outreach. Interventions delivered via the Internet have great potential to be both cost-effective and reach those at greatest risk. The Internet may provide a prime opportunity to access men who would be resistant to in person prevention efforts. To date, few systematic interventions, aside from using chat rooms to talk to gay men about

HIV and safer sex, have been developed and implemented using the Internet.

BAREBACKING

Traditionally, unprotected anal sex among gay and bisexual men was considered in the context of relapse or the inability to consistently use condoms in sexual encounters. The basic idea was that men were intending to have protected sex, but encountered situations in which they were unable to maintain their commitment to use condoms. Inherent in this view was the idea that all gay and bisexual men were already, or through intervention could learn to be, committed to practicing safer sex. While unsafe sex due to relapse from intentions to use condoms continues, "unintentional" unprotected sex behavior must be differentiated from the increasingly popular unsafe anal practices, which are "intentional" (Goodroad et al., 2000).

Intentional acts of unprotected sex have become colloquially known as "barebacking," a phenomenon that has grown in gay and bisexual male communities across the US (Gauthier and Forsyth, 1999; Goodroad et al., 2000). While the term barebacking was originally applied solely to the sexual behavior of HIV-positive gay and bisexual men, it is now equally applied to the behaviors of HIV-negative men and men who do not know their HIV status (Parsons, in press). Barebacking implies the intention on the part of the individual to seek out and engage in unprotected anal sex. Colloquially, gay and bisexual men also refer to bareback sex as "BB," "raw sex," "riding raw," or "skin to skin." Some men who engage in barebacking have integrated this into their sexual identity in that they will refer to themselves as barebackers (Parsons and Bimbi, 2004).

A review of the published literature in this area reveals only a few empirical studies. Although these studies have provided some insights into barebacking, they only begin to help us understand the phenomenon and the potential effects on the HIV epidemic.

Prevalence of Barebacking

"As long as all the people involved are taking responsibility for themselves, I don't see what the big deal is. It's not like anyone is stupid enough to think fucking without a condom is safe. So if some guy wants to bareback with me, I assume he knows what he's getting himself into. Usually, I assume he's positive too. I just can't get all worried about reinfection or any of that. And when you've lived with HIV for 20 years, the idea of a STD isn't very disturbing—you just take a few more pills or get a shot and it's gone." [45-year-old White gay man from Austin]

Halkitis et al. (2003a) examined barebacking in a large sample of gay and bisexual men surveyed through a brief street-intercept survey in New York City in 2002. Most of the participants (86%) indicated that they were familiar with the term barebacking as it relates to the sexual practices of gay and bisexual men, and of those 46% reported barebacking with at least one sexual partner in the past three months. Barebacking did not differ by race/ethnicity or sexual identity. Serostatus, however, played a major role in barebacking. HIV-positive men were more than twice as likely to report barebacking (61% versus 42%) and reported a significantly greater number of bareback sex partners, compared to HIV-negative men. Serosorting was evident, with positive men reporting barebacking more often with other positive partners. Similarly, HIV-negative men were more likely to bareback with what were perceived to be seroconcordant sex partners. Nonconcordant bareback sex, however, was reported by both HIV-positive and HIV-negative participants. Of those reporting barebacking, 29% reported attending a bareback sex party that they had learned about on the Internet; HIV-positive men were more likely to have attended such a party. The majority of men felt that the Internet facilitated finding sex partners interested in barebacking. Although this study contributes much to our understanding of barebacking, and particularly barebacking among HIV-positive gay and bisexual men, it is limited by the researchers not providing a common definition of "barebacking" to participants, which may have led to some misinterpretation on the part of the respondents.

Mansergh et al. (2002) conducted an assessment of barebacking, which they specifically defined for participants as having "intentionally set out to have unprotected anal sex with someone other than a primary partner (a primary partner is someone who you live with or have seen a lot and to whom you feel a special emotional commitment)." Interview data were collected from gay and bisexual men in San Francisco recruited from a variety of venues in 2000–2001. Similar to Halkitis et al. (2003a), the majority of participants (70%) reported familiarity with the term barebacking; sociodemographic differences were noted, with white, gay-identified, and participants with higher levels of education and income more likely to be aware of the term. Among those familiar with the term, 14% reported barebacking in the previous two years and differences by serostatus were apparent; 22% of HIV-positive men had barebacked versus 10% of HIV-negative men. Specific information was obtained regarding the last barebacking experience. Like the men in New York, men in San Francisco reported some degree of serosorting, in that many of the most recent barebacking episodes involved seroconcordant partnering. However, a sizeable minority of men reported that their last barebacking experience involved unprotected insertive or receptive anal sex with partners of discordant or unknown serostatus. Barebacking under the influence of alcohol or other drugs was reported by more than half of the men, although crystal methamphetamine was the only individual drug that was more commonly reported among barebackers. Bars, dance clubs, and through friends were the most commonly cited methods of meeting bareback sex partners.

Halkitis and Parsons (2003) examined barebacking among a sample of HIV-positive gay and bisexual men seeking sex partners via the Internet. Participants from around the US and Canada were recruited and surveyed online and via email. The term barebacking was only used in the actual survey and not used in the materials used to recruit participants or to describe the study so as not to skew the sample with regard to those with strong feelings one way or the other regarding this behavior. The vast majority (84%) reported at least one episode of barebacking in the past three months; of greatest concern for HIV transmission is that 43% of these HIV-positive men reported barebacking with a known HIV-negative sex partner.

A lower proportion of men overall, and HIV-positive men specifically, in the Mansergh et al. (2002) study reported barebacking compared to those in the Halkitis et al. (2003a) study. This is particularly striking considering that in New York 61% of HIV-positive men reported barebacking in the past three months, whereas in San Francisco only 22% of HIV-positive men reported barebacking in the past two years. This substantial difference may be due to city differences, or due to the fact that data from New York was collected a year later than in San Francisco. More likely, however, these differences resulted from the nature of the assessments. In New York, men completed anonymous brief street-intercept surveys, and in San Francisco men completed interviewer-administered surveys. It is quite possible that men in New York were more comfortable reporting what has become a controversial behavior within gay communities. It is likely that the Halkitis and Parsons (2003) study of HIV-positive men recruited via the Internet documented higher rates of barebacking, compared to Halkitis et al. (2003a) and Mansergh et al.(2002) due to the methodology used. Clearly, the threat of HIV transmission or infection resulting from barebacking behavior is evident in all three studies.

Barebacking and HIV Transmission

"Barebacking feels better than having sex with a condom. Using a condom can take—I mean it's a procedure. It takes some of the excitement out of the sex. Having sex bareback makes you feel closer to the person because it's skin on skin contact. [I'd bareback] when I was feeling down and when I really wanted to try and do something exciting or have an interesting night. It's basically how well they can sell themselves. Like "Oh, I don't do this all the time" or, you know, "I'm negative and you should be too and so we should both be OK," a lot of that". [24-year-old African American gay man from New York City who recently tested HIV-positive talking about when he used to bareback]

Suarez and Miller (2001) have defined a number of neutralization techniques used by gay and bisexual HIV-positive men to justify barebacking with casual and anonymous partners. One technique involves serosorting, where HIV status is discussed prior to sexual activity and the HIV-positive man chooses to only engage in unprotected sex with other positive men. Again, as discussed previously, although this prevents the transmission of HIV to uninfected partners, concerns regarding HIV reinfection or STI co-infection persist. Another technique is to engage in "rational" risk taking, which is similar to strategic positioning described earlier in this chapter. The idea is that men will justify barebacking by engaging in the behaviors perceived to be less risky. That is, HIV-positive men will justify having anal sex without condoms provided they are the receptive rather than the insertive partner. HIV-negative men, in contrast, will justify unprotected anal sex if they are the insertive rather than the receptive partner. As has been discussed before, such "rational" risk taking makes a number of assumptions, most critical of which that both parties involved in the sexual encounter are aware of one another's HIV serostatus. HIV-positive men may also engage in some "rational" risk-taking by believing that it is acceptable to engage in barebacking when their viral loads are undetectable (Kalichman et al., 1998; Vanable et al., 2002). However, one study of positive gay men in the US found that, despite the perception that undetectable viral load results in less infectiousness, men with undetectable viral loads were actually less likely than other men to report engaging in unprotected anal sex (Vanable et al., 2003), as is the case in the UK and other places outside the US (see Chapter 9).

Then, there are individuals who use "irrational" justifications for their barebacking behaviors. For example, HIV-negative men may deny being at risk or have other irrational thoughts, such as the notion that spiritual forces or an especially strong immune system will protect them from infection if they engage in unprotected sex (Des Jarlais et al., 1997). Others think that they have inherited a genetic resistance to becoming infected with HIV, despite research showing that resistance to HIV from the homozygous CCR5 Delta-32 mutation exists in less than 1% of the Caucasian population and not at all in African-American or Asian populations (Halkitis et al., in press). Some HIV-positive men may have also developed the belief that they can not transmit the virus to their sexual partners through some similar perceptions of genetic resistance.

Such irrational beliefs may have been reinforced by multiple HIV-negative test results despite previous unprotected sex acts. HIV-positive men may have had serodiscordant relationships in which unprotected sex was practiced and the negative partner does not seroconvert, and thus they too have reinforced irrational beliefs of being unable to infect their sex partners. Suarez and Miller (2001) also point to the likelihood of irrational justifications for barebacking among gay and bisexual youth. Young men are likely to have limited experience with HIV, have not witnessed the devastating effects of AIDS, or hold generally pessimistic attitudes regarding their future, and as such will engage in barebacking with little concern.

There are, however, other justifications for barebacking made by both those involved in public health and those involved in barebacking. The risk in barebacking could be a response to burnout from safer sex messages of the past 20 years (Parsons, in press; Wolitski *et al.*, 2001). Halkitis et al. (2003a) found that half of gay and bisexual men believed that barebacking had emerged as a result of "boring" safer sex campaigns and 46% attributed it to fatigue about the AIDS epidemic. As mentioned earlier, optimism about the effectiveness of HIV treatments may permit some men to be less concerned about HIV transmission and infection, and thus facilitate their decision to bareback. For some men, sex without a condom has become an increasingly important behavior, as it enhances intimacy, wholeness, and connectedness. The most common reasons given for barebacking in the Mansergh et al. (2002) study were to have greater physical stimulation and to feel emotionally closer or connected more; a minority of HIV-positive (10%) and HIV-negative men (17%) reported doing something "taboo" or "racy" as a primary reason for barebacking. Like most risky behaviors, the more benefits one perceives regarding the behavior, the more likely one is to bareback (Halkitis *et al.*, 2003a). The positive effects of barebacking, including enjoyment, feeling closer to your partner, and increased stimulation during sex may overshadow the potential risks.

Barebacking and HIV Prevention

"In order to reach barebackers, prevention workers must become culturally competent and knowledgeable enough to understand why some men have created social identities based on their unprotected sex. What we need is a set of non-condom guidelines for barebackers to reduce the potential harm associated with their sex. This model of harm minimization, neither romanticizing nor vilifying barebackers, would be tailored to men who have made firm decisions to forgo condom use. In the same vain as needle exchange, perhaps we can reduce the potential for damaging consequences associated with barebacking in spite of a refusal to use condoms." [Michael Scarce, gay activist and author, in a 1998 article in the New York Blade]

Existing HIV prevention interventions are aimed at changing behavior in motivated individuals. HIV-positive gay and bisexual men who identify as barebackers are unlikely to be interested in such interventions. As such, an intervention approach that could be utilized with gay and bisexual men who bareback, as well as other less motivated persons, is urgently needed as we move into the next era of the AIDS prevention. Such an approach will have to be sensitive to the developing cultural norms regarding barebacking. Both HIV-positive and HIV-negative men who perceive that their peers are more accepting of unprotected sex are more likely to identify themselves as a barebacker (Parsons and Bimbi, 2004). Additionally, interventions must target the yet unidentified factors that are contributing to barebacking ambivalence. Many gay and bisexual men, regardless of serostatus, report that although they do not purposely seek out unprotected sex, they accept that it may happen (Parsons and Bimbi, 2004). That is, although they do not intentionally look for bareback sex or identify themselves as a barebacker, they will engage in sex without condoms.

A brief counseling approach that incorporates a style that is client-centered, and non-judgmental, such as Motivational Interviewing (Miller and Rollnick, 2002), may hold great promise for working with HIV-positive men who engage in barebacking. The idea behind Motivational Interviewing is that the provider helps to create discrepancy between the client's goals and their actual behavior, or what the client is doing versus what the client wants to be doing. Contrasting the feelings that HIV-positive gay and bisexual men have about not wanting to infect others, with desires for a quick sexual release while escaping thoughts of HIV, may help to motivate men to use strategies to reduce HIV transmission (Parsons, in press). Targeting men who bareback for this type of intervention while they are in sexually charged environments, such as public and commercial sex venues, circuit parties, or Internet chat rooms, seems particularly appropriate, as this may be an ideal time to explore discrepancy and issues of ambivalence regarding condom use among HIV-positive gay and bisexual men.

Microbicides for use in anal sex would be a potential alternative to condoms for men who engage in barebacking but who do have some concerns regarding HIV or STI transmission or infection. These chemical compounds have been shown to protect against HIV in animal models, and two microbicides are under investigation in large effectiveness trials (Tabet *et al.*, 2003). A number of trials with gay and bisexual men have evaluated the acceptability and feasibility of rectal microbicides for HIV and STI prevention. Overall, the majority of gay HIV-negative men in six US cities reported a willingness to participate in rectal microbicide studies, particularly those men reporting higher frequencies of receptive anal sex acts (Gross *et al.*, 1998). Other studies have shown that rectal microbicides would be acceptable and desirable to Latino men who have sex with men in New York City (Carballo-Dieguez *et al.*, 2000) and ethnically diverse gay and bisexual men in Los Angeles (Rader *et al.*, 2001). Men with more negative attitudes about condoms are more likely to use a rectal microbicide (Marks *et al.*, 2000), suggesting that men who bareback may be willing to consider this prevention alternative.

Gay communities have been divided, to some degree, over barebacking with those who support and those who condemn such behavior. In March of 2001, following a year of heated and emotional debate pro and con, Gay.com removed bareback chat rooms from their popular online service. Some communities are responding to barebacking with increased outreach efforts, while others remain ambivalent about barebacking or resist taking sides. Washington DC is enhancing their free condom distribution program, and expects to dispense half a million condoms in 2004. In West Hollywood, however, condoms are available in only about half the gay bars, and in New York City outreach workers handing out condoms have been asked to leave gay bars and clubs. Bowls of free condoms, which used to be a given in most gay bars in metropolitan areas, are either gone completely or placed in less conspicuous locations than on the bar. Some gay community leaders do not seem to want to get involved as involvement may hurt business; others may fear being accused of "blaming the victim" as characterized by the beginning of the epidemic when prevention programs targeting HIV-positive persons were non-existent. Efforts should be made to involve community leaders in addressing barebacking and how such behavior has the potential to facilitate a new wave of HIV cases in gay communities. It is interesting to note that barebacking has resulted in a unique subculture of men who would not have been accepted by the gay communities at the time before effective HIV treatments when HIV was perceived as a death sentence and when men were spending more time attending funerals than looking for sex partners in bareback chat rooms.

CLUB DRUGS

"Well, I think that if it's like a major party, I probably would do Tina. I would start with it because it gives you a lot of energy. Or maybe no, actually no, I wouldn't do Tina. I would do it later when I'm like really getting tired or like when everybody's going but you don't want to miss the party, so that would be the right time to do it. I'll probably start with one or a couple hits of ecstasy and a few bumps of K all the way throughout the whole night. And then later on I'd probably do Tina and then come home and do the after hours with K. That would be like a long party weekend." [25-year-old Latino man from New York City]

A number of studies have confirmed the explosion in club drug use in the US, particularly among gay and bisexual men in large urban areas. The term "Club Drugs" refers to a diverse group of drugs with the commonality that they are frequently used at dance clubs, sex clubs, circuit parties, and raves, and they are frequently used in combination with one another. Club drugs facilitate social disinhibition and are used to heighten sexual experiences (Romanelli *et al.*, 2003). Typically, the following drugs are considered in this capacity: Cocaine hydrochloride (Cocaine or coke), gamma-hydroxybutyrate (GHB or G), Ketamine (K or "Special K"), Methamphetamine (speed, crystal, or Tina), methylenedioxymethamphetamine (MDMA or "Ecstasy"), and nitrate inhalants ("poppers").

Ron Stall and his colleagues (2001) documented the early emergence of some club drugs in a probability telephone sample of gay and bisexual men from New York City, San Francisco, Los Angeles, and Chicago conducted in 1996–1998. Nitrate inhalants were the most commonly used club drugs (20% reporting use in the past six months), followed by cocaine (15%), ecstasy (12%), and methamphetamines (9%). Neither ketamine nor GHB were specifically assessed in this study, showing how rapidly new drugs can come on the scene. Geographical differences were identified, with methamphetamines more commonly used in Los Angeles and San Francisco, cocaine more commonly used in New York City, and the use of multiple drugs more common among men residing in San Francisco and New York. Use of multiple drugs and more frequent drug use were significantly more likely to be reported by HIV-positive men, and more frequent attendance at public and commercial sex venues were associated with multiple drug use.

At present there is very little data to fully evaluate the social, psychological or physical harm associated from using club drugs in combination, yet we know that patterns of use often include combining two or more drugs to achieve the desired effects. "Trail Mix" is a popular term that grew out of the urban gay circuit party and dance club scene, and refers to the use of more than one club drug at a time. The term itself conveys the casualty with which these drugs are used and the perception of them as having few consequences.

Club Drug Use and Unprotected Sex

"[Using these club drugs] definitely for me reduces my inhibitions and kind of reduces my want and need to be protected and have safe sex, and makes me kind of not think about it. I'm only in it for the action. I'm only in it for the dick. And it's like, if I get it protected, if I get it unprotected, it's fine. Whatever I get, I want it. And that's a bad thing." [30-year-old African American man from New York]

Club drugs may influence the sexual behaviors of users because they are commonly used in environments in which sex is the primary objective of participation, such as sex clubs or bathhouses. Halkitis and Parsons (2003) found that frequenting dance clubs and bathhouses were both significantly associated with increased club drug use, and particularly polydrug use among gay and bisexual men in New York City. Polydrug using men report significantly more acts of unprotected oral and anal sex, and use of inhalant nitrates in particular is associated with more frequent sex without condoms. A study of recent HIV seroconverters demonstrated a specific relationship between club drug use and HIV transmission: HIV seroconverters were consistently more likely to report the use of club drugs such as methamphetamine, cocaine, and nitrate inhalants than were non-seroconverters (Chesney et al., 1998). Recreational drug use places gay and bisexual men at greater risk for HIV seroconversion by increasing the likelihood of unprotected anal intercourse. This is particularly true for ecstasy and methamphetamine.

Ecstasy has been shown to be significantly related to unprotected anal sex, as well as increased frequency of one night stands, more male sexual partners, and increased visits to commercial sex venues (Klitzman et al., 2002). Klitzman et al. (2000) surveyed gay and bisexual men as they were entering gay dance clubs in New York City and found that, in the past year, ecstasy was the most commonly used drug (52%), followed by ketamine (38%), cocaine (32%), methamphetamine (20%), and nitrate inhalants (22%). Of all the drugs assessed, however, only ecstasy was significantly associated with unprotected anal sex.

Methamphetamine, in particular, has risen among club drugs in terms of its association with unprotected sex and concerns about the role it has played in the increasing HIV infections among gay and bisexual men (Semple et al., 2003; Parsons and Vicioso, in press; Romanelli et al., 2003). A recent study of methamphetamine using HIV-positive and HIV-negative gay and bisexual men in New York City found that 61% reported use during all or most of their sexual encounters (Halkitis et al., 2003b). Further, the social context of the drug was an important factor, as men who reported using methamphetamine in commercial sex venues reported more frequent overall use. HIV-positive men were more likely than negative men to report use at sex parties. If methamphetamine is inserted anally, as it was among 35% of these users in New York City, additional problems can emerge. The substance wears away at the lining of the rectum and increases the possibility of HIV transmission and infection because of damage to the rectal tissue.

Circuit Parties, Club Drugs, and Sex

"I was actually just talking about this last night with a friend of mine. They just got back from Gay Disney [an annual circuit party] and they were saying about all the fun they were having. And the first question out of my mouth was "Were you safe?" And he was like "Of course I was safe." And I was like "Yeah but you know, when you're partying like that you kind of lose track of what's really happening." A lot of times you're just so fucked up that responsibility doesn't come into the picture at all. It's the very scary reality of using drugs and using them frequently because your reality is so warped that in the heat of the moment you don't think about those things." [28-year-old White man from New York City]

The use of club drugs is substantially higher among gay and bisexual men who attend large dance clubs or circuit parties. Circuit parties attract thousands of gay and bisexual men for dancing, drug use, and sexual activity, typically over the course of an entire weekend with multiple events scheduled. Although these parties tend to attract relatively well-educated men with disposable income (admission for these parties typically costs over $100), there is much we can learn about the ways in which club drug use affects safer sex practices. Several studies have examined the men who frequent circuit parties, and have documented a consistent association between club drug use and unprotected sex.

Mattison et al. (2001; Ross *et al.*, 2003) collected data at three major circuit parties assessing club drug use at circuit parties in the past year. Ecstasy was the most common (used by 72% of the sample), followed by ketamine (60%), cocaine and nitrate inhalants (39% for each), methamphetamine (36%), and GHB (28%). Unsafe sex reported at the circuit parties was significantly related to frequent use of ecstasy, ketamine, and nitrate inhalants. The greater the number of individual drugs used, the greater the likelihood of unprotected sex. Only nitrate inhalant use, however, was significantly associated with unsafe sex over the past year (Mattison *et al.*, 2001). Men most commonly reported frequenting circuit parties to be "wild and uninhibited" (68%), to use drugs (58%), and to have sex (43%). Additional analyses revealed a significant relationship between attending circuit parties for these "sensation-seeking" oriented reasons and ecstasy, ketamine, GHB, and nitrate inhalant use, as well as with unsafe sex in the past year.

Unsafe sex was not related to more social reasons for attending (Ross *et al.*, 2003).

Mansergh *et al.* (2001) used multiple methods to sample gay and bisexual men residing in San Francisco who had attended a circuit party in the past year. The vast majority (95%) reported using at least one psychoactive drug during their most recent circuit party weekend, with 61% reporting the use of three or more drugs. In terms of individual drug use, ecstasy was the most common (75%), followed by ketamine (58%), methamphetamine (36%), GHB (25%), and cocaine (19%). Most of the men (84%) reported using these drugs on the dance floor and 63% reported use in the bathrooms at the event. One in four men reported a "drug overuse incident" in the past year, typically as a result of using GHB or ketamine. The majority of participants (67%) reported engaging in oral or anal sex during the most recent circuit party weekend, and 28% of the sample reported unprotected anal sex. Unprotected anal sex was significantly related to the number of drugs used. Additional analyses found that men who reported unprotected anal sex with serodiscordant or partners of unknown serostatus were more likely to be users of methamphetamine, nitrate inhalants and Viagra (Mansergh *et al.*, 2001). Further, unprotected sex with partners of serodiscordant or unknown status was more likely to occur at circuit parties held outside of San Francisco, suggesting that gay and bisexual men may be more inclined to engage in sexual risks when they travel to attend a circuit party in another city. Comparable to the previous study (Mattison *et al.*, 2001; Ross *et al.*, 2003), many men in the San Francisco cohort reported going to circuit parties in order to use drugs, escape everyday life, and have sex.

Men were surveyed at a circuit party outside of New York City and similar results again were obtained (Lee *et al.*, 2003). The majority (86%) reported alcohol or drug use on the day of the event, and polydrug use was common. Again, ecstasy was the most commonly used club drug (71%), followed by ketamine (53%), methamphetamine (31%), cocaine (19%), and GHB (12%). Ecstasy use was significantly related to unprotected anal sex among these men.

Clearly gay and bisexual men who frequent circuit parties report higher rates of lifetime and recent club drug use than men who do not. It is interesting though, that the rates of use for each individual club drug in these studies are remarkably similar. These circuit party attending gay and bisexual men, however, represent a somewhat unique subsample in that they are well-educated and able to afford the costs of attending these expensive events. The participants in these studies were overwhelmingly Caucasian (70–83%) and most self-reported being HIV-negative (70–83%). It is also possible that the rates of use are common across these studies, despite the geographical diversity of where the studies were each conducted, because it is essentially the same group of men attending each party. Lee and his colleagues (2003) found that although half of the participants were from the local New York City area, the average participant had traveled 802 miles to get to the party and that men reported attending an average of 3.8 circuit parties over the past year. As such, it is possible that the association between club drug use and risky sex among these men is unique to those who more frequently attend such parties. Nonetheless, it is clear that the unprotected sex that occurs at these events under the influence of club drugs has the potential to result in HIV transmission and infection. It is possible that the nature of these parties, combined with drug use creates a disinhibitory effect among men who might otherwise choose to use condoms for anal sex. The use of these drugs may lead to problems with judgment, in that men make even more errors in serosorting, by making more incorrect assumptions about the HIV status of their partners or through the diminished capacity to discuss HIV or disclose serostatus in drug-related sexual encounters. Some of these gay and bisexual men are using club drugs as a way to escape from thoughts and feelings about HIV (Romanelli et al., 2003). Gay and bisexual men who hold strong expectancies that drugs will facilitate sex and cognitive escape from thoughts about HIV risk are more likely to report sexual risk behaviors (McKirnan et al., 2001). Rather than use club drugs and then experience risky sex as a result, some men may be intentionally using these club drugs as a way to justify or reduce feelings of anxiety or distress about their decisions to engage in sex without condoms.

Prevention Issues for Club Drug Users

"What I feel about most of these workshops is that they're educational. You know what club drugs do to you—everybody knows what they do. Nobody wants to go to another workshop to know what they do. It's more about motivation. So I think maybe the workshops need to be about motivating people. We're already too educated. It's really about following what we know." [23-year-old Asian-Pacific Islander man from New York City]

While many inpatient and outpatient substance abuse programs are familiar with cocaine and methamphetamine abuse, treatment programs have less familiarity with other club drugs like GHB and ketamine. Furthermore, few treatment programs are informed about the special needs of gay and bisexual men, let alone HIV-positive gay and bisexual men. Nor do many existing drug treatment programs fully understand the social and sexual contexts in which club drugs are used. Many of these programs require abstinence in order to participate in treatment, which may not be attractive to gay and bisexual men for whom some level of drug use is such an important part of their socialization with other men. Most programs cater primarily to those with the most severe problems or those who meet criteria for drug dependence, and are unable to offer a harm reduction approach or address the different needs of those engaged in sustained recreational abuse or those meeting criteria for abuse.

While community based organizations and agencies serving HIV-positive gay and bisexual men may have a better understanding of the phenomenon of club drug use in their communities, most often their substance use programs are oriented towards a 12-step model that may be inappropriate for those experimenting with club drugs. HIV clinics may have sufficient resources to provide medical care to men living with HIV, but many lack the necessary resources to provide substance abuse treatment, and instead must rely on the use of referrals to programs outside of the clinic, many of which may have limited understanding of HIV-related issues, including the HIV risk reduction needs of HIV-positive men in order to prevent the transmission of HIV to their sexual partners. As such, the HIV-positive client is unable to obtain medical and substance abuse treatment in the same facility. Consequently, many HIV-positive gay and bisexual men may not seek help, despite the potentially life threatening consequences associated with both club drug use and unsafe sexual behaviors.

Intensive treatments for substance use may not be seen as beneficial by a large percentage of HIV-positive gay and bisexual men, for a variety of reasons. This has certainly been the case in a number of the interventions that I have been involved with. Harm-reduction strategies, on the other hand, provided in a non-judgmental environment that is sensitive to gay and bisexual issues and knowledgeable of the needs of HIV-positive men, are likely to be much more appealing, and result in better recruitment success. Retention across multiple sessions of more intensive treatments is also problematic. These issues suggest clearly the need for less intensive, brief interventions to provide harm reduction for club drug use and HIV risk behaviors among HIV-positive gay and bisexual men. This is another situation in which interventions based on principles of Motivational Interviewing could be particularly useful. Such an approach would address the needs of HIV-positive men at a variety of points of readiness to change, from those looking to abstain entirely from club drug use, to those simply looking to reduce their own health-related risks from using club drugs through harm reduction techniques. In addition, brief interventions using Motivational Interviewing to reduce the harm associated from club drug use have the potential to be integrated into HIV clinic and primary care facilities as part of comprehensive treatment of those living with HIV, because they would not require substantial resources.

CONCLUSIONS

It is critical to consider the interconnections among the contextual factors discussed in this chapter. An HIV-positive gay man may begin the evening using ecstasy, get sexually aroused and interested in sex, head to a bathhouse and engage in unsafe anal sex with several partners assuming that other gay men who frequent such venues know the risks they are taking and are there to forget about HIV and condoms anyway. An HIV-positive bisexual man may go to a park known for sexual activity in order to have anonymous sex with men without his wife finding out, and then engage in unprotected sex as a bottom thinking there is little risk to his partners because he is taking the receptive role and because his viral load is undetectable. And yet a third young HIV-positive man coming to terms with his sexual identity may get on the Internet, go into a barebacking chatroom to find someone interested in PnP, meet up with a group of men using crystal methamphetamine and engage in drug use and unsafe sex all night assuming that his partners must be HIV-positive too.

HIV-positive gay and bisexual men may turn to sexually charged venues, the use of the Internet to find sex partners, barebacking, and the use of club drugs to escape thoughts about HIV infection and the social norms and societal pressures to protect partners from HIV. It is through these experiences that HIV-positive men have an opportunity to feel liberated from the constraints of condom use, responsibility, or the need to disclose serostatus. Clearly, prevention efforts need to continue to better understand the interconnections between these contextual factors, and particularly the ways in which they can operate within the same HIV-positive gay or bisexual man. As this chapter has described, intervention approaches need to take into consideration the unique features of the venues, including bathhouses, sex clubs, public parks, and the Internet in which HIV-positive men find their sex partners. Interventions should be tailored to the unique needs of men who identify as barebackers, recognizing they are likely to lack motivation to use condoms and not be interested in traditional HIV prevention programs. The ways in which polydrug use negatively impacts the ability of HIV-positive gay and bisexual men to engage in safer sex practices needs to be considered and HIV prevention and substance use programs need to be combined to address the needs of these men.

Perhaps in direct contrast to the emerging trends of risky sex in public and commercial sex venues, the use of the Internet to find sex partners, the barebacking movement, and the accessibility of club drugs, there has been a recent emphasis on asking gay and bisexual men to protect themselves. Popular actor, writer, and gay activist Harvey Fierstein has been helping to promote gay community forums in New York City to address the recent increases in HIV infection and crystal methamphetamine use among gay men. In Seattle, gay community activists developed and published a "community manifesto" in an effort to promote new community norms geared at prevention, including urging HIV-positive men to take increased responsibility to both disclose their status to all sex partners and to not knowingly transmit HIV. In response to the number of Internet websites focused on barebacking, a new website called safesexcity.com has recently been created as a place for gay and bisexual men to meet other men committed to condom use and safer sex. Although such endeavors are not without controversy and debate, and there is a clear need to ensure that prevention efforts do not shift all the responsibility to reducing HIV infections to those living with HIV, these new efforts suggest that community-level interventions are possible.

Individual members of gay and bisexual communities are becoming increasingly involved and joining in a dialogue on how a new wave of the HIV epidemic can be addressed. Further, professionals involved in the development and implementation of HIV prevention interventions for gay and bisexual men should consider alternative harm reduction strategie that are non-judgmental in their orientation, such as Motivational Interviewing. In addition, it is time to think outside the box of traditional individual and group-level interventions, as well as to be more creative in our approach to working with HIV-positive and HIV-negative gay and bisexual men. Partnerships, even seemingly unorthodox ones are essential. In New York City, the Department of Health sponsored a program called "Hot Shots." HIV and STI testing, Hepatitis A and B vaccinations, and other health promotion efforts are provided in gay bars. The Department of Health provides the staff to conduct the testing and vaccinations. The program is hosted and sponsored by a gay porn star, working in conjunction with bar/club owners and managers. Men are encouraged to be tested and get education and information by the DIVAs (the Drag Initiative to Vanquish AIDS), a group of gay male HIV researchers and social science graduate students in matching wigs and costumes. An odd mixture, perhaps, but it works, as evidenced by the large number of men at each event who get tested for HIV and other STIs. Although such a colorful and unique initiative may not work in all communities, it effectively illustrates what is possible when prevention experts and community leaders come together to develop new approaches for HIV prevention.

ACKNOWLEDGEMENTS The author would like to acknowledge David S. Bimbi, David Frost, Jeremy Eggleston, and Chris Hietikko for their helpful comments and assistance in the preparation of this chapter.

REFERENCES

Ashton, M., Sopwith, W., Clark, P., McKelvey, D., Lighton, L. and Mandal, D. (2003). An outbreak no longer: factors contributing to the return of syphilis in Greater Manchester. *Sex. Transm. Infect.* 79:291–293.

Benotsch, E., Kalichman, S., and Cage, M. (2002). Men who have met sex partners via the internet: prevalence, predictors, and implications for HIV prevention. *Arch. Sex. Behav.* 3(2):177–183.

Binson, D., Woods, W., Pollack, L., Paul, J., Stall, R., and Catania, J. (2001). Differential HIV risk in bathhouses and public cruising areas. *Am. J. Public Health* 91:1482–1486.

Bonnel, C., Weatherburn, P., and Hickson, F. (2000). Sexually transmitted infection as a risk factor for homosexual HIV transmission: A systematic review of epidemiological studies. *Int. J. STD AIDS* 11:697–700.

Bull, S., and McFarlane, M. (2000). Soliciting sex on the internet: what are the risks for sexually transmitted diseases and HIV? *Sex. Transm. Dis.* 27(9):545–550.

Bull, S., McFarlane, M. and Rietmeijer, C. (2001). HIV/STD risk behaviors among men seeking sex with men online. *Am. J. Public Health* 91(6):988–989.

Calzavara, L., Burchell, A. N., Major, C., Remis, R. S., Corey, P., Myers, T., Millson, P., Wallace, E., and Polaris Study Team. (2002). Increases in HIV incidence among men who have sex with men undergoing repeat diagnostic HIV testing in Ontario, Canada. *AIDS* 16:1655–1661.

Carballo-Dieguez, A., Stein, Z., Saez, H., Dolezal, C., Nieves-Rosa, L., and Diaz, F. (2000). Frequent use of lubricants for anal sex among men who have sex with men: the HIV prevention potential of a microbicidal gel. *Am. J. Public Health* 90(7):1117–1120.

Catania, J., Osmond, D., Stall, R., Pollack, L., Paul, J., Blower, S., Binson, D., Canchola, J., Mills, T., Fisher, L., Choi, K., Porco, T., Turner, C., Blair, J., Henne, J., Bye, L., and Coates, T. (2001). The continuing HIV epidemic among men who have sex with men. *Am. J. Public Health* 91:907–914.

Centers for Disease Control and Prevention. (2002). Unrecognized HIV infection, risk behaviors, and perceptions of risk among young black men who have sex with men–Six U.S. cities, 1994–1998. *MMWR* 51:733–736.

Chen, S. Y., Gibson, S., Katz, M. H., Klausner, J. D., Dilley, J. W., Schwarcz, S. K., Kellogg, T. A., and McFarland, W. (2002). Continuing increases in sexual risk behavior and sexually transmitted diseases among men who have sex with men: San Francisco, Calif, 1999–2001. *Am. J. Public Health* 92:1387–1388.

Chesney, M. A., Barrett, D. C., and Stall, R. (1998). Histories of substance use and risk behavior: Precursors to HIV seroconversion in homosexual men. *Am. J. Public Health* 88(1):113–116.

Ciccarone, D. H., Kanouse, D. E., Collins, R. L., Miu, A., Chen, J. L., Morton, S. C., and Stall, R. (2003). Sex without disclosure of positive HIV serostatus in a US probability sample of persons receiving medical care for HIV infection. *Am. J. Public Health* 93:949–954.

Cooper, A., Scherer, C., Boies, S., and Gordon, B. (1999). Sexuality on the Internet: From sexual exploration to pathological expression. *Prof Psych Res Pract.* 30:154–164.

Crepaz, N., and Marks, G. (2002). Towards an understanding of sexual risk behavior in people living with HIV: A Review of social, psychological, and medical findings. *AIDS* 16:135–149.

Des Jarlais, D. C., Vanichseni, S., Marmor, M., Buavirat, A., Titus, S., Raktham, S., Friedmann, P., Kitayaporn, D., Wolfe, H., Friedman, S. R., and Mastro, T. D. (1997). "Why I am not infected with HIV": Implications for Long-Term Risk Reduction and HIV Vaccine Trials. *J. Acquir. Immune Defic. Syndr. Hum. Retrovirol.* 16:393–399.

Diaz, R. M., Stall, R. D., Hoff, C., Daigle, D., and Coates, T. J. (1996). HIV risk among Latino gay men in the Southwestern United States. *AIDS Educ. Prev.* 8:415–429.

Ekstrand, M. L., Stall, R. D., Paul, J. P., Osmond, D. H., and Coates, T. J. (1999). Gay men report high rates of unprotected anal sex with partners of unknown or discordant HIV status. *AIDS* 13:1525–1533.

Elford, J., Bolding, G., and Sherr L. (2001). Seeking sex on the internet and sexual risk behaviour among gay men using London gyms. *AIDS* 15:1409–1415.

Elwood, W. N. and Williams, M. L. (1998). Sex, drugs, and situation: attitudes, drug use, and sexual risk behaviors among men who frequent bathhouses. *J. Psychol. Human Sex.* 10:23–44.

Flowers, P., Hart, G., and Marriott, C. (1999). Constructing sexual health: Gay men and "risk" in the context of a public sex environment. *J. Health Psychol.* 4:483–495.

Fox, K. K., del Rio, C., Holmes, K. K., Hook, E. W. III, Judson, F. N., Knapp, J. S., Procop, G. W., Wang, S. A., Whittington, W. L. H., and Levine, W. C. (2001). Gonorrhea in the HIV era: A reversal in trends among men who have sex with men. *Am. J. Public Health* 91:959–964.

French, R., Power, R., and Mitchell, S. (2000). An evaluation of peer-led STD/HIV prevention work in a public sex environment. *AIDS Care* 12:225–234.

Gauthier, D., and Forsyth, C. (1999). Bareback sex, bug chasers, and the gift of death. *Deviant Behavior* 20:85–100.

Goodroad, B., Kirksey, K., and Butensky, E. (2000). Bareback sex and gay men: an HIV prevention failure. *J. Assoc. Nurses AIDS Care* 11:29–36.

Gross, M., Buchbinder, S., Celum, C., Heagerty, P., and Seage, G. (1998). Rectal Microbicides for U.S. gay men: are clinical trials needed? Are they feasible? *Sex. Transm. Dis.* 25(6): 296–302.

Halkitis, P. N., and Parsons, J. T. (2003). Intentional unsafe sex (barebacking) among HIV seropositive gay men who seek sexual partners on the internet. *AIDS Care* 15: 367–378.

Halkitis, P. N., Parsons, J. T., and Wilton, L. (2003a). Barebacking among gay and bisexual men in New York City: Explanations for the emergence of intentional unsafe behavior. *Arch. Sex. Behav.* 32:351–358.

Halkitis, P. N., Parsons, J., and Wilton, L. (2003b). An Exploratory study of contextual and situational factors related to methamphetamine use among gay and bisexual men in New York City. *J. Drug Issues* 38:413–432.

Haubrich, D., Myers, T., Calzavara, L., Ryder, K. and Medved, W. (2004). Gay and bisexual men's experiences of bathhouse culture and sex: "looking for love in all the wrong places" *Culture, Health and Sexuality* 6(1):19–29.

Halkitis, P. N., Zade, D. D., Shrem, M., and Marmor, M. (in press). Beliefs about HIV non-infection and risky sexual behavior among MSM. *AIDS Educ. Prev.*

Hecht, F. M., Grant, R., Petropoulos, C., Dillon, B., Chesney, M. A., Tian, H., Hellmann, N. S., Bandrapalli, N. I., Digilio, L., Branson, B., and Kahn, J. O. (1998). Sexual transmission of HIV-1 variant resistant to multiple reverse-transcriptase and protease inhibitors. *N. Engl. J. Med.* 339:307–343.

Hospers, H. J., Debets, W., Ross, M. W., and Kok, G. (1999). Evaluation of an HIV prevention intervention for men who have sex with men at cruising areas in the Netherlands. *AIDS Behav.* 3:359–366.

Hospers, H. J., Harterink, P., Van Den Hoek, K., and Veenstra, J. (2002). Chatters on the Internet: a special target group for HIV prevention. *AIDS Care* 4(4):539–544.

Kalichman, S. C. (2000). HIV transmission risk behaviors of men and women living with HIV/AIDS: Prevalence, predictors, and emerging clinical interventions. *Clinical Psychology: Science and Practice* 7:32–47.

Kalichman, S. C., Nachimson, D., Cherry, C., and Williams, E. (1998). AIDS treatment advances and behavioral prevention setbacks: preliminary assessment of reduced perceived threat of HIV-AIDS. *Health Psychol.* 17(6):546–550.

Kalichman, S. C., Weinhardt, L., DiFonzo, K., Austin, J., and Luke, W. (2002a). Sensation seeking and alcohol use as markers of sexual transmission risk behavior in HIV-positive men. *Ann. Behav. Med.* 24:229–235.

Kalichman, S. C., Rompa, D., Luke, W., and Austin, J. (2002b). HIV transmission risk behaviours among HIV-positive persons in serodiscordant relationships. *Int. J. STD AIDS* 13:677–682.

Kalichman, S. C., Benotsch, E. G., Weinhardt, L., Austin, J., Luke, W., and Cherry, C. (2003). Health-related Internet use, coping, social support, and health indicators in people living with HIV/AIDS: preliminary results from a community survey. *Health Psychol.* 22(1):111–116.

Katz, M. H., Schwarcz, S. K., Kellogg, T. A., Klausner, J. D., Dilley, J. W., Gibson, S., and McFarland, W. (2002). Impact of highly active antiretroviral treatment on HIV seroincidence among men who have sex with men: San Francisco. *Am. J. Public Health* 92(3):388–394.

Kim, A., Kent, C., McFarland, W., and Klausner, J. (2001). Cruising on the internet highway. *JAIDS* 28:89–93.

Klausner, J., Wolf, W., Fisher-Ponce, L., Zolt, I., and Katz, M. (2000). Tracing a syphilis outbreak through cyberspace. *JAMA* 284(4):447–449.

Klitzman, R., Greenberg, J., Pollack, L., and Dolezal, C. (2002). MDMA ('ecstasy') use, and its association with high risk behaviors, mental health, and other factors among gay/bisexual men in New York City. *Drug Alcohol Depend.* 66:115–125.

Klitzman, R., Pope, H.G., and Hudson, J. (2000). MDMA ("Ecstasy") abuse and high-risk sexual behaviors among 169 gay and bisexual men. *Am J Psychiatr.* 157:1162–1164.

Koblin, B. A., Torian, L. V., Gulin, V., Ren, L., MacKellar, D. A., and Valleroy, L. A. (2000). High prevalence of HIV infection among young men who have sex with men in New York City. *AIDS* 14:1793–1800.

Lee, S., Galanter, M., Dermatis, H., and McDowell. (2003). Circuit parties and patterns of drug use in a subset of gay men. *J. Addictive Diseases* 22(4):47–60.

Mansergh, G., Colfax, G., Marks, G., Rader, M., Guzman, R., Buchbinder, S. (2001). The Circuit Party Men's Health Survey: Findings and implications for gay and bisexual men. *Am J Pub Health.* 91:953–958.

Mansergh, G., Marks, G., Colfax, G., Guzman, R., Rader, M., and Buchbinder, S. (2002). Barebacking in a diverse sample of men who have sex with men. *AIDS* 16:653–659.

Marks, G., Mansergh, G., Crepaz, N., Murphy, S., Miller, L. and Appleby, P. (2000). Future HIV prevention options for men who have sex with men: intention to use a potential microbicide during anal intercourse. *AIDS Behav.* 4(3):279–286.

Mattison, A. M., Ross, M. W., Wolfson, T., Franklin, D., and the HNRC Group. (2001). Circuit party attendance, club drug use, and unsafe sex in gay men. *J. Subst. Abuse* 12:119–126.

McFarlane, M., Bull, S., and Rietmeijer, C. (2000). The internet as a newly emerging risk environment for sexually transmitted diseases. *JAMA* 284(4):443–446.

McKirnan, D. J., Vanable, P. A., Ostrow, D. G., and Hope, B. (2001). Expectancies of sexual "escape" and sexual risk among drug and alcohol-involved gay and bisexual men. *J. Subst. Abuse.* 13(1–2):137–154.

Mettey, A., Crosby, R., DiClemente, R., and Holtgrave, D. (2003). Associations between internet sex seeking and STI associated risk behaviours among men who have sex with men. *Sex. Transm. Infect.* 79:466–468.

Miller, W. R., and Rollnick, S. (2002). *Motivational interviewing: Preparing people for change*. 2nd ed. Guilford Press, New York.

Parsons, J. T. (in press). Motivational interviewing with gay/bisexual men who engage in barebacking. Journal of Gay and Lesbian Psychotherapy.

Parsons, J. T., and Bimbi, D. S. (2004, April). Barebacker identity and impact on risk behaviors of gay and bisexual men. Paper presented at the Western Region Conference of the Society for the Scientific Study of Sexuality: San Diego, CA.

Parsons, J. T., and Halkitis, P. N. (2002). Sexual and drug using practices of HIV+ men who frequent commercial and public sex environments. *AIDS Care* 14:815–826.

Parsons, J. T., and Vicioso, K. (in press). Brief encounters: Public and commercial sex environments. In: Halkitis, P., Gómez, C., and Wolitski, R. J., (eds.), *Positive Living: The Sexual Lives of HIV-Seropositive Gay and Bisexual Men*. American Psychological Association, Washington, D.C.

Parsons, J. T., Halkitis, P. N., Wolitski, R. J., and Gomez, C. A. (2003). Correlates of sexual risk behaviors among HIV-positive men who have sex with men. *AIDS Educ. Prev.* 15:383–400.

Parsons, J. T., Schrimshaw, E. W., Wolitski, R. J., Halkitis, P. N., Purcell, D. W., Hoff, C. C., and Gomez, C. (in press). Sexual practices of HIV seropositive gay and bisexual men: Use of harm reduction strategies in New York City and San Francisco. *AIDS*.

Rader, M., Marks, G., Mansergh, G., Crepaz, N., Miller, L., Appleby, P. and Murphy, S. (2001). Preferences about the characteristics of future HIV prevention products among men who have sex with men. *AIDS Educ. Prev.* 13(2):149–159.

Renwick, N., Halaby, T., and Weverling, G. J. (1998). Seroconversion for human herpes virus 8 during HIV infection is highly predictive of Kaposi's Sarcoma. *AIDS* 12:2481–2488.

Romanelli, F., Smith, K., and Pomeroy, C. (2003). Use of club drugs by HIV-seropositive and HIV-seronegative gay and bisexual men. *Topics in HIV Medicine* 11(1):25–32.

Ross, M., Mattison, A., and Franklin, D. (2003). Club drugs and sex on drugs are associated with different motivations for gay circuit party attendance in men. *Subst. Use Misuse* 38(8):1171–1179.

Semple, S. J., Patterson, T. L., and Grant, I. (2003). Binge use of methamphetamine among HIV-positive men who have sex with men: pilot data and HIV prevention implications. *AIDS Educ. Prev.* 15(2):133–147.

Somlai, A. M., Kalichman, S. C. and Bagnall, A. (2001). HIV risk behaviour among men who have sex with men in public sex environments: An ecological evaluation. *AIDS Care* 13:503–514.

Spengler, U., and Rockstroth, J. (1998). Hepatitis C in the patient with human immunodeficiency virus infection. *J. Hepatol.* 29:1023–1030.

Stall, R., Paul, J. P., Greenwood, G., Pollack, L. M., Bein, E., Crosby, G. M., Mills, T. C., Binson, D., Coates, T. J., and Catania, J. A. (2001). Alcohol use, drug use and alcohol-related problems among men who have sex with men: The Urban Men's Health Study. *Addiction* 96:1589–1601.

Stolte, I. G., Dukers, N. H., de Wit, J. B., Fennema, J. S., and Countinho, R. A. (2001). Increases in sexually transmitted infections among homosexual men in Amsterdam in relation to HAART. *Sex. Transm. Dis.* 77:184–186.

Suarez, T., and Miller, J. (2001). Negotiating risks in context: A perspective on unprotected anal intercourse and barebacking among men who have sex with men—where do we go from here? *Arch. Sex. Behav.* 30:287–300.

Tabet, S., Callahan, M., Mauck, C., Gai, F., Coetti, A., Profy, A., Moench, T., Sotto-Torres, L., Poindexter III, A., Frezieres, R., Walsh, T., Kelly, C., Richardson, B., van Damme, L., and Celum, C. (2003). Safety and acceptability of penile application of 2 candidate topical microbicides: buffergel and PRO 2000 Gel. *JAIDS* 33:476–483.

Tashima, K. T., Alt, E., Harwell, J., Fiebich-Perez, D. and Flanigan, T. P. (2003). Internet sex-seeking leads to acute HIV infection: a report of two cases. *Int. J. STD AIDS* 14:285–286.
Tikkanen, R., and Ross, M. (2003). Technological tearoom trade: characteristics of swedish men visiting gay internet chat rooms. *AIDS Educ. Prev.* 15(2):122–132.
Toomey, K., and Rothenberg, R. (2000). Sex and cyberspace—virtual networks leading to high-risk sex. *JAMA* 284(4) 485–487.
Valdisseri, R. (2003, Feb). Preventing New HIV Infections in the U.S.: What Can We Hope to Achieve? Paper presented at the 10th Conference on Retroviruses and Opportunistic Infections: Boston, MA.
Valleroy, L., MacKellar, D. A., Karon, J. M., Rosen, D. H., McFarland, W., Shehan, D. A., Stoyanoff, S. R., LaLota, M., Celentano, D. D., Koblin, B. A., Thiede, H., Katz, M. H., Torian, L. V., and Janssen, R. S. (2000). HIV prevalence and associated risks in young men who have sex with men. *JAMA* 282:198–204.
Van de Ven, P., Prestage, G., Crawford, J., Grulich, A. and Kippax, S. (2000). Sexual risk behavior increases is associated with HIV optimism among HIV negative and HIV positive gay men in Sydney over the Four-year period to February 2000. *AIDS* 14:2951–2953.
Van de Ven, P., Kippax, S., Crawford, J., Rawstorne, P., Prestage, G., Grulich, A., and Murphy, D. (2002). In a minority of gay men, sexual risk practice indicates strategic positioning for perceived risk reduction rather than unbridled sex. *AIDS Care* 14:471–480.
Vanable, P., Ostrow, D., McKirnan, D., Taywaditep, K., and Hope, B. (2002). Impact of combination therapies on HIV risk perceptions and sexual risk among HIV-positive and HIV-negative gay and bisexual men. *Health Psychol.* 19(2):134–145.
Vanable, P., Ostrow, D., and McKirnan, D. (2003). Viral load and HIV treatment attitudes as correlates of sexual risk behavior among HIV-positive gay men. *J. Psychosom. Res.* 54:263–269.
Vittinghoff, E., Douglas, J., Judson, F., McKirnan, D., MacQueen, K., and Buchbinder, S. P. (1999). Per-contact risk of human immunodeficiency virus transmission between male sexual partners. *Am. J. Epidemiol.* 150:306–311.
Weatherburn, P., Hickson, F., and Reid. (2003). *Gay men's use of the internet and other settings where HIV preventions occurs.* SIGMA RESEARCH,London chapter, pp. 1–26.
Wheater, C. P., Cook, P. A., Clark, P., Syed, Q., and Bellis, M. A. (2003). Re-emerging syphilis: a detrended correspondence analysis of the behaviour of HIV positive and negative gay men. *BMC Public Health* 3:34.
Wiley, D. J., Visscher, B. R., Grosser, S. Hoover, D. R., Day, R., Gange, S., Chmiel, J. S., Mitsuyasu, R., and Detels, R. (2000). Evidence that anoreceptive intercourse with ejaculate exposure is associated with rapid CD4 loss. *AIDS* 14:707–715.
Wolitski, R. J., Reitmeijer, C. A. M., Goldbaum, G. M., and Wilson, R. M. (1998). HIV serostatus disclosures among gay and bisexual men in four American cities: general pattern and relation to sexual practices. *AIDS Care* 10:599–610.
Woltiski, R. J., Valdiserri, R. O., Denning, P. H., and Levine, W. C. (2001). Are we headed for a resurgence in the HIV epidemic among men who have sex with men? *Am. J. Public Health* 91:883–888.
Wolitski, R. J., Bailey, C. J., O'Leary, A., Gomez, C. A., and Parsons, J. T. (2003). Self- perceived responsibility of seropositive MSM for preventing HIV transmission to sex partners. *AIDS Behav.* 7:363–372.
Woods, W., Binson, D., Mayne, T., Gore, L. R, and Rebchook, G. (2001). Facilities and HIV prevention in bathhouse and sex club environments. *The Journal of Sex Research* 38(1):68–74.
Woods, W., Tracy, D., and Binson, D. (2003). Number and distribution of gay bathhouses in the United States and Canada. *J. Homosex.* 44(3/4):55–70.

HIV-Positive and HCV-Positive Drug Users

Steffanie A. Strathdee and Thomas L. Patterson

INTRODUCTION

Early in the HIV/AIDS epidemic, HIV infection was recognized to be highly prevalent among certain populations who use illicit drugs. AIDS-related opportunistic infections were reported among injection drug users (IDUs) in the US in the early 1980s, leading to suspicions that were soon confirmed: the causative agent, later identified as HIV, could be transmitted through contaminated blood. These observations led to rapidly evolving public health measures to safeguard the blood supply, as well as efforts to reduce needle sharing among IDUs at the individual and community level.

During the first decade of the HIV/AIDS epidemic, it was also recognized that the nature, context and frequency of use of various licit and illicit non-injection drugs were associated with an elevated risk of HIV infection. As early as 1982, the use of amyl nitrites, or "poppers" among men having sex with men (MSM) prior to and during sexual activity was closely associated with unprotected sex and high HIV incidence (Marmor et al., 1982). Alcohol has also been shown to be associated with decreased condom use in various contexts (Leigh 2002), and among HIV-seropositive drug users receiving highly active antiretroviral therapy (HAART), poorer adherence (Lucas et al., 2001; Palepu et al., 2003). Among IDUs, cocaine injection has been consistently associated with higher risk injection behaviors such as attending shooting galleries, sharing needles and higher HIV incidence (Tyndall et al., 2003; Strathdee et al., 2001). Binging on stimulant drugs such as crack, cocaine and methamphetamine has also been associated with sexual behaviors that pose a higher risk of HIV infection, including greater numbers of partners, decreased condom use during vaginal and anal intercourse, and sex trade involvement (Edlin et al., 1994). The use of amyl nitrites, methamphetamine and club drugs is much higher among MSM compared to the general population, underscoring the need to interrupt the HIV transmission chain among MSM who and abuse these drugs, who we will denote MSM-DUs.

In this chapter, we discuss behavioral interventions that can reduce ongoing high risk behaviors among HIV-seropositive IDUs and MSM-DUs, and review the literature which has evaluated their effectiveness. It should be noted that the majority of these interventions have focused on HIV-seronegative IDUs and MSM-DUs and therefore need to be considered in this larger context; however, where possible we discuss the potential impact of these interventions among HIV-seropositive persons.

We discuss interventions for IDUs and MSM-DUs separately for several reasons. First, in the US and many other developed countries, MSM and IDUs tend to represent distinctly different demographic populations (Black et al., 2000). In the US for example, most IDUs reside in states in the Northeast, whereas a higher proportion of MSM live in the West. The link between injection drug use and poverty helps explain why a higher proportion of HIV-seropositive IDUs are African American or Hispanic compared to HIV-seropositive persons in other exposure categories. HIV-seropositive MSM are more likely to be Caucasian and college-educated than the general population (Beckitt et al., 2003; Black et al., 2000). Although MSM who inject drugs have extremely high HIV incidence and prevalence (Strathdee et al., 2001; Kral et al., 2001), few interventions have been specifically developed for this doubly marginalized subgroup.

Beyond HIV, the emergence of the Hepatitis C virus (HCV) epidemic is a major public health problem facing IDU populations (Alter 1999; Hagan and Des Jarlais, 2000), and to a lesser extent, MSM (Diamond et al., 2003). A high proportion of HIV-infected IDUs are co-infected with HCV (i.e., 25–30% among urban IDU populations in the US) (Thomas, et al., 2000, Hagan and Des Jarlais, 2000). Therefore, we briefly discuss interventions that have the potential to simultaneously reduce ongoing transmission of both viral pathogens. Finally, given the dearth of information on the effectiveness of behavioral interventions in reducing the burden of the HIV and HCV epidemic among persons already infected with either or both viruses, we describe some newer, promising interventions and offer suggestions for future studies.

THE EPIDEMIOLOGY OF HIV/AIDS AMONG
IDU POPULATIONS

According to the World Health Organization, 134 countries, regions or territories reported injecting drug use in 1999, and of these 114 (84%) reported HIV among IDUs (Ball 2002). In 1992, by comparison, only 80 countries reported injection drug use with 52 (65%) reporting HIV among IDUs (Stimson and Choopanya 1998). This represents approximately a 20% proportionate increase in less than a decade, indicating the potential for rapid diffusion of HIV as the prevalence of illicit drug injection grows. Injection drug use is now the predominant mode of HIV transmission in most of Western and Eastern Europe, North Africa, the Middle East and increasingly, in parts of Asia (Strathdee et al., 1998b; Ball 2002). Globally, it is estimated that 10% of HIV infections are attributable to injection drug use, but this proportion is increasing (UNDCP, 2000).

In the US, injection drug use accounts for approximately half of annual HIV infections on an annual basis, either directly through needle sharing between IDUs, or indirectly through sexual transmission among IDUs and their sexual partners (Holmberg et al., 1996; CDC 2002). Available figures do not reveal the extent of the impact of injection drug use on the global HIV pandemic, however, as they do not account for sexual transmission associated with having a sex partner who injects drugs and perinatal HIV transmission associated with injection drug use. US estimates from the mid-1990s indicate that 80% of HIV-infected adult heterosexuals who do not inject drugs have been infected through sexual contact with HIV-infected IDUs (Holmberg et al., 1996). Although the incidence of mother-to-child HIV transmission has decreased dramatically in developed countries due to efforts to ensure that antiretroviral therapies are offered to HIV-infected mothers, the majority of perinatally acquired HIV infections in North America can be traced back to a parent who was an IDU.

Epidemics of HIV among IDU populations demonstrate a high degree of regional and local heterogeneity (Strathdee et al., 1999). In the US for example, HIV incidence among IDUs has averaged 3% per year over the last decade in Baltimore (Nelson et al., 2002) but has remained stable at less than 1% per year in San Francisco (Kral et al., 2001). HIV incidence among IDUs in Bangkok is approximately 8% per year, whereas in Northern Thailand, HIV incidence reached 29 per 100 person years among IDUs attending a detoxification program (Celentano et al., 1999).

HIV prevalence among IDUs can stabilize at different rates. Among IDUs in San Francisco, Amsterdam, and New York, HIV prevalence leveled off at 12%, 30%, and 50% respectively (Friedman, 2000), suggesting that the extent to which HIV prevalence levels off in a given population can be attributed at least in part to the varying levels of public health responses to the epidemic. These observations highlight the need to reach HIV-seropositive IDUs with interventions that can effectively reduce their risk behaviors. Below, we discuss interventions that have been specifically aimed at prevention of HIV among IDU populations, with special mention of those shown to be effective in reducing risk behaviors among HIV-infected IDUs.

BEHAVIORAL INTERVENTIONS FOR INJECTION DRUG USERS

HIV-seropositive IDUs can transmit HIV to their partners through unsafe sex and injection behaviors and can remain vulnerable to additional blood-borne and/or sexually transmitted infections themselves through both routes. The major types of interventions aimed to reduce drug related harms include drug abuse treatment programs, needle exchange programs (NEPs), outreach and network-oriented interventions. Among HIV-seropositive IDUs, prevention of distributive needle sharing (i.e., passing on used syringes) rather than receptive needle sharing (i.e., injecting with previously used syringes) is the primary goal, as well as increasing condom use and reducing other sexual risk behaviors that can transmit HIV to others (for reviews of the interventions mentioned above see Bastos and Strathdee, 2000; Metzger and Navaline, 2003; and Semaan et al., 2002).

Drug Abuse Treatment

Since cessation of injection drug use is the only way to ensure that the probability of HIV transmission through contaminated injection equipment is reduced to zero, drug abuse treatment is the most widely endorsed intervention to reduce HIV-associated risk behaviors among IDUs (Metzger and Navaline, 2003). Over the past two decades, research has consistently shown associations between enrollment in substance abuse treatment and reductions in HIV transmission risk behaviors, which can be attributed to reductions in injection drug use (Booth et al., 1996; Metzger et al., 1993; National Consensus Development Panel, 1998). Moreover, the longer the duration of substance abuse treatment, the greater the protective effects (Metzger and Navaline 2003; National Consensus Development Panel, 1998). There is also growing evidence that drug detoxification alone is insufficient to provide protection from HIV infection unless it is followed by a longer course of treatment (Metzger and Navaline, 2003). While the majority of these studies have not focused on reductions of high risk behaviors among HIV-seropositive persons, there is no reason to believe that there would be differential effects of substance abuse treatment by HIV serostatus.

Since most IDUs in Europe and North America have tended to inject opiates, particularly heroin, either alone or in combination with other drugs, it is not surprising that among the various drug abuse treatment modalities, the most consistent reductions in HIV-related risk behaviors have been observed for medication-assisted therapies that block opiate receptors. The vast majority of the literature supports the effectiveness of maintenance programs offering methadone (Langendam et al., 1999; Metzger et al., 1993) or buprenorphine (Carrieri et al., 2003; Johnson et al., 2000). Ball et al. (1988) evaluated the impact of methadone maintenance in three US cities, showing that 60% of those enrolled ceased injection drug use for at least one year, and more than 80% of those who left treatment programs returned to injecting drugs within 12 months. These findings were replicated by subsequent studies (Ball 1988; Booth et al., 1996; Metzger et al., 1993). More recently, buprenorphine maintenance has been shown to be just as effective as methadone in reducing ongoing use of opiates (Carrieri et al., 2003; Johnson et al., 2000).

Several characteristics of opioid agonist therapies warrant important consideration in order to maximize their effectiveness in HIV-seropositive persons. First, since persons who acquired their HIV infection through sharing of contaminated syringes are likely to be more severely drug dependent than HIV-seronegative drug users, ensuring that adequate dosages of opiate agonist therapies are prescribed is paramount. Recent studies have shown that higher dosages of methadone are superior for reducing ongoing illicit drug use compared to lower dosages (Langendam et al., 1999; Johnson et al., 2000). Second, it is noteworthy that up to 40% of drug users receiving methadone experience relapse (Ball, 1988); therefore, discouraging or preventing HIV-seropositive drug users from accessing sterile injection equipment could inadvertently facilitate needle sharing. There is recent evidence from the Netherlands and Canada that "low threshold" methadone treatment which tolerates ongoing use of illicit drugs among those enrolled in drug treatment can reduce HIV risk behaviors and decrease mortality (Langendam et al., 1999; Langendam et al., 2001; Millson et al., 2002).

A third consideration to optimize opiate agonist therapies for HIV-seropositive persons is to be aware of potential interactions with HAART. For example, methadone can increase the concentration of zidovudine

(AZT) (McCance-Katz et al., 1998). Some protease inhibitors (e.g. ritonivir) may also affect uptake of methadone (McCance-Katz, 2003). An under-appreciation of these interactions in HIV-infected persons can lead to adverse side effects or toxicities and can undermine the effectiveness of drug abuse treatment.

While drug abuse treatment is considered to be an effective HIV prevention strategy, its impact has varied dramatically between and even within countries. In Amsterdam, a decline in HIV incidence among IDUs was associated with a combination of widespread access to low-threshold methadone maintenance, needle exchange and voluntary HIV testing and counseling (van Ameijden et al., 1998). Likewise, in New York City, the reversal of a major HIV epidemic that began in the early 1980's has been attributed to a combination of expanded methadone maintenance and increased access to sterile syringes and outreach (Des Jarlais et al., 2000). Between 1990 and 2001, the prevalence of HIV among IDUs entering detoxification in New York City dropped from 54% to 13% (Des Jarlias et al., 2004), and HIV incidence has decreased to less than 1% per year (Des Jarlias et al., 2000). On the other hand, the prevalence of HIV among IDUs enrolled in methadone maintenance in Baltimore has remained relatively stable, at 20–25% (Shah et al., 2000).

Unfortunately, as few as 15%–20% of active drug users in the US are enrolled in drug abuse treatment at any given time (Metzger and Navaline, 2003; Shah et al., 2000). The public health impact of substance abuse treatment has been hampered because access to these programs is severely limited. At least in the US, most communities have not adequately funded treatment services, and in some cases funding for substance abuse treatment programs has actually diminished during the course of the HIV epidemic. Additionally, the lack of third party reimbursement for substance abuse treatment limits access for some HIV-positive drug users. In one study, HIV-seropositive IDUs not receiving Medicaid were half as likely to be enrolled in methadone maintenance than those without health insurance (Shah et al., 2000). In some parts of the world, public policy restricts certain modalities of drug abuse treatment. For example, in Russia, agonist treatments for drug abuse such as methadone and buprenorphine are prohibited. In many countries in Asia which have reported explosive HIV epidemics among IDUs (e.g. Thailand, China), there is almost no access to opiate agonist therapies. It is not surprising that each of these countries is experiencing explosive HIV epidemics among IDUs.

A recent national survey of more than 400 substance abuse treatment agencies in the US found that only one in four believed that patients enrolled in drug treatment programs should be educated on strategies to reduce drug-related harm or that methadone should be offered over the long term (Rosenberg and Phillips, 2003). In another nationwide survey, only half of residential drug treatment units made HIV testing available to their patients on-site (Strauss et al., 2003). Furthermore, substance abuse treatment programs have seldom had a dual focus on injection and sexual risk reduction, which has likely accounted at least in part for reported inconsistencies in study findings of the impact of these interventions on sexual risk behaviors (Avants et al., 2000; Lollis et al., 2000). In a follow-up study of clients enrolled in methadone maintenance programs in two US states, inconsistent condom use was significantly associated with enrollment in programs where condoms were available only upon request and abstinence and monogamy between uninfected partners were promoted (MacGowan et al., 1997). These findings highlight the extent to which there are missed opportunities for identifying and offering HIV-seropositive drug users interventions to reduce their risk behaviors and provide access to HIV diagnosis and treatment.

Apart from the obvious need to expand opioid agonist treatment for HIV-positive drug users, there is also a need to expand the kinds of treatment options that are available. Co-dependence on opiates and cocaine occurs in about 60% of patients entering methadone treatment and is related to poorer prognoses. In one study, HIV-infected persons reported 20% more cocaine use and injected cocaine more than HIV negatives (Meandzija et al., 1994). Yet there are few effective drug treatments available for users of stimulants (e.g., cocaine, methamphetamine), despite the fact that HIV-seropositive stimulant users tend to be those with high risk sexual behaviors that are hardest to change. In one study, desipramine offered in combination with buprenorphine significantly reduce combined opiate and cocaine use among these dually dependent patients (Kosten et al., 2003). These effects were even more dramatic when coupled with contingency management; drug users receiving both interventions had significantly more drug-free urines (Kosten et al., 2003). Such studies are promising, but are far from achieving the same kinds of success compared to that for opiate users.

A more controversial form of drug treatment is prescription of heroin to IDUs who have failed traditional opiate agonist therapies. This approach has shown remarkable success in reducing injection drug use and its associated harms in Switzerland (Guttinger et al., 2003), where it has been adopted as part of the country's overall public health response to treating heroin addiction. Heroin maintenance trials are also underway in the Netherlands, Germany and Canada (Fischer et al., 2002). Heroin maintenance may be an appropriate treatment modality for "hard core" drug users whose behavior is hardest to change, including those who are HIV-seropositive.

Another novel approach to drug abuse treatment is that of the "therapeutic workplace" (Silverman et al., 2001). Based on the concept of contingency management which provides incentives in exchange for desired behavior changes, individuals are paid to perform jobs or to participate in job training. Salary is linked to abstinence by requiring patients to provide drug-free urine samples to gain access to the workplace. In a landmark study by Silverman et al. (2001), a therapeutic workplace environment coupled with methadone maintenance was associated with nearly a doubling of patients' abstinence from opiates and cocaine. This type of approach may be ideal for HIV-seropositive IDUs, since they could potentially receive both methadone and HAART as directly observed therapies.

Needle Exchange Programs

Needle exchange programs (NEPs) allow IDUs to exchange sterile syringes for potentially contaminated ones. An important aim of NEPs is to decrease the circulation of contaminated injection equipment, thereby reducing the spread of blood-borne pathogens in the community. Since the first NEP was introduced in Amsterdam in 1984, at least 46 regions, countries and territories reported having at least one NEP by the end of 2000 (Bastos and Strathdee, 2000). By 2002, there were 178 exchanges in 36 US states.

The overwhelming majority of studies provide strong evidence for the effectiveness of NEPs in reducing high risk injection behaviors among HIV-seronegative and HIV-seropositive IDUs. Buning et al. (1986) reported declines in needle sharing and injection frequency associated with NEP participation in Amsterdam. Other studies subsequently reported reductions in HIV incidence, Hepatitis B virus (HBV) and Hepatitis C virus (HCV) infections (Coutinho, 1998; Des Jarlais et al., 1995, 1996; Drucker et al., 1998; Hagan et al., 1995), decreased needle sharing among HIV-negative and HIV-positive persons (Bluthenthal et al., 2000; Vertefeuille et al., 2000) decreases in syringe re-use, and increased rates of entry into drug treatment programs (Heimer, 1998; Shah et al., 2000; Strathdee et al., 1999). Despite variations between programs, a recent international comparison showed that in 29 cities with established NEPs, HIV prevalence decreased on average by 5.8% per year, but increased on average by 5.9% per year in 51 cities without NEP (Hurley et al., 1997). There appears to be no published evidence that NEPs can cause negative societal effects, such as increases in drug use, discarded needles, crime or more permissive attitudes towards drugs among youth (Doherty et al., 2000; Marx et al., 2001).

A second important aim of NEPs is to provide crucial ancillary services to IDUs who are typically out of reach of traditional health care services and prevention programs. Many NEPs provide other sterile equipment or paraphernalia that facilitates safer injection (e.g. cottons, cookers, water, bleach) as well as male and female condoms. NEPs have served as a pivotal entry point for drug treatment and rehabilitation for both HIV-seropositive and HIV-seronegative drug users, provided that adequate numbers of treatment slots are available (Heimer et al., 1998; Shah et al., 2000; Strathdee et al., 1999). In many settings, NEPs tend to attract higher risk IDUs who engage in riskier behaviors compared to IDUs that tend to obtain syringes from other sources (Hahn et al., 1997; Schechter et al., 1999). In San Francisco, IDUs who later began attending NEP had higher HIV incidence rates than those who never attended (Hahn et al., 1997), suggesting that NEPs may be an ideal venue to offer additional "second tier" interventions to HIV-seropositive IDUs. In fact, some NEPs provide on-site HIV testing and counseling, screening for medical conditions such as STDs and TB, provision of HBV and HAV vaccines, abscess care, overdose prevention materials and multivitamins. Altice et al. (2003) recently reported that provision of HAART to HIV infected IDUs attending mobile NEPs was feasible.

Yet in both developed and developing countries, there exist intentional and unintentional barriers to the provision of sterile syringes to IDUs. Although global expansion of NEPs has occurred since the first NEP was introduced two decades ago, NEPs exist in less than half of the countries reporting HIV among IDUs and coverage of these programs is typically low (Strathdee et al., 2001). In the US, the reasons for this are largely political. A federal ban on US funding for NEPs was enacted in 1988, which has been upheld despite the conclusions of several US government commissioned reports which have specifically called for a lifting of the ban (US Government Accounting Office 1993; Office of the Surgeon General, 1998; NIH 1997). The ban clearly has taken a toll. In a recent assessment of syringe access in 50 states, it was considered that 16 have only retail access to sterile syringes, 9 have only NEPs, 22 have no "clearly legal" form of syringe access, and 3 have no legal form of syringe access at all (Burris et al., 2002). A national policy of funding NEPs, including pharmacy sales and syringe disposal in the US was estimated to cost $34,278 per HIV infection averted, which is well below the lifetime costs of treating an individual's HIV infection (Lurie et al., 1998).

Community Outreach

Community based outreach utilizes former IDUs and/or peers to create a liaison between the drug using community and HIV education or drug abuse treatment. In most cases, participation in street-based outreach interventions is followed by office-based HIV testing and counseling.

Community outreach has been demonstrated to be a crucial component held in common by five cities that consistently maintained low stable HIV prevalence rates among IDU populations (Des Jarlais et al., 1995). An advantage to outreach is that it is more economical and easy to implement in developing countries. Kumar et al. (1998) showed a community-based outreach program was associated with significant decreases in the frequency of injection drug use and needle sharing after 18 months of follow-up in Madras, India.

Most outreach interventions are associated with significant decreases in the frequency of drug use (Stevens et al., 1998) and re-use of needles (Kotranski et al. 1998), as well as increased use of bleach for purposes of syringe disinfection (Rietmeijer et al., 1996; Siegal et al., 1995). In Chicago, an extensive outreach intervention based on peer leaders was associated with a significant decline in HIV incidence over a four-year period (Weibel et al., 1996). While outreach is considered to be an important component of a community's response to reducing HIV risk behaviors, it has been seldom shown to generate a strong sustained effect in the absence of other HIV interventions.

Network-Oriented Interventions

Early successes with behavior change among drug users exposed to various kinds of outreach interventions led to more sophisticated interventions involving IDUs' social networks. Researchers working in this area postulated that the sharing of injection equipment is embedded in social processes that promote and reinforce HIV risk behaviors (Des Jarlais, 1989). In a study of HIV among drug users in Colorado Springs HIV was harbored in small, connected "core groups" of individuals with no demonstrated links to the general population, suggesting that social influence among drug using networks could also be protective (Potterat et al., 1999). Lessons learned from the observed community-wide HIV risk reduction among gay men in San Francisco provide support for the hypothesis that social influence can be an important approach to behavioral risk reduction (Dowsett, 1993).

Early in the HIV epidemic, research on drug use patterns demonstrated the relationship between adolescent drug use and peer influence (Brooks et al., 1989). Friedman et al. (1987) found that friends' HIV risk behaviors were the strongest predictors of behavior change; perception of friends' risk behavior was a stronger determinant of risk reduction than was knowledge about AIDS, education level, or personal knowledge of somebody with AIDS. In a study of behavior change among IDUs in Brazil,

Thailand, Scotland, and the US, talking about AIDS with drug using friends was consistently associated with reduction in self-reported risk behaviors (Des Jarlais et al., 1995). In one of the only studies of disclosure among US HIV-infected IDUs and their social networks, Latkin et al. (2001) found that people tended to disclose to network members who were also HIV-infected and were not drug users.

While social influence factors have been given more attention by HIV prevention researchers in European countries compared to the US, few have utilized experimental design and pre- and post-test assessment (Rhodes and Hartnol, 1996). Recently, attention has focused on network-based strategies of HIV prevention which are based upon the personal networks of IDUs. Personal networks include people an IDU may have a social relationship with, such as an injecting partner, a sex partner or a family member. Building upon HIV behavior change models that include social influence components (e.g., Fisher and Fisher, 1992), Latkin and colleagues demonstrated that among HIV-seronegative drug users, personal network-based interventions can decrease needle sharing and use of shooting galleries, and increase bleach disinfection (Latkin et al., 1995, 1996, 1998).

These promising findings prompted subsequent intervention studies, such as The SHIELD (Self-Help In Eliminating Life-threatening Disease) study conducted in Baltimore, which was a randomized trial targeting members of the drug using community and 1–3 members of their risk (drug user or sexual) networks, 20% of whom were HIV-seropositive (Latkin et al., 2003). Drug users randomized to the intervention were three times more likely than control participants to report greater reduction in drug-related risk behaviors after six months and were four times more likely to report increased condom use with casual partners. More recently, the US CDC sponsored a multi-site peer mentor intervention among HIV-seropositive current and former IDUs, called INSPIRE (Intervention for Seropositive Injectors—Research and Evaluation). This integrated behavioral intervention aimed to increase uptake of HIV care and decrease injection and sexual risks, results from which are forthcoming.

Interventions to Reduce Sexual Risk Behaviors among Injection Drug Users

Recent studies suggest that the role of sexual HIV transmission between IDUs and from IDUs to non-drug users has been overlooked. In studies from San Francisco (a city of low HIV prevalence among IDUs) and Baltimore (a city of high HIV prevalence among IDUs) sexual risk factors have played an important role in HIV transmission (Kral et al., 2001;

Strathdee and Sherman 2003). Although sexual behaviors among HIV-seropositive IDUs have been less well studied, Tun et al. (2003) recently showed that among sexually active HIV-seropositive IDUs, two thirds engaged in unprotected sex and approximately half also reported sharing needles in the previous six months.

IDUs can also function as an HIV transmission bridge to the general population through sexual contact with non-drug using sexual partners (Gyarmathy et al., 2002). HIV epidemics among injectors in certain regions have become "generalized," reaching well beyond the IDU community. In the Ukraine, Burma, Thailand and parts of India, Vietnam and China, HIV prevalence among the general population has surpassed 1%, which has been closely linked to sexual transmission from IDUs (Strathdee, 2003). Although injection drug use may be seen as characterizing responses to the epidemic among drug users during the past 20 years, Metzger and Navaline assert that sexual risks associated with drug use may well define the prevention research agenda of the future (Metzger and Navaline, 2003). Interventions addressing the sexual risk behaviors of drug users are especially relevant to HIV-seropositive drug users, since they can have the direct benefit of reducing the risk of acquiring new STIs, while offering the indirect benefit of protecting the sexual partners of drug users.

Prevention efforts directed toward IDUs generally have shown greater success in reducing injection risk behavior than sexual risk behavior, since interventions focused on reducing sexual risks have generally had lower effect sizes (McMahon et al., 2001; Warner et al., 2001; Prendergast et al., 2001). In a meta-analysis, Semaan et al. (2002) examined the effectiveness of 33 US-based HIV intervention studies in reducing the sexual risk behaviors of drug users by reducing unprotected sex or increasing the use of male condoms. Their analysis focused on studies with measured behavioral or biological outcomes, experimental designs or certain quasi-experimental designs. Compared to no intervention, there was a 40% reduction in risk associated with interventions to reduce sexual risks. Compared to other HIV interventions, there was modest additional benefit. These findings were similar to a previous meta-analysis of 16 studies which included weaker study designs, but nevertheless reported an identical cumulative effect size (Cross et al., 1998). In both meta-analyses, there appeared to be no experimental studies focusing on the sexual behaviors of HIV-seropositive drug users.

Understanding which types of interventions are most effective in reducing sexual risk behaviors among drug users is even more complex. Unlike interventions focused on reducing injection-related risks, there is little data that indicates which interventions focused on sexual behaviors among drug users work best, and under what circumstances. This may not be altogether surprising, since more than half the studies examined in the meta-analysis by Semaan et al. (2002) did not mention the behavioral theories, models or mechanisms hypothesized to be associated with sexual risk reduction. Levels of drug users' condom use with their main partner may remain low because the underlying constructs that need to be changed are personal, interpersonal, and social (Auerbach and Coates, 2000; Semaan et al., 2002). Indeed, a study by Friedman et al. (1994) found that higher rates of condom use among drug users existed among HIV serodiscordant partners; these authors suggested that altruism and sex partner pressure may explain these findings.

A review by van Empelen et al. (2003) concluded that the most successful interventions to reduce sexual risks among drug users were those based on Social-Cognitive Theory or the Diffusion of Innovations Theory. These interventions tended to feature inclusion of peers, modeling and rehearsal of skills, social support enhancement and skills building. Of interest was the finding that community-level interventions showed greatest sustainability. However, fewer than 5% of intervention studies aimed at reducing sexual risks among drug users randomize at the community level (Semaan et al., 2002).

Although the number of studies which are theoretically based is limited, it is clear that some interventions can successfully reduce sexual risks among drug users. Developing interventions with a stronger theoretical basis which generate effects of higher magnitude will be needed to achieve significant community-wide reductions in drug users' sexual risk behaviors.

APPLICATIONS TO HCV-SEROPOSITIVE IDUs

HCV incidence among IDUs is consistently higher than that of HIV, due at least in part to its greater transmissibility; HCV is ten times more infectious than HIV when spread through the parenteral route (Gerberding 1995). Worldwide, HCV prevalence among IDUs can be as high as 90% (Hagan and Des Jarlais 2000), whereas HCV incidence ranges between 13 and 22 per 100 person-years (Garfein et al. 1998; van Beek et al. 1998) and is highest among the susceptible pool of young IDUs. Furthermore, 20–30% of IDUs in the US are co-infected with HIV and HCV, which can complicate the treatment of both infections. HIV infection can hasten the progression of HCV disease progression, although it remains controversial whether or not the reverse is true (Thomas et al., 2000).

HCV infection can result in serious liver disease including cirrhosis and hepatocellular carcinoma. Approximately 80–85% of HCV infections result in a chronic carrier state where patients are infectious and capable of transmitting the virus to others (Alter, 1999). In some settings, morbidity and mortality attributable to HCV infections among IDUs could exceed that for HIV, since both infections are highly prevalent among drug users (Hagan and Des Jarlais 2000). Since HCV is often acquired before HIV among IDU populations, interventions that effectively reduce high risk transmission behaviors among HCV-infected IDUs could also have a significant impact on HIV prevention (Garfein et al., 1996).

In comparison to HIV, there is limited awareness of HCV among drug users, as evidenced by the coverage of voluntary testing and counseling for both infections. In a recent study of ten publicly funded methadone maintenance treatment programs in Baltimore approximately 20% of IDUs tested HIV-seropositive but 80% were aware of their infection and had sought care. On the other hand, 91% of these IDUs tested HCV-positive but three quarters had not previously been tested and were thus unaware of their infection (Loughlin et al., 2004). Clearly, IDUs will require improved counseling and testing strategies for HCV infection as well as accessible HCV medical care. However, testing and counseling for HCV infection is unlikely to have a dramatic effect on transmission risk behaviors in the absence of other interventions. In a recent study of young HCV-seropositive IDUs who had been made aware of their infection through pre- and post-test counseling, there was no significant reduction in the proportion who engaged in needle sharing after three months (Ompad et al., 2002). These findings signal an urgent need for preventive interventions with rigorous evaluations, since prevention of HCV infection may prove much more difficult than HIV prevention.

Although few empirical studies have evaluated interventions focused on HCV-seropositive IDUs, one such multicenter study is underway. Referred to as the Study to Reduce Intravenous Exposures (STRIVE), this study uses a peer-mentor approach to reduce injection related risk behaviors (e.g., distributive needle sharing) and facilitate access to HCV care.

Even in the absence of effective behavioral interventions to reduce transmission behaviors among HCV-seropositive IDUs, important prevention messages should be shared with these patients. Regardless of the route of their infection, all people with HCV should be counseled to abstain or at least reduce their alcohol use, since alcohol can accelerate progression to HCV-related liver disease (Thomas et al., 2000). Additionally, these patients should be offered vaccines for both Hepatitis A and B, since these infections can further compromise the liver. As with HIV infection, behavioral interventions may best be offered to HCV-seropositive drug users in the context of substance abuse treatment programs, where it has been shown that uptake and adherence to HCV therapies can be improved (Sylvestre et al., 2002).

THE EPIDEMIOLOGY OF MSM WHO USE DRUGS

MSM comprise up the largest number of reported US AIDS cases and represent the largest group of new AIDS cases each year in the US. In the year 2000, an estimated 42% of AIDS diagnoses were among MSM, including those who inject drugs (CDC, 2002). In addition, there are elevated HIV risks for MSM who also use drugs beyond the risks from either sex or drug use alone. This is true whether individuals are drug injectors or non-injectors who use substances such as methamphetamine. In addition, drug-using MSM may serve as a bridge for the transmission of HIV to their female or male sex partners (Strathdee et al., 2001). While there is evidence that behavioral interventions to reduce sexual risk behavior among HIV-negative MSM are effective, interventions designed to prevent secondary transmission of HIV are rare, despite continued high-risk behavior among HIV-positive individuals (Kalichman et al., 2002; Valleroy et al., 2000). In high prevalence settings, such as communities with high numbers of IDUs, even if the prevalence of risk behavior is low, there is a potential for sustained HIV transmission.

The group of drugs that are most prevalent in the MSM community has been labeled 'club drugs' (see Chapter 4). While there is no consensus on which drugs should fall within this class, the most common psychoactive agents encompassed by the term are: ecstasy (3, 4-methylenedioxy-methamphetamine or MDMA), GHB (gamma hydroxybutyrate), ketamine, LSD (lysergic acid diethylamide), PCP (pencyclidine), Rohypnol (flunitrazepam), and probably the most commonly used are methamphetamines. There is a growing concern among health promotion experts in the intersection between this class of drugs and sexual risk behaviors (Vastag, 2001), and the venues in which they are taken like raves, circuit parties, or night clubs. These drugs may be ingested, snorted, or taken anally or vaginally and some are also injected (e.g., methamphetamine, ketamine). The pharmacologic actions range from stimulant/hallucinogenic (MDMA) with desired effects for users of sensory hallucinations, heightened perception and sensory awareness; to stimulant/non-hallucinogenic (e.g., methamphetamines) with a desired effect similar to cocaine and libido enhancement; to depressant (e.g., GHB) with the desired effect of ataxia, sedation, euphoria and increased libido.

Though the use of these drugs is spreading rapidly in North America, their prevalence has been greatest on the west coast. For example, drug treatment data in California suggests that approximately one-third of all admissions are for methamphetamine use (Greenblatt and Gfoerer, 1998). Even in studies where the prevalence of methamphetamine use has been low, there remains a strong association between unprotected anal sex among MSM who use other drugs. In a recent study by Beckett et al. (2003), who compared the relationship between drug use and high risk sex among three groups of HIV-seropositive persons—MSM, IDU and heterosexuals—substance use, particularly use of cocaine and poppers, was most prevalent among MSM compared to the other two groups. Substance use and current dependence were associated with being sexually active among MSM but not IDUs; marijuana, alcohol, and hard drug use were most strongly associated with being sexually active among MSM. In this study, approximately one fifth of HIV-seropositive men engaged in high-risk sexual activity.

Studies have shown that MSM of color have high HIV incidence rates and are particularly in need of focused interventions (Valleroy et al., 2000). In a national study of young MSM, Valleroy et al. (2000) showed the highest HIV prevalence among African American MSM, which was closely linked to injection drug use. In a study of four groups of Latino MSM, sensation seeking, self-worth, and machismo were related to substance use and unprotected anal sex (Dolezal et al., 2000). The association between substance use and unprotected sex association remained when adjusting for ethnicity, acculturation, partner type, attendance at bars, and personality variables, indicating the need to address substance use among interventions aimed at Latino MSM.

Challenges Facing Prevention for Drug Using MSM

A number of new challenges have emerged which have affected sexual and drug using behaviors among MSM and IDUs overall, and among HIV-seropositives particular. In both HIV-seropositive MSM and IDUs, there is evidence that HIV treatment optimism following the advent of HAART complicates prevention efforts in the US. For example, attitudes towards HAART including a reduced concern about HIV have been associated with unprotected anal sex among HIV-seropositive MSM (Ostrow et al., 2002). HIV treatment advances, safer sex fatigue, and the increased popularity of club drugs were commonly cited as reasons for "barebacking" in a recent study of HIV-seropositive MSM (Halkitis et al., 2003). Crawford et al. (2003) found that reduced concern about HIV mediated the relationship between sexual sensation seeking and sexual risk behavior. Among HIV-seropositive IDUs, perceiving that HIV treatments could reduce HIV transmission was significantly associated with unprotected sex (Tun et al., 2003), indicating that interventions aimed at both MSM and IDUs need to take into account the unintended consequences of the impact of HAART on sexual risk behaviors. The extent to which HIV treatment optimism may affect behaviors in developing countries is unknown, but should be carefully studied as these therapies become more widely available.

A number of drugs have also emerged recently which complicate the prevention landscape. For some MSM, Viagra is used in combination with club drugs and appears to be an emerging contributing factor to unsafe sex, potentially increasing HIV transmission. HIV care and prevention providers should target MSM who use Viagra with club drugs for enhanced education on safer sex and potentially harmful drug interactions (Chu et al., 2003).

The extent to which MSM-IDUs have been impacted by the HIV epidemic has been documented in several studies. In two studies of IDU populations with more than 10 years of follow-up, homosexual activity was associated with more than a two-fold increased risk of HIV seroconversion after adjusting for injection-related risks (Kral et al., 2001; Strathdee et al., 2001). MSM-IDUs have also been shown to frequent shooting galleries and engage in needle sharing more often than other male drug users (Strathdee et al., 1997). In a study of MSM-IDUs in Denver, 45% were HIV-seropositive, and risk behaviors were rife; 82% had primary and non-primary male partners, 20% had non-primary female partners, and 15% exchanged money or drugs for sex (Bull et al., 2002). Condom use was inconsistent and infrequent for vaginal, anal and oral sex with all types of partners. Disturbingly, HIV-seropositive MSM-IDU did not report a higher proportion of protective behaviors than those who were HIV-seronegative. These findings underscore the difficulties in targeting interventions to MSM-IDUs, a subgroup that typically does not identify with either the gay community or the IDU community.

Structural issues may also impede dissemination of interventions that have been empirically shown to reduce HIV transmission. For example, there is currently political opposition to NEPs and expansion of sterile syringe access to IDUs through pharmacies and over the counter syringe sales without a prescription. In Florida, where NEPs are illegal, researchers at the University of Miami have initiated an intervention in a shooting gallery. There is limited financial support for drug abuse treatment, despite the fact that it is the most accepted HIV prevention strategy among IDUs. There are also barriers to provision of HAART among medically-eligible IDUs and crack users at the individual, provider and system-level (Celentano et al., 2001; Metsch et al., 2001; Strathdee et al., 1998a), which in turn limits opportunities for providers to offer prevention messages to difficult to reach HIV-seropositive IDUs. Since HAART can reduce viral load to undetectable levels whereupon the probability of HIV transmission is reduced, interventions which increase uptake and adherence to HAART among drug using populations should be considered an important secondary prevention intervention.

Other characteristics of HIV-positive drug users present challenges to interventions designed to promote safer sex messages. For example, a substantial proportion of HIV-positive drug users may possess some degree of cognitive impairment in domains that could impede their ability to learn, retain, and execute HIV preventive behaviors (Ripeth et al., 2004). In addition, Galvan et al. (2003) reported that 13% of people with HIV receiving care in the US in 1996 had co-occurring psychiatric symptoms and either or both drug dependence symptoms or heavy drinking. Behavioral interventions with these groups may be complicated by neuropsychological impairment associated with both HIV and drug use. Rippeth et al. (2004) found the highest rates of impairment in HIV positive methamphetamine users (58%), less with HIV negative methamphetamine users (40%), which was higher than a HIV positive non-methamphetamine users (38%) or HIV negative non-users (18%). While not yet documented, these deficits could theoretically impair an individual's ability to learn intervention messages, or alter their behavior in the real world though impairments in judgment. In addition, since a hallmark of psychiatric disorders like schizophrenia is cognitive impairment, a combination of HIV, drugs, and psychiatric disorders could further compound this problem and create additional impairments to learning of new safer drug and sex messages.

CONCLUSIONS

Below, we suggest specific prevention messages and future research directions needed to reduce ongoing risk behaviors among HIV positive IDUs and MSM DUs.

HIV-Seropositive IDUs

International experience indicates that while IDU-associated HIV epidemics may occur with incredible rapidity, it is possible for these epidemics to be stabilized, reversed or prevented through strong, responsive public health measures. In New York City and Amsterdam, which are two cities that have essentially reversed their HIV epidemics among IDUs, there are suggestions that the IDU population is shrinking (Des Jarlais et al., 2000; van Ameijden and Coutinho 2001), indicating that interventions to prevent or delay the onset of injection drug use may be successful in thwarting the spread of HIV infection. In cities where HIV has stabilized among IDUs at a prevalence of 50% or more, complacency could reverse these trends. Interventions focusing on HIV-seropositive IDUs are therefore critically important to ensure that advances in prevention are not lost. Since existing literature shows that interventions among IDUs are more successful at reducing injection risks compared to sexual risk behaviors, risks attributable to sexual HIV transmission among IDUs and their sex partners may increase over time as the risks attributable to needle sharing decrease. This underscores the need for interventions to reduce sexual HIV transmission among IDU populations even in cases where injection risks have subsided.

To date, intervention studies among IDUs do not provide adequate information about what kinds of interventions work for various population subgroups, such as HIV-seropositive IDUs. Studies are needed in settings where the majority of IDUs are already HIV positive to determine what proportion of IDUs need to be reached by successful interventions such as outreach, drug abuse treatment, and NEPs or other behavioral interventions, and in what combinations. For example, it is not known how behavior change strategies can best be paired with biomedical approaches, such as HAART, treatment of STDs, and use of microbicides, to reduce sexual transmission of HIV and drug related risk behaviors among HIV-seropositive IDUs. An approach that integrates substance abuse treatment with treatment for HIV and behavioral interventions may prove most successful. It is also clear that future intervention trials among HIV-seropositive IDU populations need to be theoretically based and deal with both sexual behaviors and distributive needle sharing.

HIV-Seropositive Drug Using MSM

As seen in this volume, there are relatively few interventions that have specifically focused on HIV-seropositive MSM-DUs. Understanding the behaviors of these men, as well as barriers to and facilitators of risk reduction and disclosure, is essential for the development of effective interventions that encourage HIV-seropositive MSM to protect themselves and their partners from HIV and other STIs. At present there are few effective interventions that are designed to do this, and there are no proven interventions specifically for HIV-seropositive MSM. Furthermore, while there is a recognition of the growing problem of club drug use and their associated increased risk behavior, there are few interventions which focus on this class of drugs (see Chapter 4).

A number of psychological factors in non-psychiatric groups of HIV-seropositive individuals have been related to high risk sexual behavior. Kalichman et al. (2003) found that an association between sensation seeking and alcohol use in unprotected sexual contexts was accounted for by expectancies that alcohol use improves sexual performance and enhances sexual pleasure. Analyses also indicated that men living with HIV/AIDS who used alcohol in sexual contexts were characterized by greater overall frequency and quantity of drinking. Prevention interventions may be improved by tailoring messages to alcohol-using HIV-infected men, particularly by challenging beliefs and expectations that alcohol enhances sexual performance and sexual pleasure. Moreover, in a recent paper by Ross et al. (2003), drug use was significantly associated with both the sensation-seeking and social dimensions of circuit party attendance. Using a greater number of drugs, sexual activity while on drugs, and unsafe sex were more closely associated with the sensation-seeking dimension of attendance at circuit parties. This suggests that interventions which aim to modify sensation-seeking, for example using motivational interviewing techniques, may in turn reduce risky sexual behavior among MSM-DUs (Kalichman et al., 1997).

Future studies may consider using venue-based interventions to reach high risk HIV-seropositive MSM, especially those who attend raves and circuit parties which can function as commercial sex environments. In one study, differences between those who frequented these venues and those who did not emerged on several psychosocial factors, including sexual sensation seeking, depression and perceived responsibility towards protecting sexual partners from HIV infection (Parsons and Halkitis, 2002). In a study of IDUs in Puerto Rico, managers of shooting galleries were more likely to be HIV-seropositive.

Innovative, theoretically-based approaches to deliver prevention interventions to HIV-seropositive drug users are an urgent public health priority. While there have been few tested interventions for HIV-seropositive persons, those who use injection drugs, crack or club drugs appear to be particularly at risk of ongoing risk behaviors that can transmit HIV to others or lead to incident STIs. Since this group is heterogeneous, a variety of interventions will likely be needed. Integrating behavioral interventions into needle exchange programs, drug treatment programs, STI clinics and HIV primary care facilities may serve to reach many HIV-seropositive drug users, but non-conventional approaches like the use of venue-based interventions, the internet, and shooting galleries could reach a higher proportion of HIV-seropositive drug users who are hidden and at high risk of ongoing HIV and HCV transmission behaviors.

ACKNOWLEDGEMENTS   Dr. Strathdee acknowledges grant support from the National Institute on Drug Abuse (DA12568, DA09225 and DA14499), as well as the Harold Simon Chair Foundation. Dr. Patterson acknowledges grant support from the National Institute on Drug Abuse (DA012116) and the National Institute on Mental Health (MH061146).

REFERENCES

Alter, M. J., Kruszon-Moran, D., Nainan, O. V., McQuillan, G. M., Gao, F., Moyer, L. A., Kaslow, R., and Margolis, H. S. (1999). The prevalence of hepatitis C virus infection in the US, 1988 through 1994. *N. Engl. J. Med.* 341(8):556–562.

Altice, F. L., Springer, S., Buitrago, M., Hunt, D. P., and Friedland, G. H. (2003). Pilot study to enhance HIV care using needle exchange-based health services for out-of treatment injecting drug users. *J. Urban Health* 80(3):416–427.

Auerbach, J. D., and Coates, T. J. (2000). HIV prevention research: accomplishments and challenges for the third decade of AIDS. *Am. J. Public Health* 90(10):29–32.

Avants, S. K., Warburton, L. A., Hawkins, K. A., and Margolin, A. (2000). Continuation of high-risk behavior by HIV-positive drug users. Treatment implications. *J. Subst. Abuse Treat* 19(1):15–22.

Ball, A. L., (2002). Overview: Policies and interventions to stem HIV–1 epidemics associated with injecting drug use. In: Stimson, G., Des, Jarlais D. C., and Ball A. (eds.), *Drug Injecting and HIV Infection: Global Dimensions and Local Responses,* UCL Press, London, pp. 201–232.

Ball, J. C., Lange, W. R., Myers, C. P., and Friedman, S. R. (1988). Reducing the risk of AIDS through methadone maintenance treatment. *J. Health Soc. Behav.* 29(3):214–226.

Bastos, F. I., and Strathdee, S. A. (2000). Evaluating Effectiveness of Syringe Exchange Programmes: Current Issues and Future Prospects. *Soc. Sci. Med.* 51:1771–1782.

Beckett, M., Burnam, A., Collins, R. L., Kanouse, D. E., and Beckman, R. (2003). Substance use and high-risk sex among people with HIV: a comparison across exposure groups. *AIDS Behav.* 7(2):209–219.

Black, D., Gates, G., Sander, S. and Taylor, L. (2000). Demographics of the gay and lesbian population in the US: Evidence from available systematic data sources. *Demography* 37:139–154.

Bluthenthal, R. N., Kral, A. H., Gee, L., Erringer, E. A., and Edlin, B. R. (2000). The effect of syringe exchange use on high-risk injection drug users: a cohort study. *AIDS* 14(5):605–611.

Booth, R. E., Crowley, T., and Zhang, Y. (1996). Substance abuse treatment entry, retention, and effectiveness: out-of-treatment opiate injection drug users. *Drug Alcohol Depend.* 42:11–20.

Brooks, J. S., Nomura, C., and Cohen, P. (1989). A network of influences on adolescent drug users involvement: Neighborhood, school, peer, and family. *Genet. Soc. Gen. Psychol. Monogr.* 115(1):125–145.

Bull, S. S., Piper, P., and Rietmeijer, C. (2002). Men who have sex with men and also inject drugs-profiles of risk related to the synergy of sex and drug injection behaviors. *J. Homosex.* 42(3):31–51.

Buning, E. C., Coutinho, R. A., van Brussel, G. H., van Santen, G. W., and van Zadelhoff. (1986). Preventing AIDS in drug addicts in Amsterdam. *Lancet* 1:1(8495):1435.

Burris S, Vernick J, Ditzler A, Strathdee SA. (2002). The legality of selling or giving syringes to injection drug users. J Amer Pharm Assoc. 6 (Suppl 2):S13–18.

Carrieri, M. P., Rey, D., Loundou, A., Lepeu, G., Sobel, A., and Obadia, Y. (2003). The MANIF-2000 Study Group. Evaluation of buprenorphine maintenance treatment in a French cohort of HIV-infected injecting drug users. *Drug Alcohol Depend.*

Celentano, D. D., Hodge, M. J., Razak, M. H., Beyrer, C., Kawichai, S., Cegielski, J. P., Nelson, K. E., and Jittiwutikarn, J. (1999). HIV–1 incidence among opiate users in northern Thailand. *Am. J. Epidemiol.* 149:558–564.

Celentano, D. D., Galai, N., Sethi, A. K., Shah, N. G., Strathdee, S. A., Vlahov, D., and Gallant, J. E. (2001). Time to initiating highly active antiretroviral therapy among HIV-infected injection drug users. *AIDS* 15(13):1707–1715.

Centers for Disease Control and Prevention. (2002). HIV/AIDS Surveillance Report. *Atlanta, GA: Center for Disease Control and Prevention.* 14; http://www.cdc.gov/hiv/stats/harslink.htm.

Chu, P. L., McFarland, W., Gibson, S., Weide, D., Henne, J., Miller, P., Partridge, T., and Schwarcz, S. (2003). Viagra use in a community-recruited sample of men who have sex with men, San Francisco. *JAIDS* 33(2):191–193.

Crawford, I., Hammack, P. L., McKirnan, D. J., Ostrow, D., Zamboni, B. D., Robinson, B., and Hope, B. (2003). Sexual sensation seeking, reduced concern about HIV and sexual risk behaviour among gay men in primary relationships. *AIDS Care* 15(4):513–524.

Cross, J. E., Saunders, C. M., and Bartelli, D. (1998). The effectiveness of educational and needle exchange programs: a meta-analysis of HIV prevention strategies for injecting drug users. *Quality and Quantity* 32:165–180.

Des Jarlais, D. C. (1989). AIDS prevention programs for intravenous drug users: Diversity and evolutions. *Int. Rev. of Psychiatry* 1:101–108.

Des Jarlais, D. C., Hagan, H., Friedman, S. R., Friedmann, P., Goldberg, D.,Frischer, M., Green, S., Tun Ving, K., Ljungberg, B., and Wodak, A. (1995). Maintaining low HIV seroprevalence in populations of injecting drug users. *JAMA* 274(15):1226–1231.

Des Jarlais, D. C., Marmor, M., Paone, D., Titus, S., Shi, Q., Perlis, T., Jose, B., and Friedman, S. R. (1996). HIV incidence among injecting drug users in New York City syringe-exchange programmes. *Lancet* 348(9033):987–991.

Des Jarlais, D. C., Marmor, M., Friedmann, P., Titus, S., Aviles, E., Deren, S., Torian, L., Glebatis, D., Murrill, C., Monterroso, E., and Friedman, S. R. (2000). HIV incidence among injection drug users in New York City, 1992–1997: evidence for a declining epidemic. *Am. J. Public Health* 90(3):352–359.

Des Jarlais DC, Perlis T, Arasteh K, Hagan H, Milliken J, Braine N, Yancovitz S, Mildvan D, Perlman DC, Maslow C, Friedman SR. (2004). "Informed altruism" and "partner restriction" in the reduction of HIV infection in injecting drug users entering detoxification treatment in New York City, 1990–2001. J Acquir Immune Defic Syndr. 35(2):158–66.

Diamond, C., Thiede, H., Perdue, T., Secura, G. M., Valleroy, L., Mackellar, D., and Corey, L. (2003). Seattle Young Men's Survey Team. Viral hepatitis among young men who have sex with men: prevalence of infection, risk behaviors, and vaccination. *Sex. Transm. Dis.* 30(5):425–432.

Doherty, M. C., Junge, B., Rathouz, P., Garfein, R. S., Riley, E., and Vlahov, D. (2000). The effect of a needle exchange program on numbers of discarded needles: a 2-year follow-up. *Am. J. Public Health* 90(6):936–939.

Dolezal, C., Carballo-Dieguez, A., Nieves-Rosa, L., and Diaz, F. (2000). Substance use and sexual risk behavior: understanding their association among four ethnic groups of Latino men who have sex with men. *J. Subst. Abuse* 11(4):323–336.

Dowsett, G. W. (1993). Sustaining safe sex: Sexual practices, HIV and social context. *AIDS* 7(1):257–262.

Drucker, E., Lurie, P., Wodak, A., and Alcabes, P. (1998). Measuring harm reduction: the effects of needle and syringe exchange programs and methadone maintenance on the ecology of HIV. *AIDS* 12(SA):S217–S230.

Edlin, B. R., Irwin, K. L., Faruque, S., McCoy, C. B., Word, C., Serrano, Y., Inciardi, J. A., Bowser, B. P., Schilling, R. F., and Holmberg, S. D. (1994). Intersecting epidemics—crack cocaine use and HIV infection among inner-city young adults. *N. Engl. J. Med.* 331:1422–1427.

Fischer, B., Rehm, J., Kirst, M., Casas, M., Hall, W., Krausz, M., Metrebian, N., Reggers, J., Uchtenhagen, A., van den Brink, W., and van Ree, J. M. (2002). Heroin-assisted treatment as a response to the public health problem of opiate dependence. *Eur. J. Public Health* 12(3):228–234.

Fisher, J. D. and Fisher, W. A. (1992). Changing AIDS risk behavior. *Psychol. Bull.* 111:455–474.

Friedman, S. R., Des Jarlais, D. C., Sotheran, J. L., Garber, J., Cohen, H., and Smith, D. (1987). AIDS and self-organization among intravenous drug users. *Int. J. Addict.* 23: 201–219.

Friedman, S. R., Jose, B., Neaigus, A., Goldstein, M., Curtis, R., Ildefonso, G., Mota, P., and Des Jarlais, D. C. (1994). Consistent condom use in relationships between seropositive injecting drug users and sex partners who do not inject drugs. *AIDS* 8(3):357–361.

Friedman SR, Kottiri BJ, Neaigus A, Curtis R, Vermund SH, Des Jarlais DC. (2000). Network-related mechanisms may help explain long-term HIV-1 seroprevalence levels that remain high but do not approach population-group saturation. *Am J Epidemiol.* 152(10): 913–22.

Galvan, F. H., Burnam, M. A., and Bing, E. G. (2003). Co-occurring psychiatric symptoms and drug dependence or heavy drinking among HIV-positive people. *J. Psychoactive Drugs* 35(S1):153–160.

Garfein, R. S., Vlahov, D., Galai, N., Doherty, M. C., and Nelson, K. E. (1996). Viral infections in short-term injection drug users; the prevalence of the hepatitis C, hepatitis B, human immunodeficiency virus, and human T-lymphotropic virus. *Am. J. Public Health* 86:655–661.

Garfein, R. S., Doherty, M. C., Monterroso, E. R., Thomas, D. L., Nelson, K. E., and Vlahov, D. (1998). Prevalence and incidence of hepatitis C virus infection among young adults injection drug users. *J. Acquir. Immune Defic. Syndr. Hum. Retrovirol.* 8(S1):S11–S19.

Gerberging, J. (1995). Management of occupational exposure to blood borne viruses. *N. Engl. J. Med.* 332:444–451.

Greenblatt, J. C., and Gfoerer, J. C. (1998). *Methamphetamine abuse in the United States.* Substance Abuse and Mental Health Services Administration. Analysis of Substance Abuse and Treatment Need Issues, Rockville, MD.

Guttinger, F., Gschwend, P., Schulte, B., Rehm, J., and Uchtenhagen, A. (2003). Evaluating long-term effects of heroin-assisted treatment: the results of a 6-year follow-up. *Eur. Addict. Res.* 9(2):73–79.

Gyarmathy, V. A., Neaigus, A., Miller, M., Friedman, S. R., and Des Jarlais, D. C. (2002). Risk correlates of prevalent HIV, hepatitis B virus, and hepatitis C virus infections among noninjecting heroin users. *JAIDS* 30(4):448–456.

Hahn, J. A., Vranizan, K. M., and Moss, A. R. (1997). Who uses needle exchange? A study of injection drug users in treatment in San Francisco, 1989–1990. *J. Acquir. Immune Defic. Syndr. Hum. Retrovirol.* 15(2):157–164.

Hagan, H., and Des Jarlais, D. C. (2000). HIV and HCV infection among injecting drug users. *Mt. Sinai J. Med.* 67(5–6):423–428.

Hagan, H., DesJarlais, D. C., Friedman, S. R., Purchase, D., and Alter, M. J. (1995). Reduced risk of Hepatitis B and Hepatitis C among injection drug users in the Tacoma Syringe Exchange Program. *Am. J. Pub. Health* 1531–1537.

Halkitis PN, Parsons JT, Wilton L. (2003). Barebacking among gay and bisexual men in New York City: explanations for the emergence of intentional unsafe behavior. Arch Sex Behav. 32(4):351–357.

Heimer, R. (1998). Can syringe exchange serve as a conduit to substance abuse treatment? *J. Subst. Abuse Treat.* 15(3):183–191.

Heimer, R., Khoshnood, K., Bigg, D., Guydish, J., and Jungue, B. (1998). Syringe use and reuse: effects of syringe exchange programs in four cities. *J. Acquir. Immune Defic. Syndr. Hum. Retrovir.* 18(S37);18 Suppl 1:S37–44.

Holmberg, S. D., (1996) The estimated prevalence and incidence of HIV in 96 large US metropolitan areas. *Am. J. Pub. Health* 86(5):643–654.

Hurley, S., Jolley, D., and Kaldor, J. (1997). Effectiveness of needle-exchange programmes for prevention of HIV infection. *Lancet* 349:1797.

Johnson, R. E., Chutuape, M. A., Strain, E. C., Walsh, S. L., Stitzer, M. L., and Bigelow, G. E. (2000). A comparison of levomethadyl acetate, buprenorphine, and methadone for opioid dependence. *N. Engl. J. Med.* 343(18):1290–1297.

Kalichman, S. C., Heckman, T., and Kelly, J. A. (1996). Sensation seeking as an explanation for the association between substance use and HIV-related risky sexual behavior. *Arch. Sex Behav.* 25(2):141–154.

Kalichman, S. C., Kelly, J. A., and Rompa, D. (1997). Continued high-risk sex among HIV seropositive gay and bisexual men seeking HIV prevention services. *Health Psychol.* 16:369–373.

Kalichman, S. C., Weinhardt, L., DiFonzo, K., Austin, J., and Luke, W. (2002). Sensation seeking and alcohol use as markers of sexual transmission risk behavior in HIV-positive men. *Ann. Behav. Med.* 24(3):229–235.

Kalichman, S. C., Cain, D., Zweben, A., and Swain, G. (2003). Sensation seeking, alcohol use and sexual risk behaviors among men receiving services at a clinic for sexually transmitted infections. *J. Stud. Alcohol* 64(4):564–569.

Kim, A. A., Kent, C., McFarland, W., and Klausner, J. D. (2001). Cruising on the Internet highway. *JAIDS* 28(1):89–93.

Kosten, T., Oliveto, A., Feingold, A., Poling, J., Sevarino, K., McCance-Katz, E., Stine, S., Gonzalez, G., and Gonsai, K. (2003). Desipramine and contingency management for cocaine and opiate dependence in buprenorphine maintained patients. *Drug Alcohol Depend.* 70(3):315–325.

Kotranski, L., Semaan, S., Collier, K., Lauby, J., Halbert, J., and Feighan, K. (1998). Effectiveness of an HIV risk reduction counseling intervention for out-of-treatment drug users. *AIDS Educ. Prev.* 10(1):19–33.

Kral, A. H., Bluthenthal, R. N., Lorvick, J., Gee, L., Bacchetti, P., and Edlin, B. R. (2001). Sexual transmission of HIV-1 among injection drug users in San Francisco, US: risk-factor analysis. *Lancet* 357:1397–1401.

Kumar, M. S., Mudaliar, S., and Daniels, D. (1998). Community-based outreach HIV intervention for street-recruited drug users in Madras, India. *Public Health Rep.* 113(S1): 58–66.

Langendam, M. W., van Brussel, G. H., Coutinho, R. A., and van Ameijden, E. J. (1999). Methadone maintenance treatment modalities in relation to incidence of HIV: results of the Amsterdam cohort study. *AIDS* 13(13):1711–1716.

Langendam, M.W., van Brussel, G.H., Coutinho, R.A., and van Ameijden, E.J. (2001). The impact of harm-reduction-based methadone treatment on mortality among heroin users. *Am. J. Public Health* 91(5):774–780.

Latkin, C. A. (1998). Outreach in natural settings: the use of peer leaders for HIV prevention among injecting drug users' networks. *Public Health Rep.* 113(S1):151–159.

Latkin, C. A., Mandell, W., Vlahov, D., Knowlton, A., Oziemkowska, M., and Celentano, D. D. (1995). Personal Network characteristics as antecedents to needle-sharing and shooting gallery attendance. *Soc. Networks* 17:219–228.

Latkin, C. A., Mandell, W., Vlahov, D., Oziemkowska, M., and Celentano, D.D. (1996). The long-term outcome of a personal network-oriented HIV prevention intervention for injection drug users: the SAFE Study. *Am. J. Community Psychol.* 24(3):341–364.

Latkin, C. A., Forman, V., Knowlton, A., Hoover, D., Hatcher, M., and Celentano, D. D. (2001). Injection Drug Users' Disclosure of HIV Seropositive Status to Network Members. *AIDS and Behavior* 5:297–305.

Latkin, C. A., Sherman, S. G., and Knowlton, A. (2003). HIV prevention among drug users: Outcome of a network-oriented peer outreach intervention. *Health Psychol.* 22(4):332–339.

Leigh, B. C. (2002). Alcohol and condom use: a meta-analysis of event-level studies. *Sex Transm. Dis.* 29(8):476–482.

Lollis, C. M., Strothers, H. S., Chitwood, D. D., and McGhee, M. (2000). Sex, drugs, and HIV: does methadone maintenance reduce drug use and risky sexual behavior? *J. Behav. Med.* 23(6):545–557.

Loughlin, A., and Strathdee, S. A. (2004). Hepatitis C infection among drug users enrolled in methadone maintenance program. *Int. J. Drug Policy* 15: 93–101.

Lucas, G. M., Cheever, L. W., Chaisson, R. E., and Moore, R. D. (2001). Detrimental effects of continued illicit drug use on the treatment of HIV-1 infection. *JAIDS* 27(3):251–259.

Lurie, P., Gorsky, R., Jones, T. S., and Shomphe, L. (1998). An economic analysis of needle exchange and pharmacy-based programs to increase sterile syringe availability for injection drug users. *J. Acquir. Immune Defic. Syndr. Hum. Retrovirol.* 18(S1):S126–S132.

MacGowan, R. J., Brackbill, R. M., Rugg, D. L., Swanson, N., Weinstein, B., Couchon, A., Scibak, J., Molde, S., McLaughlin, P., Barker, T., and Voight, R. (1997). Sex, drugs and HIV counseling and testing: a prospective study of behavior-change among methadone-maintenance clients in New England. *AIDS* 11(2):229–235.

Marmor, M., Friedman-Kien, A. E., Laubenstein, L., Byrum, R. D., William, D. C., D'onofrio, S., and Dubin, N. (1982). Risk factors for Kaposi's sarcoma in homosexual men. *Lancet* 15(1)(8281):1083–1087.

Marx, M. A., Brahmbhatt, H., Beilenson, P., Brookmeyer, R. S., Strathdee, S. A., Alexander, C., and Vlahov, D. (2001). Impact of needle exchange programs on adolescent perceptions about illicit drug use. *AIDS and Behavior* 5(4):379–386.

McCance-Katz, E. F., Rainey, P. M., Jatlow, P., and Friedland, G. (1998). Methadone effects on zidovudine disposition (AIDS Clinical Trials Group 262). *J. Acquir. Immune Defic. Syndr. Hum. Retrovirol.* 18(5):435–443.

McCance-Katz, E. F., Rainey, P. M., Friedland, G., and Jatlow, P. (2003). The protease inhibitor lopinavir-ritonavir may produce opiate withdrawal in methadone-maintained patients. *Clin. Infect. Dis.* 37(4):476–482.

McMahon, R. C., Malow, R. M., Jennings, T. E., and Gomez, C. J. (2001). Effects of a cognitive-behavioral HIV prevention intervention among HIV negative male substance abusers in VA residential treatment. *AIDS Educ. Prev.* 13:91–107.

Meandzija, B., O'Connor, P. G., Fitzgerald, B., Rounsaville, B. J., and Kosten, T. R. (1994). HIV infection and cocaine use in methadone maintained and untreated intravenous drug users. *Drug Alcohol. Depend.* 36(2):109–113.

Metsch, L. R., Pereyra, M., and Brewer, T. H. (2001). Use of HIV health care in HIV seropositive crack cocaine smokers and other active drug users. *J. Subst. Abuse.* 13(1–2):155–167.

Metzger, D. S., and Navaline, H. (2003). Human immunodeficiency virus prevention and the potential of drug abuse treatment. *Clin. Infect. Dis.* 37(S5):S451–S456.

Metzger, D. S., Woody, G. E., McLellan, A. T., Druley, P., De Philippis, D., O'Brien, C. P., Stolley, P., and Abrutyn, E. (1993). Human immunodeficiency virus seroconversion among in- and out-of-treatment intravenous drug users: an 18-month prospective follow-up. *J. Acquir. Immune Defic. Syndr.* 6:1049–1056.

Millson, P., Challacombe, L., Strike, L., Villeneuve, P., Myers, T., Fisher, B., Shore, R., Hopkins, S., Pearson, M., and Raftis, S. July (2002). Reduction in HIV risk behaviours six months after enrollment in needle exchange based on low threshold methadone programs. XIV International AIDS Conference, Barcelona.

Nelson, K. E., Galai, N., Safaeian, M., Strathdee, S. A., Celentano, D. D., and Vlahov, D. (2002). Temporal trends in the incidence of human immunodeficiency virus infection and risk behavior among injection drug users in Baltimore, Maryland, 1988–1998. *Am. J. Epidemiol.* 156:641–653.

NIH Consensus Statement. (1997). Interventions to prevent HIV risk behaviors. 15:1–41.

National Consensus Development Panel on Effective Medical Treatment of Opiate Addiction. (1998). Effective medical treatment of opiate addiction. *JAMA* 280(22):1936–1943.

Office of the Surgeon General, Evidence-based findings on the efficacy of syringe exchange programs: an analysis from the Assistant Secretary for Health and Surgeon General of the scientific research completed since April 1998, Washington D.C. (2000); (http://www.harmreduction.org/surgreview.html).

Ompad, D. C., Fuller, C. M., Vlahov, D., Thomas, D., and Strathdee, S. A. (2002). Lack of behavior change after disclosure of hepatitis C virus infection among young injection drug users in Baltimore, Maryland. *Clin. Infect. Dis.* 35(7):783–788.

Ostrow, D. E., Fox, K. J., Chmiel, J. S., Silvestre, A., Visscher, B. R., Vanable, P. A., Jacobson, L. P., and Strathdee, S. A. (2002). Attitudes towards highly active antiretroviral therapy are associated with sexual risk taking among HIV-infected and uninfected homosexual men. *AIDS* 16:775–780.

Palepu, A., Tyndall, M. W., Li, K., Yip, B., O'Shaughnessy, M. V., Schechter, M. T., Montaner, J. S., and Hogg, R. S. (2003). Alcohol Use and Incarceration Adversely Affect HIV-1 RNA Suppression Among Injection Drug Users Starting Antiretroviral Therapy. *J. Urban Health* 80(4):667–675.

Parsons, J. T., and Halkitis, P. N. (2002). Sexual and drug-using practices of HIV-positive men who frequent public and commercial sex environments. *AIDS Care* 14(6):815–826.

Potterat, J. J., Rothenberg, R. B., and Muth, S. Q. (1999). Network structural dynamics and infectious disease propagation. *Int. J. STD. AIDS* 10(3):182–185.

Prendergast, M. L., Urada, D., and Podus, D. J. (2001). Meta-analysis of HIV risk-reduction interventions within drug abuse treatment programs. *Consult. Clin. Psychol.* 69: 389–405.

Rhodes, T. and Hartnoll, R. (eds.). (1996). *AIDS, Drugs, and Prevention: Perspectives on Individual and Community Action.* Routledge, London.

Rietmeijer, C. A., Kane, M. S., Simons, P. Z., Corby, N. H., Wolitski, R. J., Higgins, D. L., Judson, F. N., and Cohn, D. L. (1996). Increasing the use of bleach and condoms among injecting drug users in Denver: outcomes of a targeted, community-level HIV prevention program. *AIDS* 10(3):291–298.

Rippeth, J. D., Heaton, R. K., Carey, C. L., Marcotte, T. D., Moore, D. J., Gonzalez, R., Wolfson, T., Grant, I., and the HNRC group. (2004). Methamphetamine dependence increases risk of neuropsychological impairment in HIV infected persons. *J. Int. Neurospsychol. Soc.* 10:1–14.

Rosenberg, H., and Phillips, K. T. (2003). Acceptability and availability of harm-reduction interventions for drug abuse in American substance abuse treatment agencies. *Psychol. Addict. Behav.* 17(3):203–210.

Ross, M. W., Mattison, A. M., and Franklin, D. R. Jr. (2003). Club drugs and sex on drugs are associated with different motivations for gay circuit party attendance in men. *Subst. Use Misuse.* 38(8):1173–1183.

Schechter, M. T., Strathdee, S. A., Cornelisse, P. G., Currie, S., Patrick, D. M., Rekart, M. L., and O'Shaughnessy, M. V. (1999). Do needle exchange programmes increase the spread of HIV among injection drug users?: an investigation of the Vancouver outbreak. *AIDS* 13(6):F45–F51.

Semaan, S., Des Jarlais, D. C., Sogolow, E., Johnson, W. D., Hedges, L. V., Ramirez, G., Flores, S. A., Norman, L., Sweat, M. D., and Needle, R. (2002). A meta-analysis of the effect of HIV prevention interventions on the sex behaviors of drug users in the US. *JAIDS* 30(S1):S73–S93.

Shah, N., Celentano, D. D., Vlahov, D., Stambolis, V., Johnson, L., Nelson, K. E., and Strathdee, S. A. (2000). Correlates of enrollment in methadone maintenance programs differ by HIV-serostatus. *AIDS* 14:2035–2043.

Siegal, H. A., Falck, R. S., Carlson, R. G., and Wang, J. (1995). Reducing HIV needle risk behaviors among injection-drug users in the Midwest: an evaluation of the efficacy of standard and enhanced interventions. *AIDS Educ. Prev.* 7(4):308–319.

Silverman, K., Svikis, D., Robles, E., Stitzer, M. L., and Bigelow, G. E. (2001). A reinforcement-based therapeutic workplace for the treatment of drug abuse: six-month abstinence outcomes. *Exp. Clin. Psychopharmacol.* 9(1):14–23.

Stevens, S. J., Estrada, A. L., and Estrada, B. D. (1998). HIV sex and drug risk behavior and behavior change in a national sample of injection drug and crack cocaine using women. *Women Health* 27(1–2):25–48.

Stimson, G. V., and Choopanya, K. (1998) "Global Perspectives on Drug Injecting". In: Stimson, G. V., Des Jarlais, D. C., and Ball, A, (eds.), *Drug Injecting and HIV Infection: Global Dimensions and Local Responses (Social Aspects of AIDS)*, UCL Press, London, pp. 1–21.

Strathdee, S. A. (2003). Sexual HIV Transmission in the Context of Injection Drug Use: Implications for Interventions. *International Journal of Drug Policy* 14:79–81.

Strathdee, S. A., and Sherman, S. G. (2003). The role of sexual transmission of HIV infection among injection and non-injection drug users. *J. Urban Health* 80(S3):iii7–14.

Strathdee, S. A., Patrick, D. M., Archibald, C. P., Ofner, M., Cornelisse, P. G. A., Rekart, M. L., Schechter, M. T., and O'Shaughnessy, M. V. (1997). Social determinants predict needle sharing behaviour among injection drug users in Vancouver, Canada. *Addiction* 92(10):1339–1347.

Strathdee, S. A., Palepu, A., Cornelisse, P. G. A., Yip, B., O'Shaughnessy, M. V., Montaner, J. S. T., Schechter, M. T., and Hogg, R. S. (1998a). Barriers to utilization of antiretroviral therapies among HIV-infected injection drug users in a universal health care setting. *JAMA* 280(6):547–549.

Strathdee, S. A., van Ameijden, E. J. C., Mesquita, F., Wodak, A., Rana, S., and Vlahov, D. (1998b). Can HIV epidemics among injection drug users be prevented? *AIDS* 12(SA):S71–S79.

Strathdee, S. A., Celentano, D. D., Shah, N., Lyles, C., Macalino, G., Nelson, K., and Vlahov, D. (1999). Needle Exchange Attendance and Health Care Utilization Promote Entry into Detoxification. *J. Urban Health* 76(4):448–460.

Strathdee, S. A., Galai, N., Safaiean, M., Celentano, D. D., Vlahov, D., Johnson, L., and Nelson, K. E. (2001). Sex differences in risk factors for HIV seroconversion among injection drug users: a 10-year perspective. *Arch. Intern. Med.* 161:1281–1288.

Strauss, S. M., Des Jarlais, D. C., Astone, J., and Vassilev, Z. P. (2003). On-site HIV testing in residential drug treatment units: results of a nationwide survey. *Public Health Rep.* 118(1):37–43.

Sylvestre, D. L. (2002). Treating hepatitis C in methadone maintenance patients: an interim analysis. *Drug Alcohol Depend.* 67(2):117–123.

Thomas, D. L., Astemborski, J., Rai, R. M., Anania, F. A., Schaeffer, M., Galai, N., Nolt, K., Nelson, K. E., Strathdee, S. A., Johnson, L., Laeyendecker, O., Boitnott, J., Wilson, L. E., and Vlahov, D. (2000). The natural history of Hepatitis C virus infection: host, viral, and environmental factors. *JAMA* 284(4):450–456.

Tun, W., Celentano, D. D., Vlahov, D., and Strathdee, S. A. (2003). Attitudes toward HIV treatments influence unsafe sexual and injection practices among injecting drug users. *AIDS* 17:1953–1962.

Tyndall, M. W., Currie, S., Spittal, P., Li, K., Wood, E., O'Shaughnessy, M. V., and Schechter, M. T. (2003). Intensive injection cocaine use as the primary risk factor in the Vancouver HIV-1 epidemic. *AIDS* 17(6):887–893.

United Nations International Drug Control Programme and the Joint Programme on HIV/AIDS. (2000). Drug Abuse and HIV/AIDS: A devastating combination. Geneva

US General Accounting Office. (1993). Needle exchange programs: research suggests promise as an AIDS prevention strategy. Washington, DC: US Government Printing Office, (Publication no. GAO/HRD 93–60).

Valleroy, L. A., MacKellar, D. A., Karon, J. M., Rosen, D. H., McFarland, W., Shehan, D. A., Stoyanoff, S. R., LaLota, M., Celentano, D. D., Koblin, B. A., Thiede, H., Katz, M. H., Torian, L. V., and Janssen, R. S. (2000). HIV prevalence and associated risks in young men who have sex with men. Young Men's Survey Study Group. *JAMA* 284:198–204.

van Ameijden, E. J. C., and Coutinho, R. A. (1998). Maximum impact of HIV prevention measures targeted at injecting drug users. *AIDS* 12:625.

van Ameijden, E. J. and Coutinho, R. A. (2001). Large decline in injecting drug use in Amsterdam, 1986–1998: explanatory mechanisms and determinants of injecting transitions. *J. Epidemiol. Community Health* 55:356–363.

van Beek, I., Dwyer, R., Dore, G. J., Luo, K., and Kaldor, J. M. (1998). Infection with HIV and hepatitis C virus among injecting drug users in a prevention setting: retrospective cohort study. *BMJ* 317:433–437.

van Empelen, P., Kok, G., van Kesteren, N. M., van den Borne, B., Bos, A. E., and Schaalma, H. P. (2003). Effective methods to change sex-risk among drug users: a review of psychosocial interventions. *Soc. Sci. Med.* 57(9):1593–1608.

Vastag, B. (2001). Ecstasy experts want realistic messages. *JAMA* 286(7):777.

Vertefeuille, J., Marx, M. A., Tun, W., Huettner, S., Strathdee, S. A., and Vlahov, D. (2000). Decline in Self-Reported High Risk Injection-Related Behaviors Among HIV Seropositive Participants in the Baltimore Needle Exchange Program. *AIDS and Behavior* 4(4):381–388.

Warner, B. D., and Leukefeld, C. G. (2001). Assessing the differential impact of an HIV prevention intervention: who's putting the message into practice? *AIDS Educ. Prev.* 13:479–494.

Wiebel, W. W., Jimenez, A., Johnson, W., Ouellet, L., Jovanovic, B., Lampinen, T., Murray, J., and O'Brien, M. U. (1996). Risk behavior and HIV seroincidence among out-of-treatment injection drug users: a four-year prospective study. *J. Acquir. Immune Defic. Syndr. Hum. Retrovirol.* 12(3):282–289.

CHAPTER SIX

Young People Living with HIV

Amy Elkavich, Mary Jane Rotheram-Borus, Rise Goldstein, Diane Flannery, and Patricia Jones

INTRODUCTION

Gabrielle was a 17-year-old African-American woman living in Brooklyn, New York. Her boyfriend, Tony, had been in jail upstate for a year, but had recently returned home and gotten a job at the local dry-goods store. He loved her and she loved him; they had talked about a baby being the reflection of their love. When Gabrielle missed her first period and went for the pregnancy test, she found out that she was HIV positive. She was scared to tell Tony; she had had one boyfriend prior to Tony and maybe her first boyfriend was responsible for her contracting HIV. She wanted the baby, but was afraid this was the end of her relationship. How would she handle her HIV status?

Devon was a 19-year-old Latino young man who dated women, but who was also attracted to men. While he had a girlfriend, he sometimes went downtown to the public baths to check out men's bodies and, occasionally a relationship resulted. His basketball team routinely donated blood; one month he was called aside and informed that he was HIV positive. He started withdrawing from all social activities. He had told no one that he had any desires for men and certainly would tell no one that he was HIV positive.

In this chapter, we will address interventions for young people living with HIV (YPLH). Adolescents whose parents are living with HIV are also affected by their parents or siblings or family-members' infections;

however, the challenges facing those young people will be addressed in other publications (see Rotheram-Borus et al., 2001a, 2003, in press). We will: describe the epidemiology of HIV infected young people, with a special emphasis on the US; indicate the current interventions that have been designed and evaluated for YPLH; review the organization of care settings for YPLH; outline the intervention goals and components; recount the theoretical framework of current interventions (Teens Linked to Care, TLC, and Clean Living, Empowerment, Action, and Results, CLEAR); clarify the ethnographic underpinnings of the TLC and CLEAR interventions; illustrate two programs in greater detail; and review the types of adaptations that all evidence-based interventions must make to become recognized, accepted, and broadly implemented.

EPIDEMIOLOGY OF HIV/AIDS AMONG YOUNG PEOPLE

Worldwide, there are 42 million people living with HIV and more than half of them are adolescents (UNAIDS, 2003). Globally, fewer than 5% of infected teens know their HIV serostatus and few receive any treatment for their HIV infection. Since delivering antiretroviral medications and prophylactic antibiotics are high priorities, psychosocial interventions are considered a low priority. It is anticipated that detection and prevention programs will not be successful until such interventions are accessible.

In the US, more than half of new HIV cases in 2001 (approximately 20,000 of 40,000) were identified among young people under 25 years of age (Kaiser Family Foundation, 2002); over 50% of all AIDS cases diagnosed in the US in 2002 were under the age of 25 (National Institute on Allergy and Infectious Disease, 2004; Centers for Disease Control and Prevention, CDC, 2003). Unlike the situation in the developing world, young people in the US have substantial access to both HIV testing and to care for those who test seropositive for HIV. Since the introduction of highly active antiretroviral treatment (HAART), the potential life expectancy of persons living with HIV has increased dramatically. As HIV disease is transformed into a chronic illness in the developed world, there are increasing challenges for maintaining reductions in sexual and substance use related transmission acts over a lifespan (Crepaz and Marks, 2002; Heckman et al., 2003; Kalichman et al., 2002; Rotheram-Borus et al., 1996; Weinhardt et al., in press).

Subgroups at High Risk for HIV

Youth at high risk of contracting HIV are young men who have sex with men (MSM), intravenous drug users (IDU), racial and ethnic minorities, heterosexual females, hemophiliacs who have now aged out of adolescence, and runaway and homeless youth. In the US, 49% of all AIDS cases reported in 2000 among men 13 to 24 years of age were among MSM. An additional 9% were reported among young men infected through heterosexual contact, with 10% among IDUs (CDC, 2002a). Among women in the same age group, 45% of all AIDS cases reported in 2000 were attributed to heterosexual transmission, and 11% to injection drug use. Exposure category was not reported or identified for substantial proportions of cases in both males (26%) and females (43%). However, with completion of follow-up investigations, it was anticipated that most of these would be reclassified into sexual and drug use related risk (CDC, 2002a, 2002b).

Young Men Who Have Sex with Men (MSM)

For MSM, unprotected anal intercourse represents the primary HIV risk factor (Ekstrand et al., 1999). Most young MSM do not self-identify as gay or bisexual. Because being gay or bisexual is stigmatizing, these youths are often forced to seek partners and services outside their home communities; the gay-identified sites in urban centers like New York and Los Angeles are places where they are at elevated risk of encountering seropositive, and older, partners (Rotheram-Borus et al., 2000).

Heterosexual Young Women

Heterosexual youth living with HIV, both male and female, often disproportionately live in inner cities and neighborhoods with high seroprevalence rates that in large part reflect high rates of drug use. In this context, the probability of transmission of HIV is related to more frequent intercourse (Kann et al., 1998), less consistent condom use (Norris and Ford, 1998), multiple partners in short spans of time (Leach et al., 1997), and co-occurring sexually transmitted infections (CDC, 1998).

Compared to the gender distribution of HIV cases among adults, a much higher proportion of adolescents with HIV are female. Young women comprise half the incident HIV cases reported among 13- to 24-year-olds, and 61% of incident cases in 13- to 19-year-olds. Young women are at increased risk for sexually transmitted infections, including HIV, for reasons thought to be related to the cellular structure of their lower reproductive tract. In particular, the columnar epithelium of the cervix is more exposed during adolescence than adulthood and is a primary site for Chlamydia and gonococcal infections (Cates, 1990). Immune-protective factors in cervical mucus do not fully develop until several years following menarche (Cowan and Mindel, 1993).

Young Injection Drug Users (IDU)

Injection drug use, and in particular needle sharing, poses a direct risk for HIV infection, but one of low prevalence in young people (2% of high school and 1.7% of college students; Kann et al., 1998). However, another 3% report sexual contact with IDU partners (Hingson et al., 1990). Substance use, whether by injection or other routes, can disinhibit sexual behavior and impair young people's abilities to make and implement decisions to use condoms (Siegal et al., 1999), and youth who are using or abusing substances may trade sex for drugs or money to buy drugs. This indirect link of substance use to sexual transmission is more prevalent for young people than for adults (Rotheram-Borus et al., 2000).

Ethnic Minority Youth

With respect to ethnicity, young African-Americans are the most heavily affected, comprising 56% of all HIV cases reported among 13- to 24-year-olds in 34 US states with confidential HIV reporting as of 2000. Overall, African-American males are at the greatest risk because of their earlier age at sexual debut and larger numbers of sexual partners compared to their age peers of other ethnic groups (Kann et al., 1998). Young African-American and Latino MSM are at approximately 4- and 2-fold increased risk, respectively, for infection compared to their white counterparts, with recent seroprevalence estimates for MSM aged 15 to 22 years reported at 14% for African-American, 7% for Latino, and 3% for white youth (CDC, 2002a).

Runaway and Homeless Youth

Runaway and homeless youth are at 6- to 12-fold increased risk for HIV infection (2.3–12%) compared to adolescents ascertained in medical clinics (0.2–0.4%) and Job Corps (0.4%) settings, as well as the general population of youth in AIDS epicenters in California, New York, and Florida. Their excess risk reflects the increased likelihood that they are involved in drug use and bartering sex for food, drugs, or shelter (Rotheram-Borus et al., 2000, 2003).

CURRENT INTERVENTIONS DESIGNED
AND EVALUATED

It is now recognized that people living with HIV (PLH) comprise a crucial set of populations with different but overlapping needs to target in preventive interventions (del Rio, 2003; Janssen et al., 2001). There are only a few behavioral interventions tailored for adults living with HIV (Chesney et al., 1996; Kalichman et al., 2001; Kelly et al., 1993; Marks et al., 2002; Margolin et al., 2003; Parsons et al., 2000; Patterson et al., 2003; Rotheram-Borus et al., 2001a; 2003, in press). There are an additional four interventions targeted at YPLH: one for transmission behaviors for hemophiliacs (Butler et al., 2003), family-focused increases in medication adherence (Lyon et al., 2003), and adolescents and young adults, especially those who engage in substance use and abuse (Rotheram-Borus et al., 2001b, in press). A summary of the goals and methods of each of these programs is provided in Table 6.1.

Butler et al. (2003) reported outcomes among 104 HIV-positive adolescent and young adult men (12 to 25 years old) with hemophilia who participated in the Adolescent Hemophilia Behavioral Intervention Evaluation Project, designed to promote safer sex practices. Based on the transtheoretical model (Prochaska and DiClemente, 1992) and the Theory of Reasoned Action (Fishbein, 1979), the protocol consisted of two individual counseling and two peer-centered group sessions. Individual sessions focused on developing and implementing individualized behavior change plans and future goals; group activities involved stage-of-change-based discussion, skills-building exercises, practice in self-expression, communication, and problem solving, and recreational activities. Stage of change was assessed and feedback provided to participants at every session. For ethical reasons, a control group was not utilized; the intervention was evaluated using pre- to post-test comparisons.

At post-test, 79% of participants were in the action or maintenance stage for safer sex, vs. 62% at pre-test. Participants sexually active at post-test were more likely to be in the action or maintenance stage for condom use with main (68% vs. 44%) and with casual partners (77% vs. 69%) than at pre-test. Self-efficacy for all safer sex activities increased significantly over the intervention year. The proportion reporting having ever engaged in "outercourse", defined as sexual contact with neither vaginal nor anal penetration, increased from 63.7% to 72.5% (Butler et al., 2003).

Lyon et al. (2003) combined family group and peer approaches to increase antiretroviral therapy adherence in YPLH. Twenty-three YPLH 15 to 22 years old and 23 family members, or "treatment buddies," participated in 12-week groups. Sessions alternated biweekly between those for both

Table 6.1. Interventions for Youth Living with HIV

Author	Target population	Participants and follow-up	Intervention activities/ theoretical framework	Format	Design	Outcomes
Butler et al. (2003)	HIV+ adolescents with hemophilia	N = 104 Follow-up: 6 mo. Assessment immediately following intervention and at 6 mo.	Transtheoretical Model, Theory of Reasoned Action; cognitive-behavioral techniques.	Two individual and 2 peer-centered activities over one year.	Pre- to post-test, within-subject comparisons (no control group due to ethical concerns)	Significant pre- to posttest increase in percentage of participants in action or maintenance stages for safer sex and condom use w/casual partners; increased use of outercourse. Increased self-efficacy and knowledge regarding safer sex.
Rotheram-Borus et al. (2001b, 2001c).	HIV+ youth 13–24 years old.	N = 310 Follow-up: 21 mo. Assessment at 9, 15 and 21 mo.	Social Action Model; cognitive-behavioral techniques including role-plays and skill-building exercises. Module 1 targeted health maintenance; Module 2, sex and drug risk reduction; and Module 3, quality of life and mental health.	31 small group sessions over 3 modules	Quasi-experimental	*Module 1:* More positive lifestyle changes and increased use of active coping among females and increased social support coping among both genders in intervention. *Module 2:* Intervention youth reported fewer sex partners; fewer HIV–sex partners, fewer unprotected sex acts, less drug use, and less hard drug use. *Module 3:* Intervention youth reported lower global, somatization, anxiety, and phobic anxiety scores on the BSI, as well as lower levels of non-disclosure coping.

Lyon et al. (2003)	HIV+ youth and their family members/ caregivers.	23 YPLH and 23 family members Follow-up: 6 mo. Assessment at 3 and 6 mo.	Youth-only and youth + family member education sessions on HIV medications, and devices to increase adherence such as vibrating beepers and alarm watches in youth-only groups.	6 biweekly youth-only and 6 biweekly youth + family groups	Quasi-experimental	91% of youths reported increased adherence. Caregivers and youths increased their knowledge related to HIV medications and adherence heir belief in the efficacy of the medications. General health practices increased (e.g. flu shots, dental care).
Rotheram-Borus et al. (in press)	HIV+, substance-using youth 16 to 29 years old	N = 175 Follow-up: 15 mo. Assessment at 3, 6, 9, and 15 mo.	Social Action Model. Module 1 targeted health maintenance; Module 2, sex and drug risk reduction; and Module 3, quality of life and mental health.	18 individual sessions (6 sessions in each of 3 modules) delivered in person or by telephone	Randomized trial	Increased proportion of protected sex acts with all partners and with HIV-partners over time among youth in in-person intervention.

youth and their treatment buddies, and those for youth only. The curricu-
lum covered: dynamics of HIV; purpose of antiretroviral therapy; medication choices and managing side effects, nutrition, exercise, and alternative
treatments; communication with health care providers; and separating fact
from fiction. Youths tested five devices to improve adherence, including
multiple alarm watches, pillboxes, dummy beepers, calendars, and gym
bags. This pilot study used a pre- to post-test comparison to evaluate the
intervention.

At the start of the groups, 82% of YPLH were on antiretroviral treatment. Eighteen of the 23 YPLH completed the group intervention and
21 self-reported increased medication adherence following completion of
a group; participants rated the multiple alarm watch as the best aid for improving medication adherence. An unanticipated benefit was an increase
in other health behaviors, including medical and dental appointments, referrals to mental health and substance abuse treatment, and Hepatitis B
and influenza immunizations (Lyon et al., 2003).

Rotheram-Borus et al. (2001b, 2001c) described outcomes of a preventive intervention for YPLH, Teens Linked to Care (TLC), outlined in greater
detail below. Small cohorts to either the intervention or to a lagged control
condition assigned a total of 310 HIV-positive youths 13 to 24 years old; 73%
in the intervention condition attended at least one session. If one session
was attended, about 70% of youth completed the intervention. Based on social action theory (Ewart, 1991), the 31-session intervention was delivered
to small groups of participants in three modules. Module 1 targeted adjustment to and coping with one's serostatus, health maintenance routines,
issues of stigma and disclosure, and participation in health care decisions.
Module 2 targeted sexual and substance-related risk, and Module 3 focused
on reducing emotional distress and improving quality of life. Subsequent to
Module 1, the number of positive lifestyle changes and active coping styles
increased significantly more often among females in the intervention than
among females in the control condition. Social support coping increased
significantly among both genders in the intervention as compared to those
in the control condition. Following Module 2, intervention youth reported
82% fewer unprotected sex acts, 45% fewer sex partners, 50% fewer HIV-
negative sex partners, and 31% less substance use on a weighted index
than those in the control condition. Outcomes of Module 3 included significantly lower global, somatization, anxiety, and phobic anxiety scores
among YPLH in the intervention than in the control condition. In addition,
YPLH in the intervention condition reported significantly lower levels of
nondisclosure coping than did YPLH in the control condition.

Because 27% of YPLH randomized to the intervention did not attend any sessions, Rotheram-Borus et al. (in press) adapted TLC, targeting

barriers to group participation including changes in schedule, stigma associated with group participation in an HIV-related setting, and transportation, as well as the need to combine young MSM, women, and heterosexual males in groups due to small numbers of YPLH living in most geographic regions, despite very different issues affecting each subpopulation. Based on the results obtained in TLC (Rotheram-Borus et al., 2001a, 2001b), further tailoring was required because some YPLH were not involved in substance use or abuse. Project CLEAR (Rotheram-Borus et al., in press) consists of 18 individual sessions delivered either in person or by telephone in three modules. One hundred seventy-five substance-using YPLH were randomized to individual in-person intervention, individual telephone intervention, or delayed control conditions. In-person sessions were attended by 85% of youth. Intention-to-treat analyses demonstrated that, compared to the control condition, in-person intervention was associated with a significantly greater proportion of protected sexual encounters across all partners and with HIV-negative partners at follow-up (Rotheram-Borus et al., 2004a).

A second cohort of 189 youth living with HIV who have engaged in recent substance use was recruited and received the intervention in individual sessions, telephone delivery, or a delayed intervention. Reductions in anonymous sex partners, reductions in the number of partners, and increases in condom use are significant for the individual delivery format. There were substantial increases in condom use (109%) and a decrease in the number of partners (149%) for the telephone group compared to the no-treatment control condition; however, the sample size of 60 youth was small and such increases were not statistically significant. In this second study, it appears that individual sessions are a more effective delivery strategy than are groups.

ORGANIZATION OF CARE FOR YPLH

There are regional differences in the organization of care for YPLH. In the US, New York has the highest rates of HIV infection (CDC, 2002). Treatment services are more often incorporated into large medical facilities on the east coast. For example, in New York City, there are five primary Adolescent AIDS Clinic sites: Montefiore Hospital, Mount Sinai, Kings County Hospital, Harlem Hospital, and Columbia Presbyterian Medical Center in Spanish Harlem. By contrast, services for YPLH on the West Coast are delivered by community-based agencies. In Los Angeles, which has the second highest rate of HIV infection (CDC, 2002), HIV services for YPLH are more often located in West Hollywood in clinics serving homeless and gay-identified youth, backed up with hospital-based care by Children's Hospital. Young people and adult clients are often not served by the same agencies. Incorporating services to provide for all YPLH's needs, including social services, housing referrals, and transportation, as well as general medical and mental health care, in one facility is highly desirable, as adolescents prefer easy access and a single visit to a facility or clinic to numerous visits or appointments at a number of facilities (Advocates for Youth, 2002; Johnson et al., 2003; Martinez et al., 2003). By accommodating the unique needs and preferences of YPLH, service providers can increase retention in care, leading to better clinical outcomes (Johnson et al., 2003) and potentially improved cost efficiency.

GOALS

Especially with the increased lifespan in the developed world, YPLH face three prevention challenges that will persist over time: 1) maintaining physical health, including being assertive with their health care providers, staying current on advances in HIV treatment and care, and adhering to medications and medical regimens; 2) reducing transmission risk behaviors, particularly as new partnerships evolve and perceptions of infectivity decrease with decreasing viral loads; and 3) promoting and maintaining a high quality of life and positive mental health (Rotheram-Borus and Miller, 1998). To ignore any of these three issues is likely to result in reemergence of risk over time. For example, the stressors associated with an HIV positive diagnosis can lead to mental health problems, including depression, in YPLH. Mental health problems in turn can compromise YPLH's ability to institute and sustain health-maintaining behaviors, as well as their ability to reduce transmission acts (Johnson et al., 2003; Martinez et al., 2003). Furthermore, an immunization approach to prevention is likely to result in relapse. Current interventions are designed for delivery in a specific dose. Yet, YPLH may live into old age: it is likely that their romantic relationships, the medical management of HIV, and the mental health consequences of a chronic illness will change over time. We need to anticipate these challenges in helping YPLH anticipate and prepare for a long-term chronic illness.

Early in the HIV epidemic, persons living with HIV, unlike persons with other potentially terminal diagnoses, were granted a range of services that were not traditionally provided: for example, child care, housing, food banks. These resources have been declining systematically over time and cutbacks have significantly impacted the treatment protocols for YPLH. YPLH present with multiple medical, psychological, economic, and social problems, including those related to pre-existing conditions such as sub-stance abuse or questions about their sexuality, housing and employment concerns (Martinez et al., 2003). Fear of stigmatization for one's HIV sta-tus can lead to stress, depression, and increased transmission acts among YPLH. These threats decrease YPLH's quality of life and increase their challenges in successfully following their health care regimens (Rotheram-Borus et al., 2001c).

Protection of others from transmission may take on reduced impor-tance for YPLH who are unable to meet basic economic or social needs, including a secure place to live, friends or family who can provide so-cial support, or resources to pay for needed medical care (Martinez et al., 2003). One out of seven HIV-infected adolescents is without medical in-surance, significantly limiting their access to health care (Advocates for Youth, November, 2002). Because of lack of adequate insurance coverage, many YPLH do not receive necessary care until they experience physical symptoms indicating that the illness has progressed significantly (Huba et al., 2000; Martinez et al., 2003). Homelessness increases the risk of trad-ing sex for money and shelter (Rotheram-Borus et al., 1991), unprotected sex, and failure to follow medical routines (Live Positive, 2004; Rotheram-Borus et al., 1991, 2003). Therefore, while resources for YPLH have been declining for "wraparound services", the need for such services remains.

In addition to resources for basic survival and security, disclosure is a key issue to YPLH and often involves disclosure of drug use or sex-ual orientation, in addition to HIV status. YPLH's relationships with their families and friends may be jeopardized with disclosure (Rotheram-Borus and Miller, 1998). For gay, lesbian, bisexual, transgender, and questioning youth, who may already be coping with stigma surrounding their sexual-ity, HIV positive status can increase stigma and feelings of social isolation. Disclosing their HIV positive status to potential sexual partners and tak-ing the necessary precautions to decrease transmission risk are difficult maneuvers for YPLH, as they may fear rejection and abandonment. Main-taining and enhancing positive social support thus appears to be critical to successful transmission risk reduction efforts with YPLH.

THEORETICAL FRAMEWORKS FOR PREVENTIVE INTERVENTIONS

The theoretical perspectives underlying most HIV prevention in-terventions, including those for YPLH, have been dominated by varia-tions on social-cognitive theory (Bandura, 1986): the health belief model (Rosenstock et al., 1994), theory of reasoned action (Fishbein, 1979), theory of planned behavior (Ajzen, 1991), AIDS risk reduction model (Catania et al., 1990), transtheoretical model of behavior change (Prochaska and DiClemente, 1992), and information-motivation-behavioral skills model (Fisher and Fisher, 1992). Interventions informed by these frameworks utilize cognitive-behavioral principles both to build and practice specific skills such as correct condom use, needle cleaning, and medication adherence; and to encourage youth to develop attitudes and intentions favorable to risk reduction. Attitudes regarding risk among youth can be influenced by their self-concept and the norms and stereotypes they perceive in the social groups with which they identify. Both their own negative personal stereotypes, and perceived peer group opposition to protected sex, HIV testing, medical regimen adherence, and other health behaviors are important barriers to successful behavior change. Youth are assisted in challenging and reframing perceptions, thoughts, and feelings that constitute barriers to prevention activities, and in developing self-efficacy with respect to their abilities to carry out the desired behaviors.

A limitation common to these frameworks is that, in their primary focus on cognitive processes and behavioral skills, they give little attention to the role of emotion in sexuality and the meanings of sexual acts to the participants (Rosenthal et al., 1998). Another concern is their limited attention to the role of contextual factors, including social environment characteristics such as gender role expectations, stigma and discrimination related to ethnic and sexual minority status (Brown et al., 2003). Stigma and discrimination can influence individuals' perceptions of risk, their ability to assess their own needs for health care, and their decisions about whether and when to seek services or implement protective behaviors. For example, Peterson et al. (1993) suggest that fear of being stereotyped as gay or bisexual influences black men to use condoms less often. It is therefore critical to take into account the ways in which YPLH identify with particular social groups, and the consequences to them of those social identities, in addressing their perceptions of risks and the factors influencing these perceptions.

Many health-related behaviors, including substance use and abuse (e.g., Jessor et al., 1991; Kandel et al., 1992) and sexual risk acts (Rotheram-Borus et al., 2000), follow developmental trajectories, which may be gender and ethnicity specific (Rotheram-Borus et al., 2000). Youths start with activities they perceive to be less risky, such as cigarette smoking or alcohol use, and then may move on to higher-risk activities such as marijuana use and eventually hard drug use. Individuals may accurately perceive that they are engaged in high-risk behavior but continue to engage in the activity. Health behaviors, including those related to HIV risk, are multifactorially determined (DiClemente and Wingood, 2003). Behavior change is often a

protracted, nonlinear process, in which "slips" as well as full-blown re-
lapses to the target behavior are common (Marlatt and Gordon, 1984).
Intensive interventions, involving multiple sessions that are spread
out over time and include repeated opportunities to practice the new
skills learned in the intervention, are required (Rotheram-Borus and Miller,
1998). Prevention interventions for YPLH need to be cast in a broad framework relevant to their interests, including popular youth culture in general
and their own social networks' values and beliefs in particular. Ideally, prevention messages would also be reiterated and reinforced through multiple
channels outside the sessions, such as popular television programs, entertainment events, video games, music, and other venues in which YPLH are
likely to be found, such as schools, churches, and after school programs. In
addition, because intervention effects often decay over time, it is necessary
to incorporate relapse prevention skills and build in mechanisms for maintenance or "booster" activities (Marlatt and Gordon, 1984; Rotheram-Borus
et al., 2003).

ETHNOGRAPHIC STUDY OF HIV POSITIVE YOUTH

As part of our ongoing intervention development work, we conducted
an ethnographic study with 86 YPLH in New York, San Francisco, and
Los Angeles (Luna and Rotheram-Borus, 1999). Through the collection of
life histories and repeated interviews with young gay men, injecting drug
users, and young women, we identified the personal, social and environmental components of the HIV positive adolescent experience and investigated these contextual influences on YPLH's life choices. Several issues
relevant to adolescents that required attention in the design of the intervention were identified. First, roles as peer educators often led to lower self-
esteem, conflicts with health care providers (those trying to help youth),
unreasonable expectations and poor peer-modeling. YPLH often acquired
HIV when experiencing periods of drug abuse or mental health problems;
their lives had periods of instability. Community-based agencies helped
youth to assume more responsibility by hiring young people as HIV advocates. In such roles, YPLH delivered AIDS 101 lectures, led small groups
about living with HIV, and shared their life history as a warning to other
youth not to experience similar problems. Yet, the level and types of support provided to peer leaders often appeared inadequate.
Yet, the level and types of support provided to peer leaders often appeared inadequate. When becoming peer leaders, young people related
to their health care providers as employers, as well as providers. When
the "patient" could not live up to expectations as "employees", which role

was more important? Young gay men, presenting to high school audiences, sometimes lied about their sexual orientation in order to be more acceptable to the audience; again, how can being an advocate be validating when it forces hiding of oneself? Finally, if a period of relapse occurred, an employee could initiate a relationship with a counselee and risk transmitting the virus to another young person. These were difficult challenges faced by agencies utilizing YPLH as peer advocates.

Second, almost all young people experienced challenges to consistent medical regimen adherence. Many turned to their culturally based 'folk' beliefs or myths. Recent research suggests that persons living with HIV frequently use alternative medicines. Curanderos, card readers, massage, and other forms of healing were common, especially among young women. The beliefs of YPLH often led them to adopt unusual health practices: for example, feeding their babies half breast milk and half formula in order to maintain optimal health. Beliefs grounded in cultural practices are common, and usually not assessed by health care providers. In order to effectively intervene with YPLH, it is critical to monitor such beliefs and help counter any beliefs that are likely to lead to sub-optimal health care.

Third, there was substantial variability in risk behaviors and sociodemographic profiles, particularly substance use, between YPLH in suburban and urban areas. The primary concerns of young women were fundamentally different from young men. Among young women, two subsets were identified. One subgroup lived in drug-infested neighborhoods, but reported low levels of sexual risk behavior and few sexual relationships over their lifetimes. These women did not know that their partners were currently or had been injection drug users. They characteristically learned of their infection through routine testing in connection with pregnancy or childbirth. For them, adaptation to their serostatus depended heavily on the meaning of HIV within their ongoing familial, social, and sexual relationships. A second subset comprised partners of IDUs, who themselves were often homeless and experienced psychological distress as well as multiple behavior problems. Their histories included repeated victimization and bartering of sex to meet basic survival needs. For them, and similar to IDUs, successful adaptation to life with HIV depended upon stopping their own substance abuse and developing strong support systems for a stable, drug-free lifestyle (Rotheram-Borus and Miller, 1998; Rotheram-Borus et al., 1996).

Finally, methamphetamine was the drug of choice. HIV positive adolescent substance abusers typically tweaked (were high on methamphetamine for two or three days in a row) and only sought health care when they were "coming down" from drugs. For the first six months after initiation of methamphetamine use, young people experienced increased sexual desire and inability to engage in sexual activities. However, following this initial period, a prolonged difficulty in raising sexual desire and an ability to engage in sexual relationships emerges. The shifts in sexual behavior patterns over time appeared strongly related to acquiring HIV infection, based on young people's reports. Across treatment settings, there was limited access to substance abuse treatment and, sometimes, negative attitudes of adolescent healthcare providers to substance abuse treatment, decreasing the possibility of clinical interventions for high-risk HIV-positive youth.

Based on these qualitative data, interventions for YPLH must: a) emphasize the importance of ongoing support for young people, especially by clarifying roles and responsibilities; b) explore and address idiopathic belief systems grounded in alternative medicine; c) tailor programs to rural, urban, and gender subgroups; and d) identify windows of opportunity for interventions, especially methamphetamine users.

TEENS LINKED TO CARE—TLC

The TLC intervention is based on cognitive-behavioral principles and comprises 31 sessions divided into three modules, each module consisting of 8 to 12 two-hour sessions. Each module has a targeted outcome: promote healthy behavior (Module 1), reduce transmission risk acts (Module 2), and improve quality of life (Module 3). Designed for small group implementation, the intervention utilizes an interactive, participatory psychoeducational format, including scripted and unscripted role-plays of real-life situations confronting YPLH. A detailed manual is available online at http://chipts.ucla.edu for further reference (see Table 6.2; Miller and Rotheram-Borus, 1994; 1995a; 1995b).

Module 1: Promoting Healthy Behavior
(Stay Healthy)

Adherence to medical care regimens, attendance at doctors' appointments, and active participation in health care decision-making appear to be associated with increased survival time among individuals living with HIV (Remien et al., 1992). However, individuals with chronic diseases often have difficulty changing their behavior in ways necessary to manage their illnesses (Remien et al., 1992). YPLH may have particular difficulty instituting and sustaining health-promoting behaviors when they also have

Table 6.2. Outline of modules for Teens Linked to Care
intervention

Module 1: Staying healthy
Basic attitudes about living with HIV
Being HIV positive and thinking about the future
To tell or not to tell: Disclosing HIV positive status
Learning about HIV stigma and how to handle it
Finding the desire to be healthy
Why use substances? Are they coping mechanisms?
It's time to deal with substance abuse
Decreasing re-infection
Keeping cool and in control
Going to appointments
Having medication and taking it
Staying involved in your medical decisions

Module 2: Act safe
Protection for yourself and your partners
What kinds of protection are out there?
Disclosing HIV: Do I tell my sexual partner?
Condoms: Should I talk about using one?
Unprotected sex: Should I say no?
Introducing a commitment
What to do about controlling drug and alcohol urges
What to do about external triggers
What to do about internal triggers?
What to do about anxiety and anger?
What to do about drugs, alcohol and sex?

Module 3: Being together
Goals to improve quality of life: What are they?
How to be consistent: Daily routine and quality of life
Dealing with substance abuse relapse
Overview of strategies for substance abuse relapse
Keeping up your quality of life: Believe in others and yourself
Reducing potential sexual risk
Overview of strategies for substance abuse relapse
Review collective skills and goals for daily life, and reinforce a positive self-image

substance use problems. Hence, at least three of the 12 sessions deal explicitly with increasing motivation to initiate and maintain a healthy, drug-free lifestyle. Negative perceptions of HIV and living as an HIV-positive youth may serve as barriers to health-promoting behavior; therefore, the intervention addresses these barriers from the outset by encouraging hope and the formation of long term goals.

In addition to laying the groundwork for reduction or cessation of substance use, this module focuses on motivating HIV-positive youth to take responsibility for their health behaviors and introducing sexual risk reduction (Rotheram-Borus and Miller, 1998). Though risk reduction issues are addressed more fully in the second module, skills for coping with substance use and reducing harm from it, including needle cleaning, are taught here. Youths identify how they usually deal with situations involving substance use, the typical antecedents, and their behavioral responses. Reviewing daily diaries identifies behavior patterns. Storytelling is used to provide a possible social routine for changing habitual behavior patterns. For example, boys are instructed to retell the story below, so that Danny does not end up using alcohol and then having unprotected sex.

> Danny has two close friends— Claude and Jerry. They live next door. Often he hangs out over there, eats meals with them, and goes places with them. Jerry has to go out of town for a few weeks.
> One day Claude calls and asks Danny over for dinner. Claude says that he really misses Jerry.
> Danny says he would love to come. When he gets there, the table is nicely set for two and Claude is dressed in a very sexy outfit. They have drinks before dinner, and Danny thinks that the drinks are unusually strong. Dinner is wonderful. They eat and talk and drink wine. Claude keeps brushing his bare feet against Danny under the table.
> After dessert, they move to the couch and have brandy. Danny is feeling very drunk.
> Claude moves close and starts casually touching Danny. Pretty soon Danny is feeling very excited. He and Claude start kissing passionately. Soon their clothes are off, and they are doing it on the floor. Danny is too hot to even think about a condom. No condom is used.

Self-regulation skills such as stress management techniques are also introduced in this module to help YPLH develop a repertoire of positive behavioral alternatives to use in dealing with stressful situations that might otherwise trigger behaviors such as unprotected sex or substance use that could pose risks to themselves or others. A retelling of the story below outlines positive alternative behaviors available to youth:

> Danny has two close friends—Claude and Jerry. They live next door. Often he hangs out over there, eats meals with them, and goes places with them. Jerry has to go out of town for a few weeks.
> One day Claude calls and asks Danny over for dinner. Claude says that he really misses Jerry.
> Danny says he would love to come. When he gets there, the table is nicely set for two and Claude is dressed in a very sexy outfit. They have a drink before dinner, but they drink one drink each, drink it slowly, and nurse it along with some pretzels.
> Dinner is wonderful. They eat and talk but decide not to drink any more alcohol. Claude keeps brushing his bare feet against Danny under the table.
> After dessert, they move to the couch and keep talking. Danny is starting to feel turned on, but knows he wants to practice safe sex.

He tells Claude how important it is to him that they are both protected. Danny doesn't have a condom with him, but Claude says he does. Because they haven't consumed much alcohol, they're both thinking clearly and decide to take a time out. Claude finds a condom and makes sure it isn't expired. Then they go back to the couch. Claude moves close and starts casually touching Danny.

Pretty soon Danny is feeling very excited. He and Claude start kissing passionately.

Soon their clothes are off, but they make sure to put the condom on correctly before they are doing it on the floor. They have hot, but protected, sex.

Role-playing and problem-solving approaches are utilized to prepare youth for making sound decisions about whether, when, and how to disclose their serostatus. These approaches are also used in situations where youth experience stigma, particularly in dealing with negative attitudes from health care providers.

Module 2: Reducing Transmission of HIV (Act Safe)

Module 2 focuses on promoting safer sex and reduction, cessation, or maintenance of low levels of substance use. The first five sessions focus on reducing sexual transmission risk, avoiding unwanted pregnancy, and decreasing the chances of re-infection. Correct condom use is practiced and options for both disease prevention and pregnancy are reviewed. During each session, YPLH are encouraged to identify positive outcomes for difficult, real-life situations that pose ethical dilemmas, such as: dealing with pregnancy and whether or not to take medication to reduce vertical transmission risk; negotiating safer sex behavior with HIV-positive partners to avoid re-infection and other sexually transmitted diseases, and with HIV-negative partners to protect them from infection; and risking the loss of a relationship or other adverse consequences by telling someone about being HIV positive. YPLH role-play these situations and practice skills such as convincing partners to use condoms, putting condoms on anatomical demonstration models, and saying no to a potential partner who does not want to have protected sex.

The next six sessions strive to motivate YPLH to enter into treatment if they are having problems with substance use. Enrollment and graduation from a substance abuse treatment program is a major goal for YPLH in this intervention; drug treatment is vital for YPLH who may not know how to reduce transmission or make educated, safe decisions about their health. These sessions focus on breaking the cycle of substance abuse (Beck et al., 1993; Rawson et al., 1991; Shoptaw et al., 1995). YPLH are taught to identify triggers for substance use, and to stop negative thoughts about using that may lead to the belief that they need to use. YPLH are provided with tools and guidelines for monitoring their routines and substance use practices. Each session identifies positive solutions to problems introduced by YPLH in the group. This process helps address typical situations YPLH must deal with before they can commit to a substance abuse treatment program, such as: educational goals, relationship aspirations, stable housing, consistent employment and positive family relations. Once some of these issues are resolved, YPLH have a better chance of addressing their substance abuse successfully. YPLH are also taught a set of skills to counter external triggers and negative thoughts (Rotheram-Borus et al., 1991; Sarason et al., 1996; Shulman, 1989), including relaxation and assertive communication skills. Participants role-play situations which include refusal to use substances or leave a party where substance use is present. In the last session of Module 2, YPLH apply the problem solving, stress management, and assertive communication skills they have acquired by rehearsing situations involving both refusal of potential drug use and negotiation of safer sex.

Module 3: Improving the Quality of Life (Being Together)

In addition to reinforcing the behavior changes introduced in the prior modules, this eight-session module, the content of which is depicted in Table 2, focuses on increasing YPLH's life satisfaction and emotional strength. Major themes in Module 3 include: discovering a basic set of values that define their "core" selves; distancing themselves from a self-destructive identity; reducing negative emotional reactions to living with HIV; increasing perceptions of personal control; reducing self-destructive behavior, particularly for substance use; and living fully and joyously in the present moment (Rotheram-Borus and Miller, 1998). Underlying this module is the assumption that pain, loss, discouragement, and discontent are far more pervasive in YPLH's lives than feelings of joy or serenity.

In Module 3, YPLH learn to concentrate on the present moment through meditation in order to develop an awareness of each moment of life. In addition, meditation skills provide a vehicle for YPLH to gain insight into the interconnectedness and interdependence between their perceptions of their daily lives and their emotional reactions, as well as a tool that will help them overcome automatic thought processes and self-destructive behaviors. The heightened awareness that YPLH acquire concerning destructive or harmful situations and negative triggers will increase their ability to decide what they want to do in order to stabilize their health, stick to their core beliefs and values, and refrain from substance use. Recognition of control over their actions and responses to emotions and triggers will strengthen their self-efficacy in acting on the values they have identified for themselves. In addition, awareness of their life experiences on a moment-by-moment basis helps YPLH to increase their acceptance of life the way it is—HIV status, shifts in physical capacities, financial situation, home life, and relationship status. Once YPLH accept life as it is, without placing demands on themselves or others to be what they are not, YPLH are in a better position to live their lives as fully as possible, with both self-respect and respect for others.

INTERVENTION DELIVERY FORMATS

There are three general formats for interventions delivered to YPLH: small group, telephone, and individual sessions. The number of sessions and efficacy of interventions varies across delivery modality. Here we describe examples of interventions for YPLH delivered in these formats.

Small Group Delivery

The intervention described above, TLC, was developed for delivery to small groups. YPLH reported a positive experience with this format, but because attendance rates were not always optimal, it was necessary to explore alternative delivery strategies as a means of increasing intervention participation (Rotheram-Borus et al., 2001a). Schedule changes, stigma associated with group participation in an HIV-related setting, language barriers, and transportation difficulties have frequently been identified as barriers to intervention attendance (Martinez et al., 2003; Rotheram-Borus et al., in press). In addition, the relatively small size of the total population of YPLH in a given geographic area typically meant combining young MSM, women, and heterosexual males, some of whom were and others of whom were not using substances, within a single group (Rotheram-Borus et al., in press), even though some of the issues were very different for each subpopulation and required considerable tailoring of session content. Difficulties with regular attendance are also foreseeable in rural settings where there may be even fewer individuals requiring specific intervention services, creating a longer and more problematic recruitment process.

Individual Delivery

Alternative formats and modes of intervention delivery can retain the efficacy of prevention programs for YPLH while obviating many of the barriers to attendance at group sessions. Rotheram-Borus et al. (in press) have adapted the intervention described above for individual delivery. Individual sessions allow for greater tailoring of session content to the diversity of YPLH's experiences; youth with varied backgrounds and life experiences are not required to attend small group sessions that do not focus on their specific issues (Rotheram-Borus et al., in press). In addition, the one-on-one format is consistent with case management models being implemented throughout the US (CDC, 1997).

Individual sessions can be delivered both face-to-face and by telephone (Rotheram-Borus et al., in press). Intention-to-treat analyses of the randomized trial evaluating the adapted intervention demonstrated that, compared to a delayed-intervention control condition, in-person individual intervention was associated with a significantly greater proportion of protected sexual encounters across all partners and with HIV-negative partners at follow-up (Rotheram-Borus et al., in press).

Telephone Delivery

The adaptation by Rotheram-Borus et al. (in press) of their CLEAR intervention for YPLH (Rotheram-Borus et al., 2001c) to individual telephone delivery attended to the concerns of youth both about the security of environments in which they disclose their HIV status and about transportation difficulties. The telephone as a mode of intervention delivery also makes sessions accessible to participants with children, who might not be able to find a babysitter or the money to pay for one, as well as those who are too ill to leave their homes without discomfort. An intervention delivered via telephone enables participation by clients with these and other barriers to in-person attendance. An intervention that does not threaten the privacy of YPLH, particularly in rural settings, and that imposes minimal logistical requirements on clients, has a greater chance of successful participant retention and efficacy (Rotheram-Borus et al., in press).

Internet Delivery

The Internet and other advances in computing technology have opened up a plethora of information and expedited communication for individuals and groups all over the world. Computer-assisted psychoeducation has been provided to patients with phobias (Gosh and Greist, 1988), depression (Selmi et al., 1990), obesity (Agras et al., 1990), eating disorders (Andrewes et al., 1996), and diabetes (Glasgow et al., 1995). Based on these successes, computer-based interventions have been widely advocated for health education and prevention (Burnett et al., 1989; Orlandi et al., 1990; Sampson and Kruboltz, 1991; Schinke et al., 1990), though as yet there are few positive models of computer-aided HIV prevention.

Using the Internet, friends can write to each other and receive replies almost immediately, while groups have meetings without individual members leaving their homes. Students are successfully completing academic coursework over the World Wide Web via "distance education" programs (Gurak and Lannon, 2004). The use of the Internet for intervention delivery carries numerous potential benefits. For example, perhaps more than telephone sessions, it eliminates barriers posed by confidentiality concerns as well as discomfort with group settings, interpersonal avoidance, and denial. In addition, the intervention can be programmed to be responsive specifically to YPLH's unique risk patterns; youth exhibiting particular triggers for unprotected sex or substance use can be referred to activities that target that trigger. Targeting the content of the intervention with this level of specificity may increase its effectiveness.

Additionally, the individualized attention that characterizes one-on-one counseling can be simulated through the use of interactive multimedia programming. The computer is able to control output and feedback such that the branching and decision making process is dependent on the user's choices or responses, personalizing the experience. Since computers are considered objective and accurate, a computer's ability to respond and give selective, personalized feedback creates intense attraction to the intervention and suggests that youth would be likely to engage with it (Bosworth et al., 1983). Internet-based interventions also provide the opportunity for participants with sufficiently fast Internet connections and powerful computer systems to download personal copies of intervention materials. For participants whose Internet access is not fast enough or whose computers are not powerful enough, these materials can be burned onto CDs or DVDs and made available through community-based agencies or by mail.

ADAPTATION OF EVIDENCE-BASED INTERVENTIONS

All evidence-based interventions have manuals, detailed examples of implementation protocols and detailed scripts that can be used as positive models. Manuals are usually large, boring, and not presented in an attractive, marketable format. Most evidence-based interventions will need

Table 6.3. Non-specific elements of evidence-based interventions

	Efficacious Facilitators
Provide HOPE for change	Shape behaviors over time
Redefine challenges	Demonstrate Affect/Behavior/Cognition
Provide vocabulary	Provide choices
Are prepared	Reward
Establish predictability	
	Consumers
Believe hope to change	Acquire anticipatory awareness of risk
Construct new meaning	Change routines to be prepared for challenges
Value desired behaviors	Adopt value of consistency over time
Identify ranked challenges	Imitate behavior
Generalize change over time	

extreme format makeovers in order to be recognized, accepted, and broadly implemented.

In the interventions described in this chapter, we developed an initial intervention that was condensed and adapted into different formats. However, we still have a need for CD-ROM delivery formats, videotape for intervention sessions (not scripts that are long and require literacy skills), effective strategies for selection and training of facilitators, and workbooks that are highly attractive to the target population.

In addition to the problem in formats of the delivery of efficacious interventions, there are many non-specific factors that influence the delivery of evidence-based interventions. Table 6.3 outlines non-specific factors that are necessary for the implementation of evidence-based interventions. The list of these non-specific factors comes from a review of existing HIV prevention manuals for young people: Street Smart, Safe Choices, Becoming a Responsible Teen, Community Popular Opinion Leader, and Be Proud, Be Responsible (see Jemmott and Jemmott, 2000). A synthesis of the non-specific factors identified in this review is presented below.

While preventive and therapeutic interventions address different populations, there are three outcomes implicit in all interventions: (1) participation in the intervention, (2) changing the target behavior, and (3) maintaining the change over time. In the review, most interventions do not specifically address outcomes 1 and 3; researchers merely offer incentives to get participation and the follow-up period is not long enough to challenge maintenance. However, the intervention's goals were consistently clear in each program about the target behavior; in fact, goals were outlined for each session and each segment of each session, as well as for the overall intervention. Each group meeting indicated the specific goals and changes desired within the session, across sessions, and after the termination of the group. Each of the programs defined the intervention context as key to behavior change, attempting to create a safe, supportive group environment. Once established, the group environment was used to reward positive norms, values, and behaviors among group members. Group cohesion, humor and refreshments were integrated into all interventions, appealing to basic rituals for joining with others.

At the first session of group interventions, rules and guidelines are specified by the group leaders, often inviting participants to create rules to increase their comfort attending groups. All intervention groups modeled democratic and consensus models of operation, in contrast to authoritarian. The leaders are instructed to provide compliments and to avoid judgmental statements or impatience. Self-disclosure is valued, modeled, and requested by participants. Cooperative groups are formed to accomplish many of the activities, with the specific goal to enhance cohesion. Many prompts are used (cards, signs, tokens, games) in order to disseminate information, with didactic teaching minimized. Almost all manuals instruct their leaders to be selective and to utilize the language relative to group members' ethnicity, age, gender, and life experiences. When video demonstrations are used, it is to enhance awareness of "people like us" who are coping with similar life stressors. All leaders created a sense of relevance and motivation to participate in the intervention by using handouts outlining the goals of the intervention; each intervention is quite explicit about the behaviors to be addressed at each group meeting and the final outcomes to be addressed in the group.

While behaviors were the stated goal of the intervention and it was important to specify behavioral outcomes, there were a variety of outcomes and issues embedded in the training related to enhancing and shifting capacities for the self, social identity, gender roles, and community reference group. Several interventions had activities aimed at improving self-worth and self-respect (e.g., exercises stating, "I deserve respect"), enhancing values around self-protection (care about my own health), and cultivating the ability to differentiate and be separate from others (e.g., resist group pressure, set limits on the behaviors of significant others), as well as outlining future goals that enhance the motivation for self-preservation (e.g., caring about the future of my unborn children, having vocational aspirations that require positive health). Building on enhancing these beliefs and attitudes towards oneself, promoting a healthy reference group and shifting the social identity and roles (usually roles as advocates) of participants were also addressed in sessions.

Within the group, leaders specified that the group was the supportive environment needed to implement different self-protective behaviors; enhancing group cohesion was building these norms. Almost all interventions actively lobbied for youth to adopt the social role of health advocate, even though this topic was the basis of only one intervention (community opinion leader). The advocacy for a healthy community charged participants to spread the word to others and to protect the community from harm. In particular, helping one's group, despite the lack of caring and protection by the broader society, attempted quite specifically to mobilize ethnic pride. Several interventions also helped youth establish a set of pro-health values and a set of rules for dealing with potential high risk situations (e.g., always carry a condom, do not enter a private space without talking about sex, etc). Many of these components of the intervention were not an explicit part of the theories on which the program was designed, nor were there evaluations on how or whether the program shifted these intervention components.

A variety of strategies and techniques were directed at mobilizing the traditional social cognitive beliefs and skills associated with HIV behavior change: self-efficacy ("I am capable of using condoms"), perceived vulnerability ("This could happen to me"), negative perceptions of the outcome of infection ("AIDS would destroy my future"), enhanced personal control of HIV ("AIDS is preventable by me"), assertiveness skills, identification of triggers for risk situations, awareness of feelings and the ability to control sexual attractiveness, and problem solving of specific risk situations. Some groups were more cognitive than others; some interventions emphasized affective awareness and self-control; still others were more behavioral. Nevertheless, the commonalities across these adaptations were apparent.

CONCLUSIONS

As YPLH look forward to increased length and quality of life due to the successes of HIV treatment, the need for preventive services will increase, and will highlight the advantages of early detection. YPLH will need support in incorporating new skills, values, and motivations when learning to live with HIV. These skills, tools, and values will help them make and act on healthy choices for themselves, potential sexual partners, friends, family, and society. Appropriately tailored interventions addressing health, mental health, and transmission risk reduction will aid YPLH with many different tools to live long, productive, safe, and high-quality lives. As choices related to sexual intimacy, relationships, and substance use resurface as regular parts of YPLH's lives, interventions tailored for youth living with HIV may appropriately include partners, as some issues to be addressed may include risk within long-term relationships and protection with primary partners. Current prevention projects with YPLH will explore Internet-based curricula to make interventions broadly accessible and additional maintenance components will sustain desired behavior changes over time.

REFERENCES

Advocates for Youth, *Issues at a glance: Serving HIV-positive youth, 2002*, Washington D.C. (November 2002); http://www.advocatesforyouth.org.

Agras, W. S., Taylor, C. B., Feldman, D. E., Losch, M., and Burnett, K. (1990). Developing computer assisted therapy for the treatment of obesity. *Behav. Ther.* 21:99–109.

Ajzen, I. (1991). The theory of planned behavior.*Organ. Behav. Hum. Decis. Process* 50:179–211.

Andrewes, D. G., O'Connor, R., Mulder, C., McLennan, H. D., Weigall, S., and Sy, S. (1996). Computerized psychoeducation for patients with eating disorders. *Aust. N. Z. J. Psychiatry* 30:492–497.

Bandura, A. (1986). *Social foundations of thought and action: A social cognitive theory*. Prentice-Hall, Englewood Cliffs, NJ.

Beck, A., Wright, F., Newman, C., and Liese, B. (1993). *Cognitive therapy of substance abuse*. Guilford Press, New York.

Bosworth, K., Gustafson, D., Hawkins, R., Chewning, B., and Day, T. (1983). Adolescents, health education, and computers: The Body Awareness Resource Network (BARN). *Health. Ed. Microcomp.* 14:48–60.

Brown, L., Macintyre, K., and Trujillo, L. (2003). Interventions to reduce HIV/AIDS stigma: what have we learned? *AIDS Educ. Prev.* 15(1):49–69.

Burnett, K. F., Magel, P. E., Harrington, S., and Taylor, C. B. (1989). Computer assisted behavioral health counseling for high school students. *J. Couns. Psychol.* 36:63–67.

Butler, R. B., Schultz, J. R., Forsberg, A. D., Brown, L. K., Parsons, J. T., King, G., Kocik, S. M., Jarvis, D., Schulz, S. L., Manco-Johnson, M., and CDC Adolescent HBIEP Study Group. (2003). Promoting safer sex among HIV-positive youth with haemophilia: Theory, intervention, and outcome. *Haemophilia* 9(2):214–222.

Catania, J. A., Kegeles, S. M., and Coates, T. J. (1990). Towards an understanding of risk behavior: An AIDS risk reduction model. *Health Ed. Q.*17:53–72.

Cates, W., Jr. (1990). The epidemiology and control of sexually transmitted diseases in adolescents. In: Schydlower, M. and Shafer, M. A. (eds.), *AIDS and other sexually transmitted diseases*. Hanley and Belfus, Philadelphia, pp. 409–427.

Centers for Disease Control and Prevention (CDC), *HIV Prevention Case Management*. National Center for HIV, STD and TB prevention, 1997, Atlanta, GA, (September 1997); http://www.cdc.gov/hiv/pubs/hivpcmg.htm.

Centers for Disease Control and Prevention (CDC) (1998). *Prevention and treatment of sexually transmitted diseases as an HIV prevention strategy*. Atlanta, GA.

Centers for Disease Control and Prevention (CDC), *Young People at Risk: HIV/AIDS among America's Youth, 2002*, Atlanta,GA(May2002a); http://www.cdc.gov/hiv/pubs/facts/youth.pdf.

Centers for Disease Control and Prevention (CDC), *HIV/AIDS among U. S. Women: Minority and Young Women at Continuing Risk, 2002*, Atlanta, GA (May 2002b); http://www.cdc.gov/hiv/pubs/facts/women.pdf.

Centers for Disease Control and Prevention (CDC) (2003). Advancing HIV prevention: New strategies for a changing epidemic—US, 2003. *MMWR* 52(15):329–332.

Chesney, M., Folkman, S., and Chambers. D. (1996). Coping effectiveness training for men living with HIV: preliminary findings. *Int. J. STD AIDS* 7(S2):75–82.

Cowan, F. M., and Mindel, A. (1993). Sexually transmitted diseases in children: Adolescents. *Genitourin. Med.* 69:141–147.

Crepaz, N., and Marks, G. (2002). Towards an understanding of sexual risk behavior in people living with HIV: A review of social, psychological, and medical findings. *AIDS* 16:135–149.

del Rio, C. (2003). New challenges in HIV care: Prevention among HIV-infected patients. *Top. HIV Med.* 11(4):140–144.

DiClemente, R. J., and Wingood, G. M. (2003). Human immunodeficiency virus prevention for adolescents: windows of opportunity for optimizing intervention effectiveness. *Arch. Pediatr. Adolesc. Med.* 157(4):319–320.

Ekstrand, M. L., Stall, R. D., Paul, J. P., Osmond, D. H., and Coates, T. J. (1999). Gay men report high rates of unprotected anal sex with partners of unknown or discordant HIV status. *AIDS* 13(12):1525–1533.

Ewart, C. (1991). Social Action Theory for a public health psychology. *Am. Psychol.* 46:931–946.

Fishbein, M. (1979). A theory of reasoned action: Some applications and implications. *Nebr. Symp. Motiv.* 27:65–116.

Fisher, J. D., and Fisher, W. A. (1992). Towards changing AIDS-related risk behavior. *Psychol. Bull.* 111:455–474.

Glasgow, R. E., Toobert, D. J., Hampson, S. E., and Noell, J. W. (1995). A brief office-based intervention to facilitate diabetes dietary self-management. *Health Educ. Res.* 10:467–478.

Gosh, A., and Greist, J. H. (1988). Computer treatment in psychiatry. *Psychiatr. Ann.* 18:246–250.

Gurak, L. J., and Lannon, J. M. (2004). *A concise guide to technical communication.* Pearson Education Inc, New York.

Heckman, T. G., Silverthorn, M., Waltje, A., Meyers, M., and Yarber, W. (2003) HIV transmission risk practices in rural persons living with HIV disease. *Sex. Transm. Dis.* 30(2):134–136.

Hingson, R., Strunin, L., and Berlin, B. (1990). Acquired immunodeficiency syndrome transmission: Changes in knowledge and behavior among teenagers. Massachusetts statewide survey, 1986 to 1988. *Pediatrics* 85:24–29.

Huba, G. J., Melchior, L. A., Woods, E. R., Panter, A. T., Feudo, R., Schneir, A., Trevithick, L., Wright, E., Martinez, R., Sturdevant, M., Remafedi, G., Greenberg, B., Tierney, S., Wallace, M., Goodman, E., Tenner, A., Marconi, K., Brady, R. E., and Singer, B. (2000). Service use patterns of youth with, and at high risk for, HIV: A care typology. *AIDS Patient Care STDs* 14(7):359-3-79.

Janssen, R. S., Holtgrave, R. O., Shepherd, M., Gayle, H. D., and DeCock, K. M. (2001). The serostatus approach to fighting the HIV epidemic: Prevention strategies for infected individuals. *Am. J. Public Health* 91(7):1019–1024.

Jemmott, J.B. and Jemmott, L.S. (2000). HIV risk reduction behavioral interventions with heterosexual adolescents. *AIDS* 14 (suppl 2):S40–52.

Jessor, R. (1991). Risk behavior in adolescence: a psychosocial framework for understanding and action. *J. Adolesc. Health* 12(8):597–605.

Johnson, R. L., Botwinick, G., Sell, R. L., Martinez, J., Siciliano, C., Friedman, L. B., Dodds, S., Shaw, K., Walker, L. E., Sotheran, J. L., and Bell, D. G. (2003). The utilization of treatment and case management services by HIV-infected youth. *J. Adolesc. Health* 33S:31–38.

Kalichman, S. C., Rompa, D., Cage, M., DiFonzo, K., Simpson, D., Austin, J., Luke, W., Buckles, J., Kyomugisha, F., Benotsch, E., Pinkerton, S., and Graham, J. (2001). Effectiveness of an intervention to reduce HIV transmission risks in HIV-positive people. *Am. J. Prev. Med.* 21(2):84–92.

Kalichman, S. C., Rompa, D., Luke, W., and Austin, J. (2002). HIV transmission risk behaviours among HIV-positive persons in serodiscordant relationships. *Int. J. STD AIDS* 13(10):677–682.

Kandel, D. B., Yamaguchi, K., and Chen, K. (1992). Stages of progression in drug involvement from adolescence to adulthood: further evidence for the gateway theory. *J. Stud. Alcohol* 53(5):447–457.

Kann, L., Kinchen, S. A., Williams, B. I., Ross, J. G., Lowry, R., Hill, C. V., Grunbaum, J. A., Blumson, P. S., Collins, J. L., and Kolbe, L. J. (1998). Youth risk behavior surveillance—US, 1997. *MMWR* 47(3):1–89.

Kelly, J. A., Murphy, D. A., Bahr, G. R., Kalichman, S. C., Morgan, M. G., Stevenson, L. Y., Koob, J. J., Brasfield, T. L., and Bernstein, B. M. (1993). Outcome of cognitive-behavioral and support group brief therapies for depressed, HIV-infected persons. *Am. J. Psychiatry* 150(11):1679–1686.

Leach, M. P., Wolitski, R. J., Goldbaum, G. M., and Fishbein, M. (1997). HIV risk and sources of information among street youth. *Psychology, Health, and Medicine,* 2(2):119–134.

Live Positive, Living *with HIV/AIDS: Challenges for HIV positive youth,* 2004, Toronto, Ontario (2004); http://www.livepositive.ca/positivelife/livingwith/challanges.html.

Luna, G. C., and Rotheram-Borus, M. J. (1999). Youth living with HIV as peer leaders. *Am. J. Community Psychol.* 27(1):1–23.

Lyon, M. E., Trexler, C., Akpan-Townsend, C., Pao, M., Selden, K., Fletcher, J., Addlestone, I. C., and D'Angelo, L. J. (2003). A family group approach to increasing adherence to therapy in HIV-infected youths: results of a pilot project. *AIDS Patient Care STDs* 17(6):299–308.

Margolin, A., Avants, S. K., Warburton, L. A., Hawkins, K. A., and Shi, J. (2003). A randomized clinical trial of a manual-guided risk reduction intervention for HIV-positive injection drug users. *Health Psychol.* 22(2):223–228.

Marks, G., Richardson, J. L., Crepaz, N., Stoyanoff, S., Milam, J., Kemper, C., Larsen, R. A., Bolan, R., Weismuller, P., Hollander, H., and McCutchan, A. (2002) Are HIV care providers talking with patients about safer sex and disclosure?: A multi-clinic assessment. *AIDS* 16(14):1953–1957.

Marlatt, G. A., and Gordon, J. R. (1984). *Relapse Prevention: Maintenance strategies in the Treatment of Addictive Behaviors.* Guilford, New York.

Martinez, J., Bell, D., Dodds, S., Shaw, K., Siciliano, C., Walker, L. E., Sotheran, J. L., Sell, R. L., Friedman, L. B., Botwinick, G., and Johnson, R. L. (2003). Transitioning youths into care: Linking identified HIV-infected youth at outreach sites in the community to hospital-based clinics and or community-based health centers. *J. Adolesc. Health* 33S:23–30.

Miller, S., and Rotheram-Borus, M. J. (1994). *Staying healthy: A training manual for youth.* Department of Psychiatry, Division of Social and Community Psychiatry, University of California, Los Angeles.

Miller, S., and Rotheram-Borus, M. J. (1995a). *Act safe: A training manual for youth.* Department of Psychiatry, Division of Social and Community Psychiatry, University of California, Los Angeles.

Miller, S., and Rotheram-Borus, M. J. (1995b). *Being together: A training manual for youth.* Department of Psychiatry, Division of Social and Community Psychiatry, University of California, Los Angeles.

National Institute on Allergy and Infectious Diseases, *HIV/AIDS statistics,* 2004, Bethesda, MD (January 2004); http://www.niaid.nih.gov/factsheets/aidsstat.htm.

Norris, A. E., and Ford, K. (1998). Moderating influences of peer norms on gender differences in condom use. *Applied Developmental Science* 2(4):174–181.

Orlandi, M. A., Dozier, C. E., and Marta, M. A. (1990). Computer-assisted strategies for substance abuse prevention: Opportunities and barriers. *J. Consult Clin. Psychol.* 58: 425–431.

Parsons, J. T., Huszti, H. C., Crudder, S. O., Rich, L., and Mendoza, J. (2000). Maintenance of safer sexual behaviours: Evaluation of a theory-based intervention for HIV seropositive men with haemophilia and their female partners. *Haemophilia* 6(3):181–190.

Patterson, T. L., Shaw, W. S., and Semple, S. J. (2003). Reducing the sexual risk behaviors of HIV+ individuals: Outcome of a randomized controlled trial. *Ann. Behav. Med.* 25(2):137–145.

Peterson, J. L., Catania, J. A., Dolcini, M. M., and Faigeles, B. (1993). Multiple sexual partners among blacks in high-risk cities. *Fam. Plan. Perspectives* 25(6):263–267.

Prochaska, J. O., and DiClemente, C. C. (1992). Stages of change in the modification of problem behaviors. *Prog. Behav. Modif.* 28:183–218.

Rawson, R., Obert, J., McCann, M. and Scheffey, E. (1991). *The neurobehavioral treatment manual.* The Matrix Center, Beverly Hills, CA.

Remien, R. H., Rabkin, J. G., Williams, J. B., and Katoff, L. (1992). Coping strategies and health beliefs of AIDS long-term survivors. *Psychol. Health* 6:335–345.

Rosenstock, I. M., Strecher, V. J., and Becker, M. H. (1994). The health belief model and HIV risk behavior change. In: DiClemente, R. J. and Peterson, J. L. (eds.), *Preventing AIDS: Theories and methods of behavioral interventions. AIDS prevention and mental health,* Plenum Press, New York, pp. 5–24.

Rosenthal, D., Gifford, S., and Moore, S. (1998). Safe sex or safe love: Competing discourses? *AIDS Care* 10:35–47.

Rotheram-Borus, M. J. and Miller, S. (1998). Secondary prevention with HIV-positive youth. *AIDS Care* 10(1):17–34.

Rotheram-Borus, M. J., Miller, S., Koopman, C., Haignere, C. and Selfridge, C. (1991a). *Adolescents living safely: AIDS awareness, attitudes and actions.* Department of Psychiatry, Division of Social and Community Psychiatry, University of California, Los Angeles.

Rotheram-Borus, M. J., Koopman, C., Haignere, C., and Davies, M. (1991b). Reducing HIV sexual risk behaviors among runaway adolescents. *JAMA.* 266:1237–1241.

Rotheram-Borus, M. J., Murphy, D. A., and Miller, S. (1996). Intervening with adolescent girls living with HIV. In: O'Leary, A. and Jemmott, L. S. (eds.), *Women and AIDS: Coping and Care,* Plenum Press, New York, pp. 87–109.

Rotheram-Borus, M. J., O'Keefe, Z., Kracker, R., and Foo, H. H. (2000). Prevention of HIV among adolescents. *Prev. Sci.* 1(1):15–30.

Rotheram-Borus, M. J., Lee, M. B., Gwadz, M., and Draimin, B. (2001a). An intervention for parents with AIDS and their adolescent children. *Am. J. Public Health* 91:1294–1302.

Rotheram-Borus, M. J., Lee, M. B., Murphy, D. A., Futterman, D., Duan, N., Birnbaum, J. M., Lightfoot, M., and the Teens Linked to Care Consortium. (2001b). Efficacy of a preventive intervention for youth living with HIV. *Am. J. Public Health* 91:400–405.

Rotheram-Borus, M. J., Murphy, D. A., Wight, R. G., Lee, M. B., Lightfoot, M., Swendeman, D., Birnbaum, J. M., and Wright, W. (2001c). Improving the quality of life among young people living with HIV. *Eval. Program Plann.* 24:227–237.

Rotheram-Borus, M. J., Song, J., Gwadz, M., Lee, M., van Rossem, R., and Koopman, C. (2003). Reductions in HIV risk among runaway youth. *Prev. Sci.* 4(3):173–187.

Rotheram-Borus, M. J., Swendeman, D., Comulada, W. S., Weiss, R. E., and Lightfoot, M. (in press). Prevention for substance using HIV positive young people: Telephone and in-person delivery. *JAIDS.*

Rotheram-Borus, M. J., Wong, F. L., Goldstein, R. B., Remien, R. H., Morin, S. F., Weinhardt, L. S., Johnson, M. O., Steward, W. T., Kelly, J. A., Lightfoot, M., and Correale, J. (2004a). Associations of Highly Active Antiretroviral Therapy and Risk Patterns among People Living with HIV. *Manuscript Submitted for Publication.*

Sampson, J. P., and Kruboltz, J. D. (1991). Computer assisted instruction: A missing link in counseling. *J. Couns. Dev.* 69:395–397.

Sarason, I. G., Pierce, G. R., and Sarason, B. R. (eds.), (1996). *Cognitive interference: Theories, methods, and findings.* Mahwah, NJ, Lawrence Erlbaum.

Schinke, S. P., Orlandi, M. A., Gordon, A. N., Weston, R. E., Moncher, M. S., and Parms, C. A. (1990). AIDS prevention via computer-based intervention. *Computers in Human Services* 5:147–156.

Selmi, P. M., Klein, M. H., Greist, J. H., Sorrel, S. P., and Erdman, H. P. (1990). Computer-administered cognitive behavioral therapy for depression. *Am. J. Psychiatry* 147:51–56.

Shoptaw, S., Rawson, R., Blum, M., and Obert, J. (1995). *Outpatient drug treatment for HIV-positive substance abusers.* The Matrix Center, Beverly Hills, CA.

Shulman, G. D. (1989). Experience with the Cocaine Trigger Inventory. *Adv. Alcohol Subst. Abuse* 8:71–85.

Siegel, H. A., Li, L., Leviton, L. C., Cole, P. A., Hook, E. W. III, Bachmann, L., and Ford, J. A. (1999). Under the influence: Risky sexual behavior and substance abuse among driving under the influence offenders. *Sex. Transm. Dis.*26(2):87–92.

UNAIDS. (2003). UNAIDS (2003) AIDS epidemic update, December. Available from http://www.unaids.org/en/default.asp.

Weinhardt, L. S., Kelly, J. A., Brondino, M. J., Rotheram-Borus, M. J., Kirshenbaum, S. B., Chesney, M. A., Remien, R. H., Morin, S. F., Lightfoot, M., Ehrhardt, A. A., Johnson, M. O., Catz, S. L., Benotsch, E. G., Hong, D. S., and Gore-Felton, C. (in press). HIV transmission risk behavior among men and women living with HIV in four U. S. cities. *JAIDS.*

CHAPTER SEVEN

Interventions in Community Settings

Lisa R. Metsch, Lauren K. Gooden, and David W. Purcell

INTRODUCTION

During the first two decades of the AIDS epidemic, HIV prevention messages typically targeted uninfected, at-risk persons with the aim of averting the acquisition of HIV. Recently, public health practitioners have recognized the importance of developing intervention strategies for persons living with HIV to prevent HIV transmission to uninfected persons as well as to protect infected persons from acquiring other STDs or potential reinfection with HIV (CDC, 2003b; Institute of Medicine [IOM], 2001; National Institutes of Health [NIH], 2002). One of the four key strategies outlined in CDC's prevention initiative, "Advancing HIV Prevention: New Strategies for a Changing Epidemic," directs efforts towards preventing new infections by working with persons diagnosed with HIV and their partners (CDC, 2003b). This additional prevention strategy is predicated on the notion that each infection begins with someone already infected and therefore, primary prevention would be strengthened by focusing some of our prevention resources on HIV-positive persons.

Community-based organizations (CBOs), AIDS Service Organizations (ASOs), health departments, and other HIV prevention practitioners are now faced with the challenge of broadening their HIV prevention approach and strategies. How are communities throughout the US responding to this new challenge? Is this really a new phenomenon or have selected communities been addressing prevention with people living with HIV for some time? What types of prevention strategies are being used and are CBOs and health departments replicating interventions that have been shown effective in research? What are the potential barriers and facilitators faced by CBOs and health departments in implementing interventions addressing prevention with people living with HIV? Do these barriers and facilitators vary in different regions or types of communities in the US? What resources are available to assist CBOs, ASOs, and local health departments?

Answers to these questions form the content of our chapter. We begin the chapter with a review of promising interventions designed for people living with HIV that have been rigorously tested in community-settings. Although some of these interventions are discussed in other chapters in this volume, we describe their results from a community perspective. Next, we address the practices, perceived barriers and facilitators, and recommendations for launching prevention strategies in the community for people living with HIV. Our chapter concludes with an overview of resources available to assist CBOs and health departments and provides some overall recommendations.

We rely on multiple sources of data for this chapter. First, we conducted a literature review to identify published behavioral prevention interventions for persons living with HIV that were tested in community settings. Our definition of community-settings is broad and refers to non-HIV medical care settings (discussed in Chapter 8), including CBOs, HIV/AIDS service organizations, health departments, drug treatment and methadone maintenance programs, needle exchange programs, and STD clinics. Second, we conducted telephone interviews with 45 of 52 National Alliance of State and Territorial AIDS Directors (NASTAD) or their designates between December 15, 2003 and January 15, 2004.[1] These individuals direct the HIV/AIDS health care, prevention, education, and supportive services efforts for their state or territory's health departments and often have close contact with many of the CBOs and local health departments in their areas. In some cases, designates selected by the directors were directors of CBOs that have implemented prevention strategies. These interviews were brief (averaging 20 minutes in length) and we asked questions about what CBOs and other agencies in their state or area are currently doing regarding prevention with HIV-positive persons, what are the barriers and facilitators to implementing these interventions, and what recommendations they had for agencies just starting programs for this population.

---

[1] There is a total of 72 NASTAD programs within 60 distinct states and territories. 52 above represents those directors in the 50 states, Washington D.C. and Puerto Rico. Some states have more than one NASTAD member and we combined their interviews. We did not contact NASTAD members outside the US with the exception of Puerto Rico.

In reporting on the responses and suggestions of the NASTAD members we do not identify any specific states; however, when appropriate, we report issues that appear to be particularly relevant for specific types of communities (e.g., rural) or regions of the US. While the responses given in these interviews may not reflect the full range of community-based prevention work that is occurring in specific communities, they do provide some indication of the types of prevention strategies being attempted and the potential barriers and facilitators that have been experienced. The information in this chapter should be viewed as part of an evolving process, as prevention for HIV-positive persons is new in many areas of the country. It is our hope that the information presented here will assist CBOs and other agencies in implementing these intervention strategies in their local areas.

TESTED INTERVENTIONS ADDRESSING PREVENTION FOR PEOPLE LIVING WITH HIV/AIDS

To date, there have only been four behavioral interventions specifically designed for HIV-positive individuals that have been tested, shown to be effective, and published in peer reviewed journals (Kalichman et al., 2001; Rotheram-Borus et al., 2001; Rotheram-Borus, Murphy, et al., 2001; Margolin et al., 2003; Fogarty et al., 2001). The effective interventions vary in their format and duration—three are group interventions and one is a mixed individual and group intervention. Another widely-used intervention is prevention case management, an intensive intervention that combines case management with intensive risk reduction (CDC, 1997a, 1997b, 2003a; Purcell et al., 1998). In addition, there are a number of other interventions for HIV-positive persons now being tested in community settings. Many of these interventions were presented at an NIH/CDC/Health Resources and Services Administration (HRSA)-sponsored meeting focusing on prevention with HIV-positive persons that took place in July, 2003. Brief overviews and information on how far the research has proceeded for each of these interventions can be found at: http://ari.ucsf.edu/policy/pwp_presentations.htm.

Group-Level Interventions for HIV-Positive Persons

Since the beginning of the HIV epidemic in the US, support groups have been one of the most common strategies used by community-based organizations and HIV/AIDS service organizations to meet the psychosocial needs of their HIV-positive clientele. However, very few of these group interventions have been rigorously tested against control groups. In the 1980s and early 1990s, many of the research-based group interventions designed for HIV-positive persons focused on improving mental health, reducing stress, providing social support and skills for coping with HIV rather than on decreasing risk behavior (Blanch et al., 2002; Coates et al., 1989; Lechner, 2003; Perry et al., 1991; Rotheram-Borus et al., 2001a, 2001b). A few of these early studies measured whether this type of program changed risk behaviors. Some found that a support group format was effective in decreasing sexual risk behaviors even though the focus was primarily on mental health and coping (Kelly et al., 1993).

As new, more successful HIV medications began to be used in the late 1990s risk reduction interventions for HIV-positive persons became a major focus of research and programmatic interest. In one study, Kalichman et al., (2001) recruited HIV-positive men and women (74% African American, 22% White and 4% other ethnicities) from AIDS services and infectious disease clinics and randomly assigned them to one of two group-level conditions. The primary intervention consisted of a skills-based behavior-change intervention to reduce HIV-transmission risk that focused on strategies for practicing safer sexual behaviors, developing coping skills, developing skills to maintain safer sex, and enhancing decision-making skills for disclosure of HIV status to families, friends, and sex partners. In developing this intervention, careful consideration was given to establishing relationships with local CBOs, and four HIV-positive individuals from the community were recruited to serve as community consultants (Kalichman et al., in press). The health maintenance, comparison intervention consisted of general group support and health information. Both intervention conditions consisted of five group sessions with two 120-minute sessions per week conducted over a 2.5-week period. The groups were conducted within a community-based organization and co-facilitated by one male and one female facilitator, one of whom was an HIV-positive peer counselor. Six months after the intervention ended, participants who received the cognitive-behavioral intervention reported less unprotected intercourse and greater condom use than did the participants in the comparison group (Kalichman et al., 2001).

It is important to note that this intervention was tested and found successful with gay and bisexual men as well as heterosexual men and women (52% gay, 9% bisexual and 39% heterosexual). Groups were conducted separately by gender and men were also given the option to attend gay/bisexual groups or heterosexual groups. Since demonstrating its effectiveness, this intervention, named *Healthy Relationships*, and the materials necessary to implement it have been compiled into a user-friendly package to facilitate and simplify implementation in community settings. Regional training on *Healthy Relationships* is available through the CDC's Diffusion of Effective Behavioral Interventions (DEBI) Project described in detail later in this chapter.

A second study incorporated prevention efforts into the structure of existing substance abuse treatment programs. Margolin and colleagues (2003) recruited male and female, HIV-positive injection drug users (IDUs, 49% African American, 36% White and 16% Hispanic) who were entering an inner-city methadone treatment program and randomly assigned them to one of two interventions, each of which was embedded within a standard substance abuse treatment program lasting 6 months. Participants in the comparison intervention received daily methadone, weekly individual substance abuse counseling, case management, and a 6 session HIV risk-reduction intervention. The harm-reduction intervention included everything in the comparison condition plus manual-guided group psychotherapy sessions held twice a week for two hours each. The study found that people assigned to the harm-reduction intervention reported lower addiction severity scores at follow-up and were less likely to engage in unprotected sex or needle sharing behaviors. Additionally, of the study participants who had been prescribed antiretroviral medications, significantly more who were assigned to the harm-reduction intervention reported 95% or greater adherence to their medications during the treatment phase of the study than did those in the comparison intervention.

Since demonstrating its effectiveness, the harm reduction intervention and the materials necessary to implement it have been compiled into a user-friendly package entitled, *Holistic Harm Reduction Program (HHRP).* Regional training on the program is also available through CDC's DEBI Project and the intervention manual is available from the researchers at http://info.med.yale.edu/psych/3s/training.html).

Finally, a third intervention, *Teens Linked to Care (TLC),* by Rotheram-Borus and colleagues (Rotheram-Borus et al., 2001a, 2001b) from the University of California at Los Angeles, targeted HIV-positive youth aged 13–24. The TLC intervention is described in detail in Chapter 6. HIV-positive youth were recruited from hospital-based adolescent medical clinics and community-based agencies and assembled into small groups (cohorts), which were then sequentially assigned to an intervention or control condition. The control condition consisted of standard of care at the recruitment sites plus receipt of the intervention at the conclusion of the study. The intervention condition was an intensive 31-session, three-module intervention designed to decrease HIV transmission behaviors, help HIV-positive youth maintain health care regimens and improve their quality of life. The first module (12 sessions), "Staying Healthy," emphasized a strong HIV education component and counseled study participants on coping with HIV. Findings showed an increase in positive coping styles among study participants in various domains as well as improved health outcomes in females (Rotheram-Borus et al., 2001b). The second module (11 sessions), "Act Safe," focused on educating the teens about changing high-risk sexual and drug-using behaviors. Those who attended this intervention reported fewer unprotected sexual acts, fewer sex partners, fewer HIV-negative partners, and less substance abuse (Rotheram-Borus et al., 2001b). The third module (8 sessions), "Being Together" focused on improving quality of life. Those who participated in the intervention condition demonstrated significantly lower levels of emotional distress, physical symptoms of distress, anxiety, and phobic anxiety than did participants in the control condition (Rotheram-Borus et al., 2001a). This intervention was tested effective with youth from various risk groups, although most of the young men (88%) were gay or bisexual. The first two modules were tested among males (72%) and females. Additionally, most (64%) of the youth were minorities (27% African American and 37% Latino). The third module was tested with a subset of these youth.

Since demonstrating the effectiveness of the three modules, the intervention and materials have been compiled into a user-friendly package entitled, *Teens Linked To Care (TLC)*. Regional training on the program is also sponsored by CDC's DEBI Project. Additionally, based on new findings from the study of the three modules and on scientific advances in HIV care, the 31-session intervention has been restructured and shortened to an 18-session intervention. This restructured intervention is entitled *CLEAR: Choosing Life: Empowerment, Action, and Results Intervention for Youth Living with HIV* and can be delivered in either one-on-one telephone sessions or in-person sessions. The manuals for both the *TLC* and *CLEAR* interventions are available from the researchers (http://chipts.ucla.edu).

Individual-Level Interventions for HIV-Positive Persons

Individual-level interventions may be appropriate for persons who require more intensive services than can be provided by a group setting or other prevention settings. Studies that have evaluated the effectiveness of individual-level interventions have reported mixed results. Two studies of individual-level interventions for HIV-positive persons found no differences in risk-reduction behaviors between the intervention group(s) and the comparison group (Patterson et al., 2003; Sorensen et al., 2003). In a study that found no differences in risk reduction between peer-based case management and usual care (Sorenson et al., 2003), the authors proposed that their findings may have been due to the brevity of contact between the peer case managers and the participants, or to the extensive services for HIV-positive persons available in San Francisco which may have made it harder for their intervention to make a difference in the risk behavior of the participants.

In the study of an individual-level intervention with favorable results, Fogarty and colleagues (2001) randomized HIV-positive women (91% African American) recruited from hospital-based and community-based HIV care settings and informal referrals to one of two 6-month interventions. The comparison condition provided comprehensive reproductive health services including health education and counseling on relevant topics. The enhanced condition included comprehensive reproductive health services plus peer advocate services where HIV-positive peer advocates worked with the women individually or in groups to share information on condom use with their primary and secondary partners, and information on contraceptive use. Optional support groups met weekly while individual sessions occurred on an as-needed basis. The women in the enhanced intervention reported improved consistency in condom use, perceived condoms as more advantageous, and increased their level of self-efficacy for condom use at follow-up compared with women in the comparison condition. The authors suggested four reasons for the intervention's success. First, women reported a preference for interacting with HIV-positive peers. Second, there was a close collaboration with case managers and community referral agencies due to the high unmet needs of participants. Third, behavior change messages were tailored to address current motivations, intentions, and partner characteristics. Finally, intervention messages for the peers were reinforced by medical care providers, and most participants were in care.

Prevention Case Management

In some cases, a more intensive intervention may be necessary to meet the specialized needs of HIV-positive persons with multiple medical, social, and economic challenges. Prevention case management (PCM) combines individual HIV risk-reduction with case management to provide intensive on-going support (CDC, 1997a, 1997b, 2003a; Purcell et al., 1998). This intervention is typically reserved for HIV-positive or high-risk HIV-negative persons having or likely to have difficulty initiating or sustaining practices to reduce or prevent HIV transmission (Purcell et al., 1998).

PCM is characterized by highly-trained staff, small case loads, the need to triage clients into services, development and revision of client-specific risk reduction plans, and specific protocols to define the ongoing relationship between PCM and other case management systems. In the fall of 2003, CDC funded nine CBOs as part of a two-year demonstration project to evaluate different models of PCM for HIV-positive persons and make recommendations based on field testing. A variety of documents exist to support agencies in evaluating whether PCM is an appropriate service for their organization and to assist them in developing a PCM program (CDC, 1997a, 1997b; Purcell et al., 1998; San Francisco Department of Public Health, 2000; UCSF, n.d.).

CURRENT PRACTICES REGARDING PREVENTION WITH HIV-POSITIVE PERSONS IN COMMUNITY SETTINGS

While only a handful of states have fully developed prevention programs for HIV-positive persons, our telephone interviews with NASTAD members revealed that most states are beginning to develop a variety of programs and support mechanisms for local CBOs. For example, several states reported having been engaged in prevention with positives work for many years and said that they are well-prepared for CDC's prevention strategy focusing on working with HIV-positive persons. Approximately five states indicated that they have had ongoing efforts focusing on prevention for people living with HIV/AIDS since the mid-1980s. One large state has produced a manual on this topic. Approximately ten states indicated that they have been working in this area for the past five years. All but two of the remaining directors indicated that they were rapidly gearing up for this additional prevention strategy and that efforts had begun in their states. Virtually all the NASTAD members agreed that prevention for people living with HIV/AIDS represented a worthwhile addition to existing prevention activities.

In addition, state directors indicated that their offices were doing a variety of activities to assist CBOs in conducting interventions to address prevention with HIV-positive individuals. The majority indicated that they were engaged in providing training and technical assistance to CBOs in their states. Various topics were addressed in these trainings including HIV treatment education, harm reduction strategies, focused counseling and motivational interviewing, and methods of working with issues associated with disclosure of HIV status to partners. In many cases, NASTAD interviewees spoke about coordinating these training sessions with national training resources offered by CDC (described later in this chapter) and the HRSA-funded AIDS, Education, and Training Centers (AETCs). Many state directors indicated that they were disseminating requests for proposals in the next year that focused on prevention for people living with HIV/AIDS and that they were making this a priority area for funding. Several states indicated that they had established state-wide taskforces to ensure that they receive input on how to best address prevention for HIV-positive individuals. Additionally, there was a strong recommendation that there be heavy involvement of persons living with HIV on these types of taskforces.

Intervention Practices in Community-Based Organizations

Because there are only a handful of interventions that have been tested and shown to be effective for HIV-positive persons, in our telephone interview we were interested in their current use of interventions focusing on prevention with persons living with HIV. We found that there was a wide variety of practices ranging from a few states reporting no efforts targeting HIV-positive persons to some states reporting that CBOs were replicating effective interventions. Many states reported that CBOs were delivering more than one type of intervention.

Prevention Case Management (PCM)

NASTAD interviewees reported that PCM was the most widely used intervention by CBOs, with 32 (71%) of the 45 states/territories implementing this approach. State directors indicated that their offices were receiving a large number of requests from CBOs to receive PCM training and that a majority planned to continue supporting PCM training. Seven directors indicated that there was confusion in their states about how PCM differs from traditional case management. Three states (in low HIV prevalence areas) indicated that PCM was too costly and one state indicated that their CBOs currently relied on licensed psychologists to deliver this intervention. Eight NASTAD members indicated that they felt that PCM was not well-defined. One state director for an area that was funded by CDC as a demonstration site indicated that this funding brought together several agencies and enabled them to receive training and implement PCM in a high quality manner. He also indicated that this experience facilitated staff coming together to enhance networks among staff in this state.

Effective Interventions

Ten (22%) NASTAD directors reported that CBOs in their states were using effective interventions to address prevention for people living with HIV. This number should increase as new funding initiatives from CDC, HRSA, and other federal agencies require CBOs to conduct interventions that have been rigorously tested and published in the peer-reviewed scientific literature. *Healthy Relationships* (Kalichman et al., 2001) was the intervention most frequently reported being used by CBOs in individual states (six states). NASTAD interviewees reported that several CBOs in their states were trying to adapt other effective interventions that had not been specifically designed for persons living with HIV, but were recommended in CDC's Compendium of HIV Prevention Interventions with Evidence of Effectiveness (CDC, 1999). Examples of these interventions include SISTA (DiClemente & Wingood, 1995) for inner city women, Mpowerment (Kegeles et al., 1996) for gay and bisexual men, and VOICES (O'Donnell et al., 1998) for Hispanic and African American heterosexual adults.

Other Group and Individual Interventions

Several states indicated that they were using group (23, 51%) or individual (8, 18%) interventions that had been developed by individual CBOs but had not yet been rigorously evaluated. In some cases, CBOs were conducting interventions that had been tested, but the outcome results were not yet available. Fourteen NASTAD members indicated that many CBOs were frustrated with the limited number of effective interventions available and hoped that more options would be available in the near future.

No Interventions

Only two (4%) directors indicated that there are no current efforts toward implementing prevention interventions for persons living with HIV in their states. Notably, these states are comprised of predominantly rural communities and are located in low HIV prevalence areas. One of these state directors indicated that HIV/AIDS cases are dispersed throughout his state, that most of the communities are between 70 and 100 miles apart, and that transportation is a major barrier to conducting interventions with persons living with HIV. He indicated that there is not a CBO in his state that is willing to coordinate these efforts or to work outside the traditional work hours to travel to clients to conduct such interventions. Another director expressed similar concerns and indicated that no CBO in his state wants to be stigmatized by an association with providing HIV services. The concerns of these rural NASTAD directors are well represented in the literature. Reduced access to HIV medical care as well as mental health and social services is commonly cited as a barrier to receiving care and services for HIV-positive individuals living in rural areas (Rural Center for AIDS/STD Prevention, 2001). Additionally, AIDS-related stigma is another barrier to HIV-positive individuals' access to care in rural communities (Rural Center for AIDS/STD Prevention, 2002; Heckman et al., 1998), so it is not surprising that CBOs providing HIV prevention services in such geographic areas may feel stigmatized as well.

BARRIERS TO IMPLEMENTING PREVENTION WITH PEOPLE LIVING WITH HIV/AIDS

While most of the NASTAD members agreed that prevention with HIV-positive persons was a good intervention strategy, they provided helpful insights into potential barriers that may make implementation of these strategies more difficult. Table 7.1 presents some of the most frequently

Table 7.1. Potential barriers and facilitators to implementing HIV prevention for people living with HIV/AIDS identified by NASTAD interviewees

	N	%
Barriers		
Recruitment and retention of persons living with HIV for interventions	22	49
Stigma and discrimination associated with disclosure		
Focus on prevention given all the other needs of persons living with HIV		
Maintaining confidentiality		
Legal repercussions		
Lack of resources (funding, staff, training)	23	51
Not enough effective interventions available at this time	14	31
Lack of integration between care and treatment	6	13
Facilitators[1]		
Involving persons living with HIV in all aspects of intervention work	12	27
Strong linkages with care settings	11	24
Collaboration with other CBOs and health departments	3	7
Adopting a harm reduction approach	2	4
Using interventions with a holistic approach	3	7
Having a plan to deal with legal issues from the beginning	1	2

[1] Several NASTAD members did not describe facilitators nor give any recommendations for CBOs who were getting started in this area.

mentioned barriers to implementing and conducting prevention interventions with HIV-positive individuals that were raised in the interviews. Previous studies have recognized multiple barriers facing CBOs in implementing evidence-based interventions. These barriers include lack of understanding about what is considered an appropriate evidence-based intervention, limited resources, lack of community readiness, challenges in adapting and tailoring the intervention to meet the needs of the local population, and lack of attention to the technology transfer process (Mitchell et al., 2002).

Recruitment and Retention of Persons Living with HIV for Interventions

NASTAD members expressed various concerns about recruitment and retention of persons living with HIV for interventions. Several members believed that this was a marketing challenge because focusing on prevention for HIV-positive persons may cause persons living with HIV to feel further stigmatized. There were concerns about how to attract people for interventions and how to address fears of disclosure and discrimination. Many states indicated that people still have difficulty with disclosing their status and that many people attend medical care clinics, but beyond that, do not want to be identified as HIV-positive. One state director indicated that an advertised meeting for persons living with HIV would draw attention to a group that already feels alienated and may not want more attention drawn to them. NASTAD members raised uncertainties about the optimal settings in which to conduct interventions. Some mentioned that many CBOs in their areas did not want to host such interventions. This was particularly the case in smaller, rural communities. In one rural state, the NASTAD member indicated that the population is very "fragile" and that someone identified as HIV-positive would be greatly stigmatized. Another state director indicated that people are terrified of acknowledging their HIV status and that it is important to proceed community by community to find support for prevention with positives.

Beyond initially recruiting individuals to interventions, there were concerns about retaining individuals in such interventions. One NASTAD member indicated that the central barrier is the lack of incentives for HIV-positive persons to get them to commit to interventions that are "ongoing, at times intensely personal and challenging." Another NASTAD member felt that some persons living with HIV might not want or be ready to deal with issues of prevention. There was a concern that it was sometimes difficult to focus on prevention given other concerns that often face persons living with HIV. Some of these other concerns may include poverty, caring for other family members with HIV, living with threats of violence, and contending with mental health problems, substance abuse, or other health problems. Some NASTAD members felt that interventions should be more holistic and integrate attention to prevention relating to these other issues. Finally, several NASTAD members expressed concerns about legal repercussions and mentioned various state criminal transmission laws and how this occasionally resulted in persons living with HIV being afraid to disclose their status or to identify their partners. There was a lack of clarity on whether CBOs may be liable if one of their clients deliberately infects others.

Lack of Resources (Funding, Staff, and Training)

Many of the NASTAD members shared concerns about needing more resources and staff to adequately fund CBOs and health departments to implement prevention interventions for people living with HIV/AIDS. Several members noted that they were asked to target a new population and change services while still receiving stable funding. One NASTAD member expressed concern about the lack of funding for medical treatment, particularly the AIDS Drug Assistance Program (ADAP), which pays for medications, and how, without adequate medical care funding, the prevention message seems to get lost. In addition to funding, several states spoke about the challenges in finding qualified intervention staff and peer educators to lead interventions. Again, in small, rural communities, it is often difficult to find individuals willing to come forward and disclose their HIV-positive status, making recruitment of peer educators more challenging in these communities than in larger urban communities.

Not Enough Effective Interventions Available at This Time

Despite numerous efforts to identify effective prevention interventions for HIV-positive individuals several NASTAD members felt that there were not enough interventions addressing prevention with positives to meet the needs of the myriad of target populations throughout the US. Some spoke about continued challenges in trying to adapt effective interventions and the need for additional (instead of stable) resources to do so. One NASTAD member who reported having difficulty with adapting interventions to meet his state's needs said that "it really isn't an inter-vention in a box," and went on to describe the difficulties in replicat-ing effective interventions. Another state director indicated that many CBOs were not comfortable working with curriculum-based programs. Another NASTAD member felt that while many of these interventions were tested in community settings, they were not tested by CBOs and, there-fore, there may be continued challenges in replicating them in real world settings.

Lack of Integration between Prevention and Care

Several NASTAD interviewees noted the lack of integration between prevention and care. One NASTAD member indicated that HIV-positive persons do not want to attend separate locations to receive services for prevention and care. This member felt that more emphasis was needed on incorporating prevention into Ryan White services. Several NASTAD members indicated that CBOs need to better align themselves with health care providers. There was a clear recognition among NASTAD members that care settings provide an ideal location for recruiting persons living with HIV for prevention interventions; however, some felt that preven-tion was often overshadowed by medical care and adherence issues in the primary care setting. This is consistent with other studies that have shown that prevention is often considered secondary to biomed-ical concerns and not a priority in the medical care setting (Duffus et al., 2003; Metsch et al., 2004; Margolis et al., 2001; Marks et al., 1999). Guidelines have been disseminated to assist providers in incorporating prevention strategies into medical settings and the US government is in-creasing resources to support clinical settings in this area (CDC, 2003b; CDC, HRSA, NIH, HIV Medicine Association of the Infectious Diseases Society of America, and HIV Prevention in Clinical Care Working Group, 2004).

Some of the barriers outlined by NASTAD members differed be-tween rural and urban communities. This is not surprising as previous studies have shown rural communities compared with their urban coun-terparts face different barriers to serving people living with HIV (Rural Center for AIDS/STD Prevention, 2001; 2002). Additionally, respondents from rural states reported some of the familiar barriers that have been reported in the HIV literature including geographic distances between pa-tients and providers, conservative political and social values contribut-ing to stigmatization, lack of resources, and concerns about privacy and confidentiality.

FACILITATORS TO IMPLEMENTING PREVENTION WITH PEOPLE LIVING WITH HIV/AIDS

While NASTAD Directors heard from many of their CBOs about barriers to conducting prevention activities for HIV-positive persons, they almost universally supported this expansion of prevention efforts in the US to include prevention with HIV-positive persons. Many NASTAD members also discussed a number of factors that would facilitate the implementation of prevention programs for HIV-positive persons as well as their integration into existing prevention activities. These facilitators of implementation are shown in the lower panel of Table 7.1.

Some NASTAD members felt that CBOs would be able to build on the infrastructures that they have already created to address the HIV prevention needs of HIV-negative individuals while other NASTAD interviewees felt that considerable restructuring of existing programs would be needed. In a recent NASTAD Newsletter article, a NASTAD director from a large state suggested that, "Doing effective prevention with positives may require rethinking traditional prevention strategies from the ground up, as well as committing to restructuring existing programs."(National Association of People Living with AIDS [NAPWA] (2003)). Almost all the interviewees recognized that there was a need to rapidly implement prevention strategies with people living with HIV/AIDS in their state and to assist CBOs in adapting to this new focus. However, several NASTAD members in rural communities commented that it is important to go slowly, to build trust in the community, and to demonstrate that these new efforts are trying to assist people living with HIV and partner with them on this issue rather than trying to further stigmatize or blame them for the spread of HIV/AIDS in their community.

Involving Persons Living with HIV in All Aspects of Intervention Work

The most frequently reported facilitator and recommendation was to partner with people living with HIV in all phases of planning, implementation, and evaluation. The majority of NASTAD members indicated that their state offices had community planning groups and/or advisory groups that are staffed with HIV-positive persons. Many NASTAD members also suggested that intervention staff be HIV-positive and/or very familiar with the needs and concerns of persons living with HIV. One NASTAD member in a high prevalence HIV state indicated that it is a strength to build on the experiences of people living with HIV who do prevention work and are able to bring their stories into their work. This motivates others who haven't gotten into care or who are not engaged in prevention services to do so. Two NASTAD members pointed out that while interventions could be delivered by persons living with HIV, it was very important that intervention staff received extensive training and have experience in counseling and conducting interventions. Notably, many of the interventions that have been shown to be effective and those currently being tested had community advisory boards whose membership included persons living with HIV.

Strong Linkages with Care Settings

The second most frequently reported facilitator was that CBOs and health departments strengthen their relationships with HIV medical care settings as this might be the most efficient setting to recruit persons living with HIV for prevention interventions. This recommendation would directly address the barrier regarding lack of integration between treatment and care previously described. Notably, care settings served as a recruitment site for several of the interventions described in the first part of this chapter.

Using Interventions with a Holistic Approach

Another suggestion was to avoid assuming that all interventions demonstrating success with HIV-negative persons will also be effective with HIV-positive persons, and that in all cases, such interventions should be tailored to meet the needs of persons living with HIV. Several NASTAD members indicated that interventions should be holistic in nature and address the multiple needs of persons living with HIV including coping with HIV, mental health needs, housing, substance abuse, HIV medical care, family issues, and prevention. One state director indicated that it was important to make interventions appealing and to avoid focusing solely on safer sexual behavior.

Adopting a Harm Reduction Approach

Another recommendation was to apply a harm reduction approach to meet people where they are in terms of their readiness to make changes in their sexual and drug use behaviors. One NASTAD member indicated that it was very important to respect individuals' right to have a healthy sex life. Similarly, another NASTAD member indicated that if abstinence is the expectation among sexually active adults, then you will lose people before you start the intervention. A few NASTAD members emphasized the importance of working with syringe exchange programs (in states where they are legal) when serving HIV-positive injection drug users.

Collaboration with Other CBOs and Health Departments

Several NASTAD members said that collaboration between CBOs and their local health department is important. One NASTAD member felt that it was important to recognize that CBOs have differing strengths and that not all CBOs addressing HIV prevention will be suited to address prevention with positives issues. One NASTAD member suggested that it would be helpful to have a master list of CBOs who are currently implementing prevention with positives programs in each state so that CBOs just getting started would have a resource directory from which to seek advice and training.

Having a Plan to Deal with Legal Issues from the Beginning

Finally, one NASTAD member suggested that CBOs should be aware of the legal issues surrounding disclosure of high risk practices. This member also recommended that CBOs have a protocol in place that outlines how they will address these issues when implementing new prevention with positive interventions in their agency.

THE VOICES OF PEOPLE LIVING WITH HIV/AIDS

Many of the facilitators and recommendations made by NASTAD members on implementing and conducting prevention with positives are consistent with the "Principles of HIV Prevention with Positives" developed by the National Association of People Living with AIDS (NAPWA, 2003). Overlapping recommendations, principles or themes include: prevention must be a joint responsibility between those who are HIV-positive and negative; prevention interventions must be appropriately targeted to meet the unique needs of HIV-positive persons; interventions must accept and respect HIV-positive persons' right to intimacy and a healthy sex life; behavior change is challenging for everyone, including people living with HIV/AIDS; stigma and discrimination are alienating and make prevention more difficult for everyone, especially HIV-positive persons; people living with HIV/AIDS must be an integral part of the planning, design, implementation and evaluation of these programs in order for them to be successful. Finally, resources and capacity-building efforts must support the development of programs geared toward HIV-positive and HIV-negative persons in order to effectively respond to the HIV pandemic.

RESOURCES FOR HIV/AIDS PREVENTION TECHNOLOGY TRANSFER AND CAPACITY BUILDING

Nearly all of the NASTAD interviewees reported that CBOs need appropriate guidance and technical assistance to meet the challenges of providing prevention interventions and services to HIV-positive individuals (with or without additional funding). Below, we summarize nationally-available resources for HIV/AIDS prevention technology transfer and capacity building. Additionally, there are resources available from many state and local sources that are not outlined in this chapter. CBOs are urged to work with their state and local health departments in designing and implementing prevention programs for people living with HIV/AIDS.

Replicating Effective Programs (REP)

The CDC's Replicating Effective Programs (REP) initiative highlights science-based behavioral intervention programs that have demonstrated effectiveness in reducing risky behaviors, such as unprotected sex, or in encouraging safer ones, such as using condoms and other methods of practicing safer sex. The REP allows original investigators and other contractors to translate their interventions into common language, packages them into user-friendly kits to make implementation easy, and then tests these packages in CBOs. These kits are designed, developed, and field-tested by researchers collaborating with community-based partners. The end products can guide prevention providers in using effective risk-reduction programs in their own settings and communities. Current REP packages target a variety of populations in a number of community settings, including: health care settings, street venues, homeless shelters, bars, and other places. Some packaged interventions employ one-on-one peer education while others use small group formats (CDC, Replicating Effective Programs Plus, 2004).

Diffusion of Effective Behavioral Interventions (DEBI) for HIV Prevention Project

As part of CDC's ongoing effort to facilitate HIV prevention technology transfer and capacity building, it has established a national-level strategy entitled, "Diffusion of Effective Behavioral Interventions (DEBI) Project." The strategy encompasses providing training and technical assistance to state and community HIV/STD program staff on evidence-based HIV/STD prevention interventions. The Academy for Educational Development's Center on AIDS and Community Health coordinates the project under the guidance of CDC's Divisions of HIV/AIDS Prevention (DHAP).

The interventions for which the DEBI project provides training and technical assistance were tested in studies using research designs that involved intervention and control groups and demonstrated their effectiveness in increasing protective behaviors and positive health outcomes (i.e., using condoms, reducing the number of sex partners and reducing contraction of STDs). To make provision of training and technical assistance and capacity building easier, the interventions and materials necessary for their implementation have been packaged into "user-friendly kits." Some of the packaged interventions generated by the REP program are part of the DEBI Project (CDC Diffusion of Effective Behavioral Interventions Project, 2004).

National Network of STD/HIV Prevention Training Centers (PTCs)

Currently, the CDC funds a group of regional centers, the National Network of STD/HIV Prevention Training Centers (PTCs), across the nation that work in partnership with health departments and universities to provide STD/HIV prevention training to prevention professionals and health providers in the public, private and community sectors. The Network provides training via four core training programs: (a) STD clinical training courses, (b) behavioral and social intervention, (c) partner services and program support training and (d) satellite broadcasts. Four of the 13 centers provide the 2nd core training program, behavioral and social intervention, and they are located in Berkeley, CA; Denver, CO; Dallas, TX; and Rochester, NY. The training provided assists prevention professionals and health providers in developing skills and strategies to help their clients prevent or reduce behaviors that place them at risk for STD or HIV infection. Upon request, some of the courses can be taught in local communities or organized to meet a regional need.

By offering a broad array of courses, the Behavioral and Social Intervention Training Core provides opportunities for STD/HIV prevention professionals and health providers to learn about behavioral science theories and behavior change models, different levels of intervention (individual, group and community), the social context of HIV risk, and provides an overview of prevention issues among individuals living with HIV. The courses also facilitate opportunities for professionals to build and practice skills such as using epidemiological data in program design, conducting program evaluation, and supporting client disclosure of HIV status. Additionally, a number of courses provide hands-on training on the implementation of specific interventions and strategies such as *Community PROMISE* (a community-level STD/HIV behavioral intervention), *Healthy Relationships* (a five-session small-group intervention for HIV-positive men and women, described above), *Prevention Case Management* (described above), *VOICES* (a group-level, single-session video-based intervention designed to increase condom use among heterosexual African-American and Latino men and women who visit STD clinics), social networking, and focus groups (CDC, National Network of STD/HIV Prevention Training Centers, 2001). The CDC is in the process of developing additional courses that are based on its *Compendium of HIV Prevention Interventions with Evidence of Effectiveness (CDC, 1999).*

Behavioral and Social Science Volunteer (BSSV) Program

Through a subcontract with the Academy for Educational Development (AED), the CDC funds another national HIV prevention technical assistance program, the Behavioral and Social Science Volunteer (BSSV) Program. The American Psychological Association (APA) Office on AIDS directs the BSSV Program. The program recruits behavioral and social science volunteers (psychologists, sociologists, anthropologists and public health experts) who are experienced in the science of HIV prevention and how to apply it, teaches them how to work with HIV prevention planners and implementers, and links them to those who request technical assistance. Technical assistance is provided for a range of topics, including: using theory to guide intervention development, identifying elements of effective interventions, adapting efficacious interventions to new settings and new populations, writing grant proposals, evaluating the effectiveness and cost-effectiveness of interventions, evaluating the community planning process, and helping CBOs use evaluation results to improve their HIV programs (Rural Center for AIDS/STD Prevention, 2002).

African American Prevention Intervention Network (APIN) and Positive Prevention Intervention Center (PIC)

The APIN is a nationwide CDC-funded project aimed at helping CBOs with designing, developing, implementing and evaluating interventions. The project is run by the Jackson State University's Mississippi Urban Research Center. The PIC is one component of the APIN and its goal is to increase use of evidence-based prevention interventions for HIV-positive persons of color. To achieve this goal, the PIC identifies effective interventions for dissemination and use by CBOs; adapts effective or "promising" interventions and services to meet the specific needs of HIV-positive persons of color; and provides a range of capacity-building assistance to CBOs and other prevention and care providers who serve HIV-positive persons of color (African American Prevention Intervention Network, n.d.).

The National Native American AIDS Prevention Center (NNAAPC)

This center provides training and capacity building services to American Indian, Alaskan Native and Native Hawaiian tribes and organizations as well as to those who serve these populations to help develop effective HIV and other STD prevention programs (The National Native American AIDS Prevention Center, 2004).

CONCLUSIONS

Clearly, there are a number of national resources to supplement local resources as CBOs and health departments strive to integrate prevention activities for HIV-positive persons into their existing programs. At the end of 2003, CDC announced a new initiative, "Human Immunodeficiency Virus (HIV) Prevention Projects For Community-Based Organizations" to fund HIV prevention projects through cooperative agreements specifically for CBOs. While the addition of prevention for people living with

HIV/AIDS to HIV prevention activities has come with some challenges and barriers, most states and CBOs have stepped up to try to meet the prevention needs of their HIV-positive clients in a thoughtful and respectful manner. As we move into the future, both local and national resources will need to continue to provide support for these efforts and continue to evaluate both technical assistance needs and the capacity building process. In all of these areas, there may be regional differences as well as different challenges for rural versus urban areas. We also need to continue conducting research on prevention interventions with HIV-positive persons, because only through these efforts, can we continue to expand both the breadth and scope of interventions available for this diverse population.

ACKNOWLEDGEMENTS   We would like to thank each University of Miami Socio-Medical Sciences Research Group staff persons who conducted key informant interviews with the NASTAD members: Tamy Kuper, Natalie Wahlay, Laurel Hall, Molly McShane, and Abby Levine. Also, special appreciation is extended to Abby Levine for coordinating the interview process. In addition, we would like to express our gratitude to Thomas Liberti, Chief of the Bureau of HIV/AIDS, Florida Department of Health, for his support and advice regarding these interviews. We would also like to thank Maggie Pereyra for her review and commentary on the chapter. Finally, we extend our utmost gratitude to the NASTAD members for their time in providing us with their honest and thoughtful commentary, which forms the core of this chapter.

REFERENCES

African American Prevention Intervention Network. (n.d.). Retrieved February 9, 2004, from http://www.apinonline.org/
Blanch, J., Rousaud, A., Hautzinger, M., Martinez, E., Peri. J., Andres, S., Cirera, E., Gatell, J., and Gasto, C. (2002). Assessment of the efficacy of a cognitive-behavioral group psychotherapy program for HIV-infected patients referred to a consultation-liaison psychiatry department. *Psychother. Psychosom.* 71:77–84.
Centers for Disease Control and Prevention (2003a). Advancing HIV Prevention: Interim Technical Guidance for Selected Interventions. Available at: http://www.cdc.gov/hiv/partners/Interim_Guidance.htm.
Centers for Disease Control and Prevention (2003b). Advancing HIV Prevention: New Strategies for a Changing Epidemic—US, *MMWR* 52(15):329–332.
Centers for Disease Control and Prevention. (2004, January 13). Diffusion of Effective Behavioral Interventions Project. Available at www.effectiveinterventions.org
Centers for Disease Control and Prevention, HIV/AIDS Prevention Research Synthesis Project. Compendium of HIV Prevention Interventions with Evidence of Effectiveness.

November 1999. Atlanta, GA: Centers for Disease Control and Prevention; Revised, [1-1-4-11].

CDC. HIV prevention case management: Literature review and current practice. (1997a); http://www.cdc.gov/hiv/pubs/pcml/pcml-toc.htm

CDC. HIV prevention case management: Guidance. (1997b); http://www.cdc.gov/hiv/pubs/hivpcmg.htm

Centers for Disease Control and Prevention, National Network of STD/HIV Prevention Training Centers. (2001). Retrieved February 9, 2004, from http://depts.washington.edu/nnptc/

Centers for Disease Control and Prevention. (2004, March 5). Replicating Effective Programs Plus. Retrieved February 9, 2004, from http://www.cdc.gov/hiv/projects/rep/default.htm.

Centers for Disease Control and Prevention, Health Resources and Services Administration, National Institutes of Health, HIV Medicine Association of the Infectious Diseases Society of America, and the HIV Prevention in Clinical Care Working Group. (2004). Recommendations for incorporating human immunodeficiency virus (HIV) prevention into the medical care of persons living with HIV. Clin Inf Dis. 38: 104–121.

Coates, T. J., McKusick, L., Kuno, R., and Stites, D. P. (1989). Stress reduction training changed number of sexual partners but not immune function in men with HIV. Am. J. Public Health 79:885–887.

DiClemente, R. J., and Wingood, G. M. (1995). A randomized controlled trial of an HIV sexual risk-reduction intervention for young African-American women. JAMA 274(16):1271–1276.

Duffus, W., Barragan, M., Metsch, L. R., Krawczyk, C., Loughlin, A., Gardner, L., Mahoney, P., Dickinson, G., and del Rio, C. (2003). Effect of physician specialty on counseling practices and medical referral patterns among physicians caring for disadvantage Human Immunodeficiency Virus-Infected Populations. Clin. Infect. Dis. 36:1577–1584.

Fogarty, L. A., Heilig, C. M., Armstrong, K., Cabral, R., Galavotti, C., Gielen, A. C., and Green, B. (2001). Long-term effectiveness of a peer-based intervention to promote condom and contraceptive use among HIV-positive and at-risk women. Public Health Rep. 116:103–119.

Heckman, T. G., Somlai, A. M., Peters. J., Walker, J., Otto-Salaj, L., Galdabini, and Kelly, J. A. (1998). Barriers to care among persons living with HIV? AIDS in urban and rural areas. AIDS CARE 10(3):365–375.

Institute of Medicine. (2001). No time to lose: Getting more from HIV prevention. National Academy Press, National Academy of Sciences, Washington D.C.

Kalichman, S. C., Rompa, D., Cage, M., DiFonzo, K., Simpson, D., Austin, J., Luke, W., Buckles, J., Kyomugisha, F., Benotsch, E., Pinkerton, S., and Graham, J. (2001). Effectiveness of an intervention to reduce HIV transmission risks in HIV-Positive people. Am. J. Prev. Med. 21(2):84–92.

Kalichman, S.C., Rompa, D., and Cage, M. (in press). Group intervention to reduce HIV transmission risk behavior among persons living with HIV-AIDS. Beh Mod.

Kegeles, S. M., Hays, R. B., and Coates, T. J. (1996). The Mpowerment project: A community-level HIV prevention intervention for young gay men. Am. J. Public Health 86(8):1129–1136.

Kelly, J. A., Murphy, D. A., Bahr, G. R., Kalichman, S. C., Morgan, M. G., Stevenson, Y., Koob, J. J., Brasfield, T. L., and Bernstein, B. M. (1993). Outcome of cognitive-behavioral and support group brief therapies for depressed, HIV-infected persons. Am. J. Psychiatry 150:1679–1686.

Lechner, S. C., Antoni, M. H., Lydston, D., LaPerriere, A., Ishii, M., Devieux, J., Stanley, H., Ironson, G., Schneiderman, N., Brondolo, E., Tobin, J. N., and Weiss, S. (2003). Cognitive-behavioral interventions improve quality of life in women with AIDS. *J. Psychosom. Res.* 54:253–261.

Margolin, A., Avants, S. K., Warburton, L. A., Hawkins, A., and Shi, J. (2003). A randomized clinical trial of a manual-guided risk reduction intervention for HIV-Positive injection drug users. *Health Psychol.* 22(2):223–228.

Margolis, A. D., Wolitski, R. J., Parsons J. T., and Gomez, C. A. (2001). Are healthcare providers talking to HIV-seropositive patients about safer sex? *AIDS* 15(17):2335–2337.

Metsch, L. R., Pereyra, M., del Rio, C., Gardner, L., Duffus, W., Dickinson, G., Kerdnt, P., Anderson-Mahoney, P., Strathdee, S., and Greenburg, A. (2004) The Delivery of HIV Prevention Counseling by Physicians at HIV Medical Care Setting in 4 US Cities. *Am. J. Public Health.* 97, 1186–1192.

Mitchell, R. E., Florin, P., and Stevenson, J. F. (2002). Supporting community-based prevention and health promotion initiatives: developing effective technical assistance systems. *Health Educ. Behav.* 29(5):620–639.

National Association of People Living with AIDS. (2003). *NAPWA's Principles of HIV Prevention with Positives.* NASTAD HIV Prevention Bulletin. December 3, 2003.

National Institutes of Mental Health. (2002). *HIV prevention in treatment settings: US and international priorities.* July 26, 2002 RFA.

The National Native American AIDS Prevention Center. (2004, February 24). Retrieved February 9, 2004, from http://www.nnaapc.org.

O'Donnell, C. R., O'Donnell, L., San Doval, A., Duran, R., and Labes, K. (1998). Reductions in STD infections subsequent to an STD clinic visit: Using video-based patient education to supplement provider interactions. *STD* 25(3):161–168.

Patterson, T. L., Shaw, W. S., and Semple, S. J. (2003). Reducing the sexual risk behaviors of HIV+ individuals: Outcome of a randomized controlled trial. *Ann. Behav. Med.* 25(2):137–145.

Perry, S., Fishman, B., Jacobsberg, L., Young, J., and Frances, A. (1991). Effectiveness of psychoeducational interventions in reducing emotional distress after human immunodeficiency virus antibody testing. *Arch. Gen. Psychiatry* 48:143–147.

Purcell, D. W., DeGroff, A. S., and Wolitski, R. J. (1998). HIV prevention case management: Current practice and future directions. *Health Soc. Work* 23:282–289.

Rotheram-Borus, M. J., Lee, M. B., Murphy, D. A., Futterman, D., Duan. N., Birnbaum, J., and the Teens Linked to Care Consortium. (2001a). Efficacy of a preventive intervention for youth living with HIV. *Am. J. Public Health* 91:400–405.

Rotheram-Borus, M. J., Murphy, D. A., Wight, R. G., Lee, M. B., Lightfoot, M., Swendeman, D., Birnbaum, J. M., and Wright, W. (2001b). Improving the quality of life among young people living with HIV. *Evaluation and Program Planning* 24:227–237.

Rotheram-Borus, M. J., Lee, M. B., Gwadz, M., and Draimin, B. (2001c). An intervention for parents with AIDS and their adolescent children. *Am. J. Public Health* 91:1294–1302.

Rural Center for AIDS/STD Prevention. (2001). *Fact Sheet: Mental Health Needs of HIV-Infected Rural Persons.* Bloomington, Indiana. (February 9, 2004); http://www.indiana.edu/~aids.

Rural Center for AIDS/STD Prevention. (2002). *Fact Sheet: AIDS and Sexually Transmitted Diseases in the Rural South.* Bloomington, Indiana. (February 9, 2004); http://www.indiana.edu/~aids.

San Francisco Department of Public Health. (2000). *HIV prevention case management: Standards and guidelines for the delivery of services in San Francisco.* Available from: Project Director, Prevention Case Management Standardization and Evaluation Project, AIDS Office, San

Francisco Department of Public Health, 25 Van Ness Ave. Suite 500, San Francisco, CA 94102, (415) 554–9031.

Sorensen, J. L., Dilley, J., London, J., Okin, R. L., Delucchi, K. L., and Phibbs, C. S. (2003). Case management for substance abusers with HIV/AIDS: a randomized clinical trial. *Am. J. Drug Alcohol Abuse* 29(1):133–150.

University of California, Los Angeles, Center for HIV Identification, Prevention, and Treatment Services. *CLEAR Choosing Life: Empowerment, action, results intervention for youth living with HIV.* [Fact Sheet]. UCLA Web site; (February 9, 2004); http://chipts.ucla.edu/projects/chipts/clear.html

UCSF. AIDS Policy Research Center. Prevention with Positives Resources. http://ari.ucsf.edu/policy/pwp.html

CHAPTER EIGHT

Interventions in Clinical Settings

Susan M. Kiene, Jeffrey D. Fisher,
and William A. Fisher

INTRODUCTION

Clinicians are uniquely well-positioned to promote health behavior change. Patients view their physicians as trusted sources of health information (Cohen, et al., 1994; Gerbert, et al., 1991; Glynn et al., 1990) and physicians generally accept health promotion and disease prevention as part of their professional role (Gemson et al., 1991; Makadon and Silin, 1995). The doctor-patient conversation is a "teachable moment" during which the patient may be particularly receptive to discussing strategies for maintaining or improving his or her health (Barzilai et al., 2001). Indeed, there is ample evidence that even a brief intervention initiated by the doctor can produce significant behavior change (Calfas et al., 1998; Nawaz et al.,1999; U.S. Department of Health and Human Services, 2000; U.S. Preventive Services Task Force, 1996).

Nonetheless, physicians engage in low rates of health behavior change counseling (CDC, 1997; Metsch et al., 2004; Nawaz et al. 1999, 2000). The health risk behaviors that have the greatest impact on public health, such as tobacco, recreational drugs, and alcohol use, are addressed in fewer than 50% of cases in which physician-delivered intervention would be appropriate (Coffield et al., 2001). Some of the disincentives to physician-delivered prevention interventions, such as the fact that prevention activities are generally not reimbursable by health insurance are possibly insurmountable (Makadon and Silin, 1995). Other barriers, such as time constraints and lack of specialized prevention training, have been addressed in the development of effective interventions that require little time to implement and equip physicians with necessary training for doing so.

In this chapter, we discuss the concept of clinician-delivered behavior change interventions aimed at promoting risk-reduction among people living with HIV/AIDS. Here, "risk behavior" will refer to either unprotected sex or the sharing of unsterilized needles during intravenous drug use—in either case, behaviors which place uninfected individuals at risk for HIV infection or that expose the HIV positive individual to other infections which, due to the HIV positive individual's compromised immune system, can have a serious impact on his or her health and quality of life (Johansen and Smith, 2002; Terrault, 2002; Janssen et al., 2001).

In making the case that using the clinical setting holds enormous potential for delivering HIV prevention interventions to HIV positive persons, the formidable personal, interpersonal, and institutional barriers that stand in the way of this type of intervention will also be considered. Means of overcoming these barriers that have been effectively applied in clinical practice will be identified. Finally, specific interventions that show promise as vehicles for clinician-delivered HIV prevention for HIV positive persons in clinical care will be highlighted.

HIV RISK BEHAVIOR AMONG PEOPLE LIVING WITH HIV/AIDS IN CLINICAL CARE

If one examines only HIV positive individuals who are receiving regular clinical care, roughly 15% continue to engage in unprotected anal or vaginal sex with HIV negative partners or partners of unknown serostatus (Fisher et al., in press; Weinhardt et al., 2004). Twenty-three percent of HIV positive patients in Fisher et al.'s study reported some form of sexual risk behavior in the prior three months, 4% reported sharing used needles or works with others, and 14% reported sexual risk behavior with a partner of HIV negative or unknown serostatus. Weinhardt et al. found, in a survey conducted in four major US cities, that 19% of HIV positive women, 16% of HIV positive men who have sex with men (MSM), and 13% of HIV positive heterosexual men reported engaging in unprotected sex with one or more HIV negative or unknown serostatus partners and 18% of IDUs reported sharing their used needles and works with others.

An additional study, which did not indicate whether unprotected sex occurred with seroconcordant or serodiscordant partners, offers data on the incidence of unprotected sex among HIV positive individuals in clinical care. In a sample of HIV positive men and women living in California, 34% reported having vaginal or anal sex without a condom at least once in the prior 3 months, and among those with two or more partners, 52% reported unprotected anal or vaginal sex (Richardson et al., 2004). The incidence of risk behavior reported in this study is comparable to rates of risky sexual behavior observed among HIV positive individuals outside of care settings.

PRIORITY TO DEVELOP INTERVENTIONS FOR HIV POSITIVE ADULTS

The task of developing, implementing, and evaluating effective and easy to disseminate behavior change interventions to promote safer sex and drug injection practices in HIV positive individuals has been designated a critical priority at this point in the HIV epidemic (CDC, 2003; NIH Consensus Panel, 1997). In response, effective HIV prevention interventions targeted at HIV positive persons have been tested (e.g., Fisher et al., 2004; Kalichman et al., 2001b; Patterson et al., 2003). However, there are very few HIV prevention interventions for persons living with HIV that have been developed specifically for delivery in the clinical care setting (Kelly and Kalichman, 2002).

The CDC (2003) has recommended that HIV prevention be integrated into routine clinical care for HIV positive persons. The US Department of Health and Human Services (1990), the Preventive Services Task Force of the American Medical Association (1990, 2000), and the American College of Physicians (1994) have joined in calling for clinicians to play a central role in promoting HIV prevention.

There is broad agreement that the clinician is well-situated to promote risk reduction among HIV positive individuals. Indeed, the clinical setting provides opportunities for repeated delivery of prevention intervention doses and there is perhaps no better venue for gaining as nearly universal access as is possible to the population of HIV positive individuals who are capable of transmitting infection to others. Due to the significant proportion of HIV positive individuals receiving clinical care, the obvious need to reach these individuals with effective interventions, and the repeated contact and established relationship that often exist between HIV positive patients and their providers, the clinical care setting is a promising setting in which to develop, test, and disseminate widely HIV prevention interventions for HIV positive individuals.

BARRIERS TO HIV PREVENTION
IN CLINICAL SETTINGS

Individual, interpersonal, and structural barriers may stand in the way of consistent provision of clinician-delivered HIV prevention interventions. Clinicians may receive little or no training in primary prevention techniques in medical school or clinical training (Calabrese et al., 1991; Makadon and Silin, 1995; McDaniel et al., 1995), and consequently lack skills necessary for this task (Calabrese et al., 1991; Valente et al., 1986). In addition, some clinicians believe their behavioral intervention attempts are generally unsuccessful (Gemson et al., 1991; Valente et al., 1986), although the literature suggests that, in fact, clinicians can be quite successful in such activities (e.g., Calfas et al., 1998; Ockene et al., 1990; Werch et al., 1996).

Physicians may also believe that their offering unsolicited prevention advice will provoke a negative reaction from the patient (Kottke et al., 1993). This belief, however, appears to be untrue. There is data to suggest that offering prevention advice may actually increase patient satisfaction (Barzilai et al., 2001). In a survey of health maintenance organization patients, a startling 92% to 98% of respondents expected help and advice regarding their health-related behavior (Vogt et al., 1998).

Even though national organizations urge practitioners to provide age-appropriate HIV/STD prevention counseling to all of their patients, compliance with this guideline is low. By some reports, fewer than 50% of providers comply. Physician discomfort with physician-patient discussion of sexuality is the most widely-cited reason for avoiding this topic in clinical care settings (Dodge et al., 2001). It is therefore unsurprising that only between 53% and 77% of physicians ever mention safer sex to their HIV positive patients (see Table 8.1), and active efforts on the part of the clinician to influence HIV risk behavior among HIV positive individuals are rare (Makadon and Silin, 1995; Marks et al., 2002; Morin et al., 2003).

Table 8.1. HIV-positive patients receiving safer-sex messages from their primary physician

% received safer-sex message	Period	N	Source
53%	6 mo.	618	Morin et al., 2003
67%	ever	839	Marks et al., 2002
68%	ever	577	Richardson et al. 2004
76.7%	ever	223	Margolis et al., 2001

Note: all data based on patient self-reports.

Discomfort with the topics of sexuality and drug use is, in part, the result of the clinician's perception that patients will respond negatively to discussion of these topics. However, this concern appears to be unwarranted. By their own accounts, patients are comfortable discussing sexual and drug use issues with their clinicians (Ward and Sanson-Fisher; 1995; Wheat et al., 1993) and regard physicians as their preferred source of HIV prevention counseling (Hazard, 1993). Providers' discomfort with sexual and drug use topics can be alleviated through training, particularly through role-playing and receiving feedback on interpersonal interactions (Epstein et al., 1998).

One approach to understanding personal barriers that may affect a physician's willingness to engage in HIV risk-reduction communications is to examine what physicians do talk about. HIV specific patient-provider discussions are more likely to cover the importance of adhering to antiretroviral medications, the patient's emotional status, diet and nutritional information, and cigarette smoking—all areas that capitalize on the typical physician's core competencies and existing referral resources—than they are the issue of HIV risk reduction. The substance of an HIV risk reduction discussion with providers also varies; in a 6-month period, 24% of patients reported discussing prevention issues in conjunction with discussion of specific sexual activities, 24% reported discussing the issue of disclosing one's HIV status to sexual partners, 27% were provided with HIV prevention reading materials, and only 7% reported having discussed the proper use of condoms (Morin et al., 2003).

The likelihood that a physician will discuss the importance of disclosing one's serostatus with potential sexual partners is particularly variable, even though this topic clearly belongs in a discussion of HIV risk reduction. According to Marks et al. (2002), the frequency with which patients receive advice about disclosure can vary from 31% to 78% between clinics. In research by Richardson et al. (2004), only 45% of HIV positive patients had been involved in a discussion of disclosure with their physicians (see Chapter 3).

It is clear that discussing with patients the importance of disclosing their HIV status to sexual partners is highly sensitive. Indeed, an HIV positive individual who discloses his or her serostatus may be vulnerable to abandonment by a partner or, in the case of women in particular, be subject to physical violence (Kalichman and Nachimson, 1999). Justifiably, physicians who lack referral resources or are not equipped to deal with the ramifications—psychological or otherwise—if a patient were to follow their recommendation may not make the recommendation in the first place (Temple-Smith et al., 1996). This highlights the importance of both training and providing an appropriate referral infrastructure. Alternatively, a provider who is sensitized to this issue through training can provide counseling strategies—such as encouraging consistent condom use—that may provide alternatives to HIV positive individuals who do not disclose their HIV serostatus to their partner.

Physicians may also avoid topics which cause them personal discomfort or that they find objectionable; heterosexual physicians may be unwilling to discuss specific sexual behaviors with their homosexual patients (Fisher et al., 1988; Wilson and Kaplan, 2000). Resident physicians' homophobia and aversion to IDUs can negatively impact the level of care that his or her patients receive (Yedidia and Berry, 1999). Ironically, disapproval of a patient with an STD who engages in unsafe sex may lead physicians to avoid raising the topic of preventive behavior with that patient (Temple-Smith et al., 1996).

Fortunately, physicians' attitudes toward treating persons with HIV can be improved through education (Makadon and Silin, 1995). Once the physician is encouraged to adopt a collaborative role in the care of his/her patient, working within this role reduces the power differential in the relationship and sensitizes the physician to the individuality of his/her patient. According to Fiske (2000), the increased salience of the individual needs and identity of the patient can directly mitigate the impact of group stereotypes on the doctor's attitudes toward the patient. According to Dovidio and Gaertner (1999), the establishment of a collaborative doctor-patient relationship can reduce prejudice by recategorizing the patient—instead of being a member of a stigmatized group, the patient becomes in a real sense a peer whose opinions and agreement are prerequisites for achieving shared treatment goals. There is, moreover, a willingness on the part of physicians to confront these personal issues if there is a benefit in terms of their interactions with their patients; 87% of physicians in one report indicated that they would welcome professional training to help increase their own comfort in caring for HIV positive patients (CDC, 1994).

More broadly, physicians vary with respect to their general interpersonal skills. This can present a barrier to the effective communication of health-related information; again, interventions exist which train physicians to ask questions more effectively and ensure that their patients have understood what they have been told (Stewart, 1995).

There are also very important structural barriers to clinician-delivered prevention work in clinical care settings. Currently, the mean duration of a doctor's visit in the US is 16 minutes (Blumenthal et al., 1999), and limitations are placed on physicians with respect to the time and resources they can devote to each patient (Calfas et al., 1998; Dietrich et al., 1994; Dickey and Kamerow, 1996; Makadon and Silin, 1995).

Admittedly, there is little that practitioners can do to overcome some of these structural barriers. The strongest case for optimism may come from recognizing that a growing body of data in the last 15 years lends powerful support to the benefits of preventive medicine, and these data may yet influence policy-makers. And, as will be seen, the time constraint on providers does not rule out the possibility of such interventions. It does, however, underscore the necessity that clinician-delivered interventions be brief in duration.

EFFECTIVENESS OF PREVENTION INTERVENTIONS IN CLINICAL SETTINGS

Although behavioral counseling by physicians does not have the same level of efficacy as specialized interventions delivered by behavior change specialists, this limitation is offset by the fact that physicians have far greater access to the general population. Taking the case of smoking cessation, physician-delivered interventions result in cessation in 5–10% of cases whereas specialists produce behavior change in 40% of cases. However, specialists only encounter the 3 to 5% of highly motivated smokers who volunteer for treatment, whereas physicians have access to 70% of the at-risk population. Hence, the potential impact of physicians on health behavior change, calculated as Impact = (Participation Rate × Efficacy), is substantially greater than that produced by behavioral specialists (Whitlock et al., 2002). Moreover, even those patients who do not exhibit behavior change following a discussion with their doctor may be more attentive to pertinent health education material that they subsequently encounter (Kreuter et al., 2000).

For a clinician-delivered prevention intervention to be successful, it is neither practical nor necessary for the provider to receive extensive training in psychological assessment and counseling. This is evidenced in a number of studies of clinician-delivered interventions, many of them quite brief and involving limited training, that have yielded favorable outcomes in terms of patient behavior change in the areas of exercise promotion (Calfas et al., 1998; Long et al., 1996), decreasing alcohol use (Werch et al., 1996), hypertension control (Grueninger et al.,1989), coronary risk reduction (Scales et al., 1998), seatbelt use, weight loss, breast self-examination (see review by Logsdon et al., 1989), and STD treatment adherence (Montesinos et al., 1990). Clinician-delivered interventions have also been shown to be effective in combating tobacco use, even though it is an addictive and notoriously intractable behavior (Kottke et al., 1992; Klein et al., 1995; Morgan et al., 1998; Ockene et al., 1990; US Department of Health and Human Services, 2000).

The opportunity for repeated contact with the target population can greatly increase the effectiveness of a behavior change intervention. Some of the demonstrated benefits of repeated contact include, (a) the opportunity for the change-agent to remind individuals of previously established goals (Whitlock et al., 2002), (b) the fine-tuning of goals and the provision of new strategies for change as the individual's circumstances change (Mandelblatt and Kanetsky, 1995; Morgan et al., 1998), (c) the repeated administration of rewards, such as praise, for the individual's successes (Whitlock et al., 2002), and, perhaps most importantly, (d) repeated contact, as assessed by the duration of the relationship, is one of the most reliable predictors of the level of trust a patient has in his or her provider (Wilson and Kaplan, 2000).

Because their health status requires regular monitoring, HIV positive individuals typically have regular, frequent contact with clinicians. These circumstances facilitate the development of a special relationship of trust between HIV positive patients and their clinicians (Gabel et al., 1994; Makadon and Silin, 1995; O'Connor et al., 1994), and led Gabel et al. (1994) to call secondary prevention of HIV transmission, via intervention with HIV positive patients, the "special province" of clinicians.

Intervention Targets Associated with HIV Risk Behavior Change

Before effective clinician-delivered HIV prevention interventions for persons living with HIV can be designed, it is necessary to understand the dynamics of HIV risk behavior among HIV positive persons.

The current analysis applies the Information-Motivation-Behavioral Skills Model of preventive behavior (IMB; Fisher and Fisher, 1992) and related research findings (e.g., review by Crepaz and Marks, 2002) to conceptualize the determinants of safer and risky sexual behavior among HIV positive persons, and to identify elements of effective prevention interventions for this population.

The IMB model provides a blueprint, identifying a set of empirically established common factors underlying a broad range of health behaviors. This model is applied by particularizing these common factors within the context of a given health behavior—a process referred to as elicitation research. For example, it is understood that, in a general sense, social norms influence the adoption of a health behavior. One goal of elicitation research is to understand and assess specific social norms governing the enactment of the behavior in a given community and leverage this knowledge to promote behavior change in that community. An intervention is designed encompassing all of the common factors identified by the IMB model, followed by rigorous intervention outcome evaluation. The

IMB model of health behavior change has been utilized in understanding HIV risk dynamics and designing HIV risk behavior change interventions in many populations, and recently has served as the basis for designing clinician-initiated interventions to promote safer sexual behavior among HIV positive persons in clinical care settings (Fisher et al., in press, 2004).

According to the IMB model, *information* that is directly relevant to HIV preventive behavior is a prerequisite of preventive action. For HIV positive persons, such information can include specific facts about HIV transmission and about HIV prevention. Information, in the IMB model, also includes HIV prevention heuristics and implicit theories of risk—simple, often incorrect, inferences based on physical appearance or cursory behavior concerning a partner's HIV status and about whether or not to engage in HIV preventive behavior with them—that may contribute to risk behavior.

Even though most HIV positive individuals have accurate HIV trans-mission information, some information deficits are relatively prevalent. In our own elicitation work, drawing on a sample of HIV positive indi-viduals in clinical care, 35% of patients thought that antiretroviral (ARV) therapy was a cure for HIV (Fisher et al., in press). We also found evidence of information heuristics that are likely to precipitate risky sexual behav-ior: 47% of HIV positive patients thought that someone who was willing to have unprotected sex with them is probably already HIV positive, and 40% thought that people who spend time in sexual "cruising" areas or in shooting galleries are most likely HIV positive. These heuristics and implicit theories—have been found to be associated with unprotected sex among people living HIV/AIDS (Kalichman, 1999; Kalichman et al., 1998; Kalichman et al., 2001a; Marks et al., 1999; Vanable et al., 2000; van der Straten et al., 2000).

It may seem obvious that behavior change can only occur if an HIV positive person has adequate HIV prevention information. However, bar-riers to clinician-initiated prevention intervention, discussed earlier, such as discomfort with sexuality, specifically impact the delivery of informa-tion. Hence, there is a clear value in systematizing the delivery of tailored, pre-defined information to patients. The effective delivery of information distinguishes effective clinician-delivered interventions from those which have less impact on patient behavior (Makadon and Silin, 1995; Whitlock et al., 2002). Fortunately, the clinic setting provides numerous complemen-tary channels for the communication of information; these include tai-lored or reinforcing prevention messages provided by multiple health care personnel (e.g., physicians, nurses, pharmacists), referrals to prevention specialists, computer information systems, videos, and voice response sys-tems (Whitlock et al., 2002).

According to the IMB model, *motivation* to engage in HIV preventive acts is a second critical determinant of HIV preventive behavior and determines whether even knowledgeable HIV positive persons will be inclined to act on what they know about HIV prevention. HIV prevention motivation includes HIV positive individuals' personal motivation to practice HIV preventive behaviors and their social motivation to engage in HIV prevention (Fishbein and Ajzen, 1975; Fisher et al., 1995). In one sample of HIV positive MSM, 41% of respondents reported that they did not use a condom because their partner did not wish to do so, while 27% who used condoms did so because of their partner's desire to practice safer sex (Fisher et al., 1998).

Among HIV positive individuals in clinical care, attitudes toward using condoms with casual and steady partners of HIV positive, HIV negative, or unknown HIV status were relatively positive and similar across partner types and serostatus of partners, with approximately 80% of persons indicating that always using condoms with different kinds of partners would be either *good* or *very good*. Normative support for condom use and intentions to use condoms in the future was similarly relatively high, but attitudes towards abstaining from sex were much less positive (Fisher et al., in press).

Beyond these findings, negative attitudes about condoms or safer sex, a hedonistic focus on short-term pleasure, and the desire to avoid thinking about one's own HIV status, are associated with HIV positive individuals' failure to engage in prevention behavior (de Vroome et al., 1998; Fisher et al., 1998; Hays et al., 1997; Kline et al., 1994). When individuals lack a firm intention to engage in HIV preventive behavior, such behavior is less likely to occur (Darrow et al., 1998; de Vroome et al., 1998; Godin et al., 1996), and this has been observed among HIV positive individuals (Fisher et al., 1998).

In the clinician-patient dialog, motivation can be developed by including the patient in the decision-making process, facilitating the patient's self-assessment of his or her own risk behavior, eliciting the patient's own reasons for considering behavior change, and reinforcing positive health behaviors where they occur (Miller and Rollnick, 1991; Rollnick et al., 2000; Morgan et al., 1998), as well as by establishing clearly defined and achievable prevention goals with the patient that provide the patient with the highest likelihood of having a success experience (Paauw and O'Neill, 1990).

In addition to HIV prevention information and HIV prevention motivation, the IMB model identifies HIV prevention *behavioral skills* as a third prerequisite of HIV preventive behavior which determine whether even well-informed and well-motivated individuals will be capable of practicing prevention effectively. The behavioral skills component of the IMB model is composed of an individual's objective ability, and perceived self-efficacy, with respect to performing HIV preventive behaviors that are involved in effective prevention practice (Bandura, 1989, 1994; J. Fisher and Fisher, 1992; Kelly and St. Lawrence, 1988).

For HIV positive individuals, behavioral skills involved in HIV prevention can include objective and perceived abilities to obtain condoms or clean needles, engage in anticipatory planning (for example, carrying condoms or keeping condoms available), negotiate and maintain abstinence from unprotected intercourse, disclose antibody status, to engage in consistent condom use or safer needle use behaviors, and do so in a fashion that disrupts valued relationships and valued outcomes as minimally as possible. Drawing again from data collected from our sample of HIV positive respondents, we found that a significant minority of participants perceived that using condoms with sexual partners would be difficult. Between 25% - 30% of participants said it would be *hard* or *very hard* to always use condoms with an HIV positive partner, compared to 23% to 26% for using condoms with an HIV negative partner and 24% to 26% for using condoms with an unknown HIV status partner (Fisher et al., in press).

Finally, psychosocial factors such as reliance on an avoidant coping style (e.g., denial, alcohol consumption, or mentally disengagement from the problem; Clement, 1992; Semple et al., 2000a, 2000b), depression (Crepaz and Marks, 2002; Kalichman, 2000), and personality factors such as impulsiveness (e.g., Semple et al., 2000a), sexual compulsivity (Hays et al., 1997; Kalichman et al., 1997), and possibly the fear of victimization by an abusive intimate partner (Kalichman and Nachimson, 1999) are also related to continued risk behavior among people living with HIV. These issues demonstrate the importance of a holistic approach to treatment, in which the resolution of pressing psychosocial issues may have to take place prior to initiating a discussion of HIV transmission risk reduction. The resolution of these issues is facilitated by having in place a comprehensive referral infrastructure.

Linking HIV Prevention with HIV Clinical Care

At present, several clinic-based interventions designed to help reduce HIV risk behavior among HIV positive individuals are being implemented and tested. These interventions are summarized below. Because these interventions represent a new area of research, outcome data are not yet available in every case.

The Healthy Living Project

The Healthy Living Project (Rotheram-Borus et al., 2003) is a multi-site intervention conducted in San Francisco, New York, Los Angeles, and Milwaukee that involves HIV positive individuals from across risk groups (study in progress at the time of this writing). Patients are recruited for the intervention at clinical care sites and either HIV positive peers or counselors deliver the 15 sessions comprising the intervention. The material covered in these 90 minute sessions include the following coping, obtaining social support (motivation), communicating effectively, and maintaining optimal health through ARV adherence and other healthy lifestyle behaviors. Of particular interest, HIV risk reduction behavioral skills are also included; specifically, training related to safer sexual behaviors, serostatus disclosure, sexual communication skills, and maintaining safer behavior. Finally, the intervention includes a structure for providing referrals for patients to outside services, such as drug abuse treatment, when necessary. This intervention represents a model suited for case management services. Should the intervention demonstrate effectiveness, its time- and labor-intensive character could pose a barrier to widespread dissemination outside of case management at the same time that it might represent a particularly useful focused and intensive approach for patients who face special challenges with respect to HIV prevention.

Partnership for Health

The Partnership for Health (Richardson et al., 2004) intervention was developed in part to implement the findings of Rothman and Salovey (1997) and others, who have shown that "framed" messages highlighting either the benefits of performing an advocated health behavior or the personal costs of not performing the behavior are differentially effective depending on specific aspects of the health behavior. This intervention asks healthcare providers to deliver an HIV prevention intervention to HIV positive patients. Providers briefly address HIV risk-reduction behaviors during each clinic visit. Each of these discussions lasts between 3 and 5 minutes and includes HIV prevention information, motivation content, and to a lesser extent behavioral skills content. Topics include: protecting one's personal health, protecting sexual partners, and disclosure of serostatus to sexual partners. This intervention was delivered at 6 HIV outpatient clinics throughout California. In two experimental conditions, providers communicated prevention messages using either an advantages (gain) frame, highlighting the benefits of engaging in the behavior, or a consequences (loss) frame, highlighting the adverse outcomes of not engaging in the behavior. Participants in the control group received an adherence to medication intervention. Providers were trained in the intervention protocol through a 4-hour training session. Intervention efficacy was evaluated at 7 months post-intervention and it was found that the loss framed intervention was effective at reducing unprotected anal or vaginal sex among MSM reporting two or more partners at baseline, compared to the control arm. However, no effects were found for participants who had only one partner at baseline.

MD 4 Life

The MD 4 Life project enlists clinical care providers to deliver an HIV risk reduction intervention for HIV positive persons (Lightfoot et al., 2004). Patients complete a 20-minute computer-assisted HIV risk behavior assessment during each clinical care visit (approximately every 3 months for 2 years) while waiting to see their clinician. Clinics are randomly assigned to either a computer-delivered intervention condition or a clinician-delivered intervention condition. Both variations are roughly based on Motivational Interviewing (MI) techniques (Miller and Rollnick, 1991) and are brief, each session lasting 5 to 15 minutes. Participants in the computer-delivered intervention receive automated feedback regarding the concordance between their self-reported values and HIV risk behavior. For example, if a patient indicates that responsibility is important to him/her, but reports high-levels of risk behavior, the feedback generated would be that potentially infecting others with HIV is not being responsible, emphasizing the discordance between the patient's values and his/her actions (motivation).

The computer also compares the patient's risk behaviors over time, provides suggestions for how a patient might change his/her behavior, and solicits an intention to reduce HIV risk behaviors. Similarly, in the provider-delivered intervention, clinicians give patients feedback on their risk behaviors in relation to the patients' self-reported values, provide behavior change recommendations, and reinforce patients' self-efficacy to change their behavior. The efficacy of these interventions to reduce HIV risk behavior among HIV positive individuals was being tested at the time of this writing.

Methadone Maintenance Programs

Another way to link HIV risk reduction with clinical care is through methadone maintenance programs. Inasmuch as injection drug users

(IDU's) are a high-risk group for HIV transmission, this is a logical avenue for gaining access to HIV positive individuals who are IDU. A recent clinical trial of HIV risk reduction interventions for HIV positive IDUs in methadone maintenance compared a standard methadone maintenance program that included an HIV risk reduction intervention based on the IMB model with the same intervention, supplemented by cognitive remediation strategies delivered in psychotherapy to enhance the ability of participants to learn and remember the intervention content (Margolin et al., 2003).

Individuals in the cognitive behavioral condition received usual methadone maintenance treatment and also participated in a 6-session HIV risk reduction intervention. Intervention content included HIV risk reduction information (including information about where to obtain condom and needle cleaning supplies, and where to exchange used needles), feedback designed to increase behavior change motivation, skills building activities to teach patients how to clean needles with bleach and how to correctly use condoms, safer sex negotiation skills, and an emphasis on teaching others in their social group about HIV risk reduction strategies and skills. Individuals in the cognitive-behavioral intervention plus psychotherapy condition participated in the 6-session intervention and attended, in addition, 2-hour long group therapy sessions twice per week for 6 months. These sessions were intended to reinforce the content of the risk reduction intervention and provide additional emotional support using cognitive remediation strategies (Miller, 1993).

The results of this clinical trial demonstrated that while both cognitive and behavioral skills model-based interventions reduced high-risk sexual and drug use behavior comparing baseline data to 3-month post-intervention follow-up, the risk reduction plus group therapy intervention was the more effective of the two (Margolin et al., 2003). These findings suggest that HIV risk reduction interventions for HIV positive individuals may benefit from providing additional support and services to help patients deal with the challenges of living with HIV and IDU. However, an alternative explanation is that because there was greater intervention dosage in the enhanced intervention, this is responsible for the greater efficacy of the supplemented intervention.

The Options Project

The Options Project is a clinician-delivered HIV risk reduction intervention for HIV positive individuals and is based on the IMB model of health behavior change (Fisher et al., in press, 2004). In the following section, detail will be provided on the development, implementation, and preliminary results of this project.

The Options Project is the result of applying the IMB model to understand the dynamics of HIV risk behavior among HIV positive individuals, developing an appropriate intervention, and assessing its outcomes. This intervention was specifically crafted to be administered to HIV positive individuals in clinical care, in order to exploit the advantages of this setting enumerated earlier. To understand risk dynamics among HIV positive patients and to design an intervention that providers would be comfortable implementing and that patients would feel comfortable *receiving*, we first conducted elicitation research with providers and with patients (described above, Fisher et al., in press).

The Options Intervention. The Options Project intervention, in brief, consists of clinicians addressing specific gaps, identified in elicitation research, in their HIV positive patients' HIV prevention information, motivation, and behavioral skills. Patient motivation to practice safer sex was enhanced using principles of MI (Rollnick et al., 2000); this approach, which has been shown to be effective in brief health behavior change interventions (Miller and Rollnick, 1991; Rollnick et al., 2000), mobilizes the patient's own competencies and behavior change goals in the context of shared decision-making between clinician and patient.

The Options Project intervention occurs on an ongoing basis and is delivered on repeated occasions over the course of HIV positive patients' clinical care. During each routine HIV care visit, a collaborative, patient-centered discussion takes place between clinician and patient. The clinician uses MI techniques to (a) introduce the topics of safer sex and safer needle use, (b) assess the patient's risk behaviors, (c) evaluate his/her readiness to change or maintain safer behaviors, (d) understand the patient's ambivalence about re-evaluating aspects of his/her own risk-reduction information, motivation, and behavioral skills, (e) elicit strategies from the patient for overcoming barriers to change, moving towards change, or maintaining change, and (f) negotiate an individually-tailored risk reduction behavior change or behavior change maintenance goal. Furthermore, the clinician is trained to ask questions of the patient as a means of verifying that the patient has understood what has been discussed.

Options Project discussions of HIV risk reduction are tailored on the basis of patient's current readiness to change his/her risk behavior. For example, a discussion with an individual who has not yet begun to think about changing his or her behavior may focus on different issues and goals than a discussion with a patient who periodically practices safer behavior. In turn, a discussion with a patient who engages in safer behavior on an ongoing basis will also have unique elements. Initial Options Project discussions can take place in 5–10 minutes for clinicians who are trained in the technique, and who have adequate referral resources for patients who need help with depression, housing issues, and other concerns. During the implementation and evaluation of the Options Project intervention, clinicians were directed to conduct the intervention at the end of every regular HIV care visit with enrolled patients for a period of 18 months. The initial intervention session with each patient was typically the longest (about 10 minutes) because more time was spent assessing the patient's risk behaviors and the dynamics of his/her behavior than in follow-up sessions. Subsequent visits were briefer ($\sim$ 5 minutes); these focused on evaluating progress toward the goal set during the previous visit, briefly reassessing risk behavior, and negotiating a new or revised goal.

The Options Study Design. The Options Project used a quasi-experimental nonequivalent control group design to evaluate intervention effectiveness within two HIV care clinics in Connecticut. The two clinics represented the two largest providers of HIV care in Connecticut: Nathan Smith Clinic (NSC) at Yale-New Haven Hospital, which served as the experimental site, and Community Care Center (CCC) at Hartford Hospital which served as the control site. These two clinics were located in the two cities in Connecticut with the largest number of reported AIDS cases. Together these two sites reported nearly 40% of the AIDS cases in the state, and at both sites the full range of HIV disease and patient populations was represented. All of the participants were HIV-infected patients receiving healthcare services at one of these two participating sites.

Patients in the experimental intervention condition were informed that they would complete four sets of computer-assisted questionnaires assessing HIV risk reduction information, motivation, behavioral skills and behavior over a period of 18 months (one questionnaire every 6 months) and would also spend a portion of each clinic visit with their clinician discussing risk behavior and how to minimize the risks associated with those behaviors. Control condition patients, on the other hand, were told that they would complete the questionnaires but would not participate in the intervention at this time. All baseline data were gathered from participants prior to implementation of the risk reduction intervention. Patients were administered the questionnaires on a laptop computer in a semi-private area of the clinic. They were paid $25 for each set of surveys completed, but received no incentive payment for participating in the intervention sessions. Patients were also told that their clinical care provider would have no access to their responses on baseline or subsequent surveys.

Options Study Findings. Based on an analysis of 18-month Options follow-up data, this brief, clinician-initiated intervention occurring at the close of a regular HIV care visit, is feasible to implement, has adequate intervention fidelity (Fisher et al., in press) and successfully assists HIV positive patients in maintaining safer behaviors and reducing the frequency of risky behaviors (Fisher et al., 2004).

Regarding intervention fidelity, a review of the data indicates that the intervention has been consistently applied, despite providers' demanding schedules, time constraints, and complex visit agendas (Fisher et al., in press). Seventy-three percent of the patient-provider meetings during the course of the intervention involved the implementation of the protocol. On those occasions when the protocol was not implemented, it was generally because other critical patient issues (e.g., serious illness) took precedence. Regarding intervention fidelity, the majority of regular patient visits have included implementation of at least 7 of the 9 intervention protocol steps, indicating that providers are delivering an adequate number of intervention protocol elements to their patients. On average, clinicians reported delivering a mean of 6.4 out of 9 intervention elements per intervention delivery. This reflects a reasonable level of intervention fidelity under clinical conditions (Fisher et al., in press).

At baseline, there were 490 patients at HIV care clinics (n = 252 experimental and n = 245 control) in the sample. Participants were ethnically diverse and predominantly of low socioeconomic status. The most frequently reported routes of HIV infection were heterosexual sex and IDU, and the majority self-identified as heterosexual. We used random coefficient (RC) regression (Cohen et al., 2003; Raudenbush and Bryk, 2002) to assess changes in risk behavior in experimental versus control participants. The only demographic variable related to risk was receiving welfare or public assistance—with those receiving assistance engaging in lower levels of risk behavior. Welfare/public assistance status was thus included in outcome analyses as a covariate. We then included the fixed effects of time, intervention condition, and the test of the intervention by time interaction. Welfare/public assistance status at baseline was included as a fixed covariate.

There was a significant effect of condition, such that there were a greater number of risk behavior episodes reported in the intervention condition as opposed to the control condition. However, essential to interpreting this data is the significant time x condition interaction. Results also indicated that there was a significant decrease in HIV risk behavior in the Options Project intervention condition over time, whereas there was no significant change over time in the control condition.

An average of 21.9 high-risk sexual events in the past 3-months was reported at baseline among participants the intervention group at baseline, which dropped to 2.7 at 18-month follow up. There was no statistically reliable change in the number of high-risk sexual events for participants in the control group from baseline to 18-month follow-up. These results provide support for the continued use of clinician-delivered risk reduction interventions aimed at HIV positive individuals (Fisher et al., in press).

Adapting Options for South Africa. Currently, the Options Project is being adapted and developed for implementation in the KwaZulu-Natal province of South Africa, which has one of the highest prevalence rates for HIV in the world (UNAIDS/WHO, 2002). Integrating prevention into care for HIV positive persons in South Africa is a timely issue, because the government has announced plans to distribute antiretroviral (ARV) medications nationally (Tshabalala-Msimang, 2003).

Implementing Options cross-culturally requires extensive elicitation work aimed at identifying unique characteristics of the health care delivery system and the cultural milieu. To this end, focus groups have been conducted in South Africa with physicians, nurses, and other health care providers, as well as with HIV positive patients (Kiene et al., 2004).

Preliminary results of these focus groups suggest that some of the same challenges faced in implementing the Options Project in the US also apply to South Africa; for example, clinicians face severe constraints on the time they can devote to each patient which is often exacerbated by language barriers, and many providers are uncomfortable discussing sexual matters. Other barriers to clinician-delivered prevention efforts are either unique to South Africa or exist to a significantly greater degree than in the US These include a profound lack of sexual decision making power among women, psychological denial of being HIV positive, mistrust of condoms, and stigma associated with HIV/AIDS (Kiene et al., 2004). Training clinicians to communicate with patients in a non-judgmental manner and enfranchise patients in the decision-making process are particular priorities for implementing such an intervention in South Africa.

It may be the case that, in adapting Options to the South African health care setting, greater reliance will be placed on a team approach than in the US implementation, including perhaps involving clinicians, HIV counselors, and nurses in the delivery of the intervention. In the South Africa focus groups, some female focus group participants voiced the belief that traditional healers (sangomas) and HIV positive counselors should be part of the team who delivers the intervention because there is widespread denial of HIV among men; "men will listen to the traditional healer and to an HIV positive male counselor who says: 'look I have HIV, it's real'. They will not believe the doctor" (Kiene et al., 2004). Such sentiments may be especially true in rural areas in South Africa. Therefore, the clinician may be a less trusted source of information than a traditional healer or a peer.

There is a major limitation to prevention efforts targeting HIV positive persons in countries in which there is a limited availability of ARV medications. Where ARV medications are scarce, individuals are less likely to seek HIV testing; hence, only a relatively small percentage of people who are HIV positive will seek clinical care (International HIV/AIDS Alliance, 2003). Under these circumstances, a clinician-delivered risk-reduction intervention aimed at HIV positive individuals will only have a limited impact on the HIV epidemic as a whole.

Fortunately, there is a strong hope that ARV medications will be soon made available to a large proportion of South Africans who are living with HIV. This development encourages a vision of positive prevention in South Africa in which clinician-delivered HIV risk prevention interventions form part of an effort to decrease the spread of HIV, while a broader public health campaign, by promoting HIV testing and providing ARV therapy to those who test positive, brings help to those who need it.

Looking more broadly at the issue of prevention work in developing or resource-poor countries, some of the lessons of primary prevention can be applied to prevention efforts aimed at HIV positive individuals. The World Health Organization (2000) has advocated the use of clinics as a cost-effective point of distribution for condoms; they also recommend that clinical care sites provide health education focusing on the provision of information about risk-factors and prevention strategies, motivation to engage in prevention behavior, and behavioral skills needed to use condoms effectively. This approach has been adapted to HIV prevention among HIV positive individuals; for example, Samraksa, a non-governmental organization in Bangalore, India, has trained doctors at STD clinics to provide condoms and prevention messages to HIV positive patients (Baksi et al., 1998). Baksi and her colleagues offer preliminary data suggesting that this project is feasible and accepted by the target population.

CONCLUSIONS

A significant minority of HIV positive individuals continue to engage in behavior that places others at risk for infection. Both the CDC and NIH have advocated prevention efforts for HIV positive persons as a critical priority to help stem the HIV epidemic, and these organizations along with the International HIV/AIDS Alliance (2003) and others have called for clinicians to play a leadership role in HIV prevention among HIV positive patients. However, a significant percentage of clinicians do not discuss HIV risk reduction with their HIV positive patients and few if any systematically employ validated behavior change intervention strategies in this context. Challenges to integrating HIV prevention into the clinical care setting include clinicians' lack of self-efficacy with respect to their role as behavior change agents, discomfort with sexual topics, and limited training and limited time to deliver prevention messages. We have also described important strengths of clinician-delivered behavior change interventions. The clinician, particularly in the US, is a highly trusted source of prevention information, and evidence from a number of health behavior-change interventions indicate that even a brief, clinician-delivered intervention can be effective in promoting change. The clinician, moreover, is in a position to mobilize a range of support services that can serve a wide variety of needs that an HIV positive individual may have and which stand in the way of change. Furthermore, it is possible to provide the clinician with powerful tools to promote behavior change that do not require him/her to undertake extensive training in psychological counseling or assessment. Critically, the clinical care setting provides repeated access to HIV positive persons in large numbers and over extended periods of time.

HIV risk behavior among HIV positive persons is associated with deficits in HIV risk reduction information, motivation, and behavioral skills, as well as psychosocial factors including depression, anxiety, alcohol dependency, or disruptions to effective coping brought on by extrinsic factors such as an abusive relationship or unstable housing. Hence, it is argued that an effective clinician-delivered intervention will identify and address a patient's gaps in information, motivation, and behavioral skills that are known to be antecedents of risk-taking. This approach, supplemented by appropriate referrals to mental health professionals to deal with psychosocial barriers to behavior change, is believed to have considerable potential.

ACKNOWLEDGEMENTS   Preparation of this chapter was supported by a grant (5RO1-MH59473-02) from the National Institute of Mental Health.

REFERENCES

American College of Physicians and Infectious Diseases Society of America. (1994). HIV infection. *Ann. Intern. Med.* 120:310–319.
American Medical Association. (2000). *Physician socioeconomic statistics.* AMA, Chicago.
Baksi, C. M., Harper, I., and Raj, M. (1998). A well woman clinic in Bangalore: One strategy to attempt to decrease the transmission of HIV infection. *Int. J. STD AIDS* 9:418–423.

Bandura, A. (1989). Perceived self-efficacy in the exercise of control over AIDS infection. In: Mays, V. M., Albee, G. W., and Schneider, S. M. (eds.), *Primary prevention of AIDS.* Sage, Newbury Park, CA, pp.128–141.

Bandura, A. (1994). Social cognitive theory and exercise of control over HIV infection. In: Di-Clemente, R.J., and Peterson, J. L. (eds.),*Preventing AIDS: Theories and methods of behavioral interventions.* Plenum Press, New York, pp. 25–59.

Barzilai, D. A., Goodwin, M. A., Zyzanski, S. J., and Stange, K. C. (2001). Does health habit counseling affect patient satisfaction? *Prev. Med.* 33:595–599.

Blumenthal, D., Causino, N., Chang, Y. C., Culpepper, L., Marder, W., Saglam, D., Stafford, R., and Starfield, B. (1999). The duration of ambulatory visits to physicians. *J. Fam. Pract.* 48:264–271.

Calabrese, L. H., Kelley, D. M., Cullen, R. J., and Locker, G. (1991). Physicians' attitudes, beliefs, and practices regarding AIDS health care promotion. *Arch. Intern. Med.*151:1157–1160.

Calfas, K. J., Patrick, K., Sallis, J. F., and Wooten, W. (1998). Academic detailing and provider recruitment/training in Project PACE (Physician-based assessment and counseling for exercise). Paper presented at the Society for Behavioral Medicine annual meeting, March 25–28, New Orleans, LA.

Centers for Disease Control and Prevention (1994). HIV prevention practices of primary-care physicians—United States, 1992. *MMWR* 42:988–992.

Centers for Disease Control and Prevention (1997). Physician advice and individual behaviors about cardiovascular disease risk reduction. *MMWR* 48:75–77.

Centers for Disease Control and Prevention (2003). Incorporating HIV prevention into the medical care of persons living with HIV: Recommendations of CDC, the Health Resources and Services Administration, the National Institutes of Health, and the HIV Medicine Association of the Infectious Diseases Society of America. *MMWR* 52(RR-12)1–26.

Clement, U. (1992). Psychological correlates of unprotected intercourse among HIV-positive gay men. *J. Psychol. Human Sexuality* 5:133–155.

Coffield, A. B., Maciosek, M. V., McGinnis, J. M., Harris, J. R., Caldwell, M. B., Teutsch, S. M., and Atkins, D. (2001). Priorities among recommended clinical preventive services. *Am. J. Prev. Med.* 21:1–9.

Cohen, S. J., Havlorson, H. W., and Gosselink, C. A. (1994). Changing physician behavior to improve disease prevention. *Prev. Med.* 23:284–291.

Cohen, J., Cohen, P., West, S., and Aiken, L. (2003). *Applied multiple regression/correlational analysis for the behavioral sciences.* 3rd Ed. Erlbaum, Hillsdale, NJ.

Crepaz, N., and Marks, G. (2002). Towards and understanding of sexual risk behavior in people living with HIV: a review of social, psychological, and medical findings. *AIDS* 16:135–149.

Darrow, W. W., Webster, R. D., Kurtz, S. P., Buckley, A. K., Patel, K. L., and Stempel, R. R. (1998). Impact of HIV counseling and testing on HIV-infected men who have sex with men: the South Beach Health Survey. *AIDS and Behavior* 2:115–126.

de Vroome, E. M. M., de Wit, J. B. F., Stroebe, W., Sandfort, T. G. M., and van Griensven G. J. P. (1998). Sexual behavior and depression among HIV-positive gay men. *AIDS and Behavior* 2:137–149.

Dickey, L. L., and Kamerow, D. B. (1996). Primary care physicians' use of office resources in the provision of preventive care. *Arch. Fam. Med.* 5:399–404.

Dietrich, A. J.,Woodruff, C. B., and Carney, P. A. (1994). Changing office routines to enhance preventive care. *Arch. Fam. Med.* 3:176–183.

Dodge, W. T., BlueSpruce, J., Grothaus, L., Rebolledo, V., McAfee, T. A., Carey, J. W., and Thompson, R. S. (2001). Enhancing primary care HIV prevention: A comprehensive clinical intervention. *Am. J. Prev. Med.* 20:177–183.

Dovidio, J. F. and Gaertner, S. L. (1999). Reducing prejudice: Combating intergroup bias. *Current Directions in Psychological Science* 8:101–105.

Epstein, R. M., Morse, D. S., Frankel, R. M., Frarey, L., Anderson, K., and Beckman, H. B. (1998). Awkward moments in patient-physician communication about HIV risk. *Ann. Intern. Med.* 128:435–442.

Fishbein, M., and Ajzen, I. (1975). *Belief, attitude, intention, and behavior: An introduction to theory and research.* Addison-Wesley, Reading, MA.

Fisher, J. D., and Fisher, W. A. (1992). Changing AIDS-risk behavior. *Psychol. Bull.* 111(3):455–474.

Fisher, J. D., Kimble, D. L., Misovich, S. J., and Weinstein, B. (1998). Dynamics of sexual risk behavior in HIV-infected men who have sex with men. *AIDS and Behavior* 2:101–113.

Fisher, J. D., Cornman, D. H., Amico, K. R., Osborn, C. Y., Fisher, W. A., and Friedland, G. H. (in press). Clinician initiated HIV-risk reduction intervention for HIV+ persons: Formative research, acceptability, and fidelity of the Options Project. *JAIDS.*

Fisher, J. D., Fisher, W. A., Cornman, D., Amico, R., Bryan, A., and Friedland, G. (2004b). Clinician-initiated intervention delivered during routine clinical care reduces risky sexual behavior of HIV positive patients. Manuscript submitted for publication.

Fisher, W. A., Grenier, G., Watters, W. W., Lamont, J., Cohen, M., and Askwith, J. (1988). Students' sexual knowledge, attitudes towards sex, and willingness to treat sexual concerns. *J. Med. Educ.* 63:379–385.

Fisher, W. A., Fisher, J. D. and Rye, B. J. (1995). Understanding and promoting AIDS preventive behavior: Insights from the Theory of Reasoned Action. *Health Psychol.* 14:255–264.

Fiske, S. T. (2000). Interdependence and the reduction of prejudice. In: Oskamp, S. (ed.), *Reducing prejudice and discrimination. The Claremont Symposium on Applied Social Psychology.* Erlbaum, Mahwah, NJ, pp.115–135.

Gabel, L. L., Crane, R., and Ostrow, D. C. (1994). HIV-related disease: Family physicians' multiple opportunities for preventive intervention. *Journal of the American Board of Family Physicians* 7:218–224.

Gemson, D. H., Columbotos, J., Elinson, J., Fordyce, E. J., Hynes, M. and Stoneburner, R. (1991). Acquired immunodeficiency syndrome prevention: Knowledge, attitudes, and practices of primary care physicians. *Arch. Intern. Med.* 151:1102–1107.

Gerbert, B., Maguire, B. T., Bleecker, T., Coates, T. J., and McPhee, S. J. (1991). Primary care physicians and AIDS. *JAMA* 266:2837–2842.

Glynn, T. J., Manley, M. W., Cullen, J. W., and Mayer, W. J. (1990). Cancer prevention through physician intervention. *Semin. Oncol.* 17:391–401.

Godin, G., Savard, J., Kok, G., Fortin, C., Boyer, R. (1996). HIV seropositive gay men: Understanding adoption of safe sexual practices. *AIDS Educ. Prev.* 8:529–545.

Grueninger, U. J., Goldsten, M. G., and Duffy, F. D. (1989). Patent education in hypertension: Five essential steps. *J. Hypertens.* 7:S93–S98.

Hays, R. B., Paul, J., Ekstrand, M., Kegeles, S. M., Stall, R., and Coates, T. J. (1997). Actual versus perceived HIV status, sexual behaviours and predictors of unprotected sex among young gay and bisexual men who identify as HIV-negative, HIV-positive and untested. *AIDS* 11:1495–1502.

Hazard, L. L. (1993). Problems encountered assessing AIDS awareness among rural Mid-West high school students in a family practice setting. *South Dakota Journal of Medicine* 46: 73–75.

International HIV/AIDS Alliance, 2003, *Positive prevention: Prevention strategies for people with HIV/AIDS, Draft background paper.* (September 20, 2003); http://www.cdc.gov/hiv/partners/AHP/Positive_Prevention_IHA_Marked.pdf

Janssen, R. S., Holtgrave, D. R., Valdiserri, R. O., Shepherd, M., Gayle, H. D., and De Cock, K. M. (2001). The serostatus approach to fighting the HIV epidemic: Prevention strategies for infected individuals. *Am. J. Public Health* 91:1019–1024.

Johansen, J. D., and Smith, E. (2002). Gonorrhoea in Denmark: High incidence among HIV-infected men who have sex with men. *Acta Dermato-venereologica* 82:365–368.

Kalichman, S. C. (1999). Psychological and social correlates of high-risk sexual behavior among men and women living with HIV/AIDS. *AIDS Care* 11:415–428.

Kalichman, S. C. (2000). HIV transmission risk behaviors of men and women living with HIV-AIDS: Prevalence, predictors, and emerging clinical interventions. *Clin. Psychol. Sci. Pract.* 7:32–47.

Kalichman, S. C. and Nachimson, D. (1999). Self-efficacy and disclosure of HIV-positive serostatus to sex partners. *Health Psychol.* 18:281–287.

Kalichman, S. C., Greenberg, J., and Abel, G. G. (1997). HIV-seropositive men who engage in high-risk sexual behavior: Psychological characteristics and implications for prevention. *AIDS Care* 9:441–450.

Kalichman, S. C., Nachimson, D., Cherry, C., and Williams, E. (1998). AIDS treatment advances and behavioral prevention setbacks: Preliminary assessment of reduced perceived threat of HIV-AIDS. *Health Psychol.* 17:546–550.

Kalichman, S. C., Roffman, R. A., Picciano, J. F., and Bolan, M. (1997b). Sexual relationships, sexual behavior, and HIV infection: HIV-seropositive gay and bisexual men seeking prevention services. *Professional Psychology Research and Practice* 28:355–360.

Kalichman, S. C., Rompa, D., Austin, J., Luke, W., and DiFonzo, K. (2001a). Viral load, perceived infectivity, and unprotected intercourse [Letter to the Editor]. *JAIDS* 28:303–305.

Kalichman, S. C., Rompa, D., Cage, M., DiFonzo, K., Simpson, D., Austin, J., Luke, W., Buckles, J., Kyomugisha, F., Benotsch, E., Pinkerton, S., and Graham, J. (2001b). Effectiveness of an intervention to reduce HIV transmission risks in HIV-positive people. *Am. J. Prev. Med.* 21:181–190.

Kelly, J. A., and St. Lawrence, J. S. (1988). AIDS prevention and treatment: Psychology's role in the health crisis. *Clin. Psychol. Rev.* 8:255–284.

Kelly, J. A., and Kalichman, S. C. (2002). Behavioral research in HIV/AIDS primary and secondary prevention: Recent advances and future directions. *J. Consult. Clin. Psychol.* 70:626–639.

Kiene, S. M., Christie, S. S., Fisher, J. D., Fisher, W. A., Cornman, D., Giddy, J., and Friedland, G. (2004). The dynamics of HIV risk behavior among HIV-positive individuals in KwaZulu-Natal, South Africa. Manuscript in preparation.

Klein, J. D., Portilla, M., Goldstein, A., and Leininger, L. (1995). Training pediatric residents to prevent tobacco use. *Pediatrics* 96(2):326–330.

Kline, A., and VanLandingham, M. (1994). HIV-infected women and sexual risk reduction: The relevance of existing models of behavior change. *AIDS Educ. Prev.* 6:390–402.

Kottke, T. E., Solberg, L. I., Brekke, M. L., Conn, S. A., Maxwell, P., and Brekke, M. J. (1992). A controlled trial to integrate smoking cessation advice into primary care practice: Doctors helping smokers, round III. *J. Fam. Pract.* 34(6):701–708.

Kottke, T. E., Brekke, M. L., and Solberg, L. I. (1993). Making "time" for preventive services. *Mayo Clinic Proceedings* 63:785–791.

Kreuter, M. W., Chheda, S. G. and Bull, F. C. (2000). How does physician advice influence patient behavior? Evidence for a priming effect. *Arch. Fam. Med.* 9:426–433.

Lightfoot, M., Milburn, N. G., Rotheram-Borus, M. J., and Gunderson, G. (2004). *Prevention for positives in medical care settings*. Unpublished manuscript, University of California, Los Angeles.

Logsdon, D. N., Lazaro, C. M., and Meier, R. V. (1989). The feasibility of behavioral risk reduction in primary medical care. *Am. J. Prev. Med.* 5:249–256.

Long, B. J., Calfas, K. J., Wooten, W., Sallis, J. F., Patrick, K., Goldstein, M., Marcus, B. H., Schwenk, T. L., Chenoweth, J., Carter, R., Torres, T., Palinkas, L. A., and Heath, G. (1996). A multisite field test of the acceptability of physical activity counseling in primary care: Project PACE. *Am. J. Prev. Med.* 12(2):73–81.

Makadon, H. J., and Silin, J. G. (1995). Prevention of HIV infection in primary care: Current practices, future possibilities. *American College of Physicians* 123:715–719.

Mandelblatt, J., and Kanetsky, P. A. (1995). Effectiveness of interventions to enhance physician screening for breast cancer. *J. Fam. Pract.* 40:162–171.

Marks, G., Burris, S., and Peterman, T. A. (1999). Reducing sexual transmission of HIV from those who know they are infected: The need for personal and collective responsibility. *AIDS* 13:297–306.

Marks, G., Richardson, J. L., Crepaz, N., Stoyanoff, S., Milam, J., Kemper, C., Larsen, R. A., Bolan, R., Weismuller, P., Hollander, H., and McCutchan, A. (2002). Are HIV care providers talking with patients about safer sex and disclosure?: A multi-clinic assessment. *AIDS* 16:1953–1957.

Margolin, A., Avants, S. K., Warburton, L. A., Hawkins, K. A., and Shi, J. (2003). A randomized clinical trial of a manual-guided risk reduction intervention for HIV-positive injection drug users. *Health Psychol.* 22:223–228.

Margolis, A. D., Wolitski, R. J., Parsons, J. T. and Gomez, C. A. (2001). Are healthcare providers talking to HIV-seropositive patients about safer sex? *AIDS* 15:2335–2337.

McDaniel, J. S., Carlson, L. M., Thompson, N. J., and Purcell, D. W. (1995). A Survey of Knowledge and attitudes about HIV and AIDS among medical students. *College Health* 44(1):11–14.

Metsch, L. R., Pereyra, M., del Rio, C., Gardner, L., Duffus, W., Dickinson, G., Kerdnt, P., Anderson-Mahoney, P., Strathdee, S., and Greenburg, A. (2004). The Delivery of HIV Prevention Counseling by Physicians at HIV Medical Care Setting in Four U.S. Cities. *Am. J. Public Health.* 94:1186–1192.

Miller, L. (1993). *Psychotherapy of the brain injured patient.* New York: Norton.

Miller, W. R., and Rollnick, S. (1991) . *Motivational interviewing: Preparing people to change addictive behavior.* Guilford Press, New York.

Montesinos, L., Frisch, L. E., Greene, B. F., and Hamilton, M. (1990). An analysis of and intervention in the sexual transmission of disease. *J. Appl. Behav. Anal.* 23(3):275–284.

Morgan, G. D., Goldstein, M. G., and Bartlett, S. (1998). Teaching behavioral medicine counseling to health care providers. Seminar presented at the Society for Behavioral Medicine annual meeting, March 25–28, New Orleans, LA.

Morin, S. F., Koester, K. A., Maiorana, A., McLaughlin, M., Myers, J. J., Steward, W. T., Vernon, K., and Chesney, M. A. (2003). *Missed opportunities: Prevention with HIV infected patients in clinical care settings.* Unpublished manuscript: University of California, San Francisco.

National Institutes of Health Consensus Panel (1997). *National Institutes of Health consensus development statement on interventions to prevent HIV risk behaviors.* Bethesda, MD: NIH Office of Medical Applications Research.

Nawaz, H., Adams, M. L., and Katz, D. L. (1999). Weight loss counseling by health care providers. *Am. J. Public Health* 89:764–767.

Nawaz, H., Adams, M. L., and Katz, D .L. (2000). Physician-patient interactions regarding diet, exercise, and smoking. *Prev. Med.* 31:652–657.

Ockene, J. K., Kristeller, J., Goldberg. R., Amick, T. L., Pekow, P. S., Mosmer, D., Quirk, M., and Kalan, K. (1990). Increasing the efficacy of physician-delivered smoking interventions: a randomized clinical trial. *J. Gen. Intern. Med.* 6:1–8.

O'Connor, P. G., Selwyn, P. A., and Schottenfeld, R. S. (1994). Medical care for injection-drug users with human immunodeficiency virus infection. *New Engl. J. Med.* 331:450–459.

Paauw, D., and O'Neill, J. F. (1990). Human immunodeficiency virus and the primary care physician. *J. Fam. Pract.* 31:646–650.

Patterson, T. L., Shaw, W. S., and Semple, S. J. (2003). Reducing the sexual risk behaviors of HIV positive individuals: Outcome of a randomized control trial. *Ann. Behav. Med.* 25:137–145.

Preventive Services Task Force of the American Medical Association. (1990). *Guide to clinical preventive services,* 2nd ed. Lippincott, Williams & Wilkins, Philadelphia.

Raudenbush, S. W., and Bryk, A. S. (2002). *Hierarchical linear models: Applications and data analysis methods.* Sage, Thousand Oaks, CA.

Richardson, J. L., Milam, J., McCutchan, A., Stoyanoff, S., Bolan, R., Weiss, J., Kemper, C., Larsen, R. A., Hollander, H., Weissmuller, P., Chou, C. P., and Marks, G. (2004). Effect of brief provider safer-sex counseling of HIV-1 seropositive patients: A multi-clinic assessment. *AIDS,* 18:1179–1186.

Rollnick, S., Mason, P., and Butler, C. (2000). *Health Behavior Change,* 2nd ed. Churchill Livingstone, Edinburgh.

Rotheram-Borus, M. J., Kelly, J. A., Ehrhardt, A. A., Chesney, M. A., Lightfoot, M., Weinhardt, L. S., Kirshenbaum, S. B., Johnson, M. O., Remien, R. H., Morin, S. F., Kertzner, R. M., Pequegnat, W., Gordon, C. M., and the NIMH Healthy Living Project Team (2003). *HIV transmission risk behavior, medication adherence, and mental health in a four-city sample of people living with HIV: Implications for HIV prevention, The Healthy Living Project.* Paper presented at the Prevention Interventions with Persons Living with HIV/AIDS: NIH/CDC/HRSA Update Conference, July 26–27, Atlanta, GA.

Rothman, A. J. and Salovey, P. (1997). Shaping perceptions to motivate healthy behavior: The role of message framing. *Psychol. Bull.* 121:3–19.

Scales, R., Lueker, R. D., Atterbom, H. A., Handmaker, N. S., and Jackson, K. A. (1998). Motivational interviewing and skills-based counseling to change multiple lifestyle behaviors. Paper presented at the Society for Behavioral Medicine annual meeting, March 25–28, New Orleans, LA.

Semple, S. J., Patterson, T. L., and Grant, I. (2000a). Psychosocial predictors of unprotected anal intercourse in a sample of HIV positive gay men who volunteer for a sexual risk reduction intervention. *AIDS Educ. Prev.* 12:416–430.

Semple, S. J., Patterson, T. L., and Grant, I. (2000b). The sexual negotiation behavior of HIV-positive gay and bisexual men. *J. Consult. Clin. Psychol.* 68:934–937.

Simoni, J. M., Mason, H., Marks, G., Ruiz, M., Reed, D., and Richardson, J. (1995). Women's self-disclosure of HIV infection: Rates, reasons, and reactions. *J. Consult. Clin. Psychol.* 63:474–478.

Stewart, M. A. (1995). Effective physician-patient communication and health outcomes: A review. *Canadian Medical Association Journal* 152:1423–1433.

Temple-Smith, M., Hammond, J., Pyett, P., and Presswell, N. (1996). Barriers to sexual history taking in general practice. *Aust. Fam. Physician* 25(S2)S71–S74.

Terrault, N. A. (2002). Sexual activity as a risk factor for hepatitis C. *Hepatology* 36(S1):S99–S105.

Tshabalala-Msimang, M. (2003). *Operational Plan for Comprehensive HIV and AIDS Care, Management and Treatment for South Africa.* Presented to the South African Cabinet (Nov 19 2003) www.gov.za/issues/hiv/careplan19nov03.htm

UNAIDS/WHO. (2002). *UNAIDS/WHO epidemiological fact sheet, South Africa.* Geneva, Switzerland: Author.

United States Department of Health and Human Services (1990). *Healthy People 2000.* U.S. Government Printing Office, Washington, D.C.

United States Department of Health and Human Services (2000). *Treating tobacco use and dependence.* U.S. Government Printing Office, Washington, D.C.

United States Preventive Services Task Force (1996). *Guide to clinical preventive services,* 2nd ed. Williams and Wilkins, Baltimore.

Valente, C. M., Sobal, J., Muncie, H. L., Levine, D. M., and Antlitz, A. M. (1986). Health promotion: physicians' beliefs, attitudes, and practices. *Am. J. Prev. Med.* 2(2):82–88.

Vanable, P., Ostrow, D. G., McKirnan, D. J., Taywaditep, K. J., and Hope, B. A. (2000). Impact of combinations therapies on HIV risk perceptions and sexual risk taking among HIV-positive and HIV-negative gay and bisexual men. *Health Psychol.* 19:134–145.

van der Straten, A., Comez, C. A., Saul, J., Quan, J., and Padian, N. (2000). Sexual risk behaviors among heterosexual HIV serodiscordant couples in the era of post exposure prevention and viral suppressive therapy. *AIDS* 14:F47–F54.

Vogt, T. M., Hollis, J. F., Lichtenstein, E., Stevens, V. J., Glasgow, R., and Whitlock, E. (1998). The medical care system and prevention: The need for a new paradigm. *HMO Practice* 12:5–13.

Ward, J., and Sanson-Fisher, R. (1995). Prevalence and detection of HIV risk behavior in primary care: Implications for clinical preventive services. *Am. J. Prev. Med.* 11:224–230.

Weinhardt, L. S., Kelly, J. A., Brondino, M. J., Rotheram-Borus, M. J., Kirshenbaum, S. B., Chesney, M. A., Remien, R. H., Morin, S. F., Lightfoot, M., Ehrhardt, A. A., Johnson, M. O., Catz, S. L., Pinkerton, S. D., Benotsch, E. G., Hong, D., Gore-Felton, C., and the NIMH Healthy Living Project Team. (2004). HIV transmission risk behavior among men and women living with HIV in four U.S. cities. *J Acquir Immune Defic Syndr.* 36:1057–1066.

Werch, C. E., Anzalone, D. M., Brokiewicz, L. M., Felker, J., Carlson, J. M., and Castellon-Vogel, E. A . (1996). An intervention for preventing alcohol use among inner-city middle school students. *Arch. Fam. Med.* 5:146–152.

Wheat, M. E., Devons, C., Hyman, R. B., and Solomon, S. (1993). Preventing HIV transmission: behavior and attitudes of medical house staff in a high-prevalence area. *Am. J. Prev. Med.* 9(5):307–315.

Whitlock, E. P., Orleans, T., Pender, N., and Allan, J. (2002). Evaluating primary care behavioral counseling interventions: An evidence-based approach. *Am. J. Prev. Med.* 22:267–284.

Wilson, I.B. and Kaplan, S.H. (2000). Physician-patient communication in HIV disease: The importance of visit length, gender, and physician sexual preference. *J Acquir Immune Defic Syndr.* 25;417–425.

World Health Organization (2000). HIV/AIDS: Report by the Director-General. 53rd World Health Assembly, 3/22/00.

Yedidia MJ and Berry CA. (1999). The impact of residency training on physicians' AIDS-related treatment practice: A longitudinal panel study. *Acad. Med.* 7:532–538.

CHAPTER NINE

International Perspectives

Jonathan Elford, Heiner C. Bucher,
Patrick Rawstorne, Andrea Fogarty,
Paul Van de Ven, Susan Kippax,
Maria Ekstrand, Shalini Bharat,
Jayashree Ramakrishna,
Leckness C. Simbayi, and
Seth C. Kalichman

INTRODUCTION

The burden of HIV/AIDS is shared, although not equally, by all the countries in the world. Most HIV infections occur in countries with the least resources, while most HIV prevention-related research has occurred in countries with the greatest resources. In particular, research on HIV transmission risks among people living with HIV/AIDS has primarily been reported from the US, Western Europe, and Australia. The preceding chapters in this book have strived to represent international aspects of HIV prevention for people living with HIV infection, but in many cases there has just not been enough empirical work to characterize the challenges and opportunities for HIV prevention with infected populations outside the US. This chapter therefore seeks to fill this gap. Contributions for this chapter were sought from researchers working in countries located on four continents; Europe, Australia, Asia, and Africa. Although by no means representing all perspectives from all countries, their perspectives shed light on the cultural boundaries of what we know and point us in the direction of what must be learned.

UNITED KINGDOM: JONATHAN ELFORD,
CITY UNIVERSITY, LONDON

There are nearly 50,000 people living with HIV in the UK, about a third of who are undiagnosed (Health Protection Agency, 2003a). Since the early 1980s, gay men have been the group at highest risk of acquiring HIV in the UK. They currently account for nearly half the people with HIV in this country (Health Protection Agency, 2003b). However, in the last five years there has been a rapid rise in new diagnoses of heterosexually-acquired HIV; these now exceed the number of new diagnoses among men who have sex with men (MSM). In 2002, there were 3305 new diagnoses of heterosexually-acquired HIV in the UK compared with 1691 as a result of sex between men (Health Protection Agency, 2003c). Nearly three-quarters of the new diagnoses due to heterosexual transmission were in people from Africa. People with heterosexually-acquired HIV now account for 40% of all those living with HIV in the UK (Health Protection Agency, 2003b).

This section is divided into two parts to reflect the evolving epidemiology of HIV in the UK: the first part considers gay men, the second part considers people from African communities living with HIV in the UK.

Gay Men

Information on the sexual behavior of gay men living with HIV in the UK comes from two sources: behavioral surveillance conducted annually among gay men in community settings such as bars, clubs, gyms, Gay Pride and, more recently, the Internet; and research conducted among HIV positive gay men attending outpatient treatment clinics in public hospitals. In all locations, men are asked to complete self-administered questionnaires to provide information on their sexual behavior including unprotected anal intercourse (UAI) in the previous 3 or 12 months. For behavioral research, it is important to distinguish seroconcordant UAI—that is, unprotected anal intercourse where both partners are HIV positive—from non-concordant UAI—where one partner is positive and the other is either negative or of unknown HIV status (Elford, et al., 2001a). Non-concordant UAI clearly presents a risk for HIV transmission.

Although the UK surveys among gay men were conducted in a variety of settings, including bars, clubs, gyms, clinics, Pride events, and the Internet they all came up with similar findings: (a) a substantial proportion of HIV positive gay men reported sexual behavior with a high risk of HIV transmission; (b) HIV positive men were more likely to report high risk sexual behavior than HIV negative or never-tested men; (c) taking highly

active antiretroviral therapy (HAART) was not associated with high risk
sexual behavior among gay men living with HIV; (d) HIV positive men may
be using the Internet to meet other HIV positive men for unprotected sex.

London Gyms

In a survey of over 800 gay men attending London gyms in 2002, 15%
said they were HIV positive. Of these HIV positive men, 42% reported non-
concordant UAI in the previous three months. HIV positive men were significantly more likely to report non-concordant UAI than HIV negative or
never-tested men (42% vs. 19%, Bolding et al., 2002). In univariate analysis,
using the Internet to look for sex, younger age, HIV treatments optimism
and recreational drug use were all associated with non-concordant UAI
among HIV positive men. There was, however, no association with ethnicity, education, employment, taking HAART or having an undetectable
viral load. In multivariate analysis the only factor that remained significant
was seeking sex on the Internet.

Between 1998–2002 the percentage of HIV positive men reporting non-
concordant UAI increased significantly from 20% to 42% (see Table 9.1). A
similar trend was seen among HIV negative and never tested men (Bolding
et al., 2002; Elford et al., 2002, 2003, 2004a). The increase in non-concordant
UAI occurred only with casual partners. In 1998, 15% of HIV positive men
reported non-concordant UAI with a casual partner, increasing to 41% by
2002. There was no change in high risk behavior with a main partner alone
(1998, 4%; 2002, 1%; see Table 9.1). These trends over time highlight the
importance of distinguishing sexual risks with a main partner from risks
that occurs with casual partners (Elford et al., 1999, 2001a).

While the increase in high-risk sexual behavior has coincided with the
availability of highly active antiretroviral therapy (HAART) it is unlikely
that optimism in the light of new HIV treatments can explain this upward
trend. This is because the increase in high risk sexual behavior was seen
equally among those who were optimistic in the light of new HIV therapies
and those who were not (Elford et al., 2002; Elford et al., 2003). If the increase
in high risk behavior had been caused solely by HIV optimism we would
have expected to see the rise predominantly, if not exclusively, among HIV
positive gay men who were optimistic with little if any increase among
other men. This was not the case. Furthermore, less than half the HIV
positive men expressed optimism in the light of new HIV therapies; the
majority appeared to be realistic rather than optimistic about the benefits
of these new drugs (International Collaboration on HIV Optimism, 2003).

HIV positive men were also more likely to report an STI than other
men. Nine percent of HIV positive men reported syphilis in the previous

Table 9.1. Sexual risk behaviour of HIV positive gay men surveyed in London gyms 1998–2002 (United Kingdom)

No. of HIV positive men surveyed each year	1998 N = 118		1999 N = 101		2000 N = 120		2001 N = 116		2002 N = 121		test for a trend
	n	%	n	%	n	%	N	%	n	%	p
Number (%) of men reporting non-concordant UAI											
Total	23	19.5	20	19.9	25	20.9	50	43.1	51	42.1	<0.001
With a casual partner	18	15.3	15	14.9	23	19.2	45	38.8	50	41.3	<0.001
With main partner alone	5	4.2	5	5.0	2	1.7	5	4.3	1	0.8	0.6
Number (%) of men reporting concordant UAI											
Total	14	11.9	10	10.0	24	20.0	19	16.4	18	14.9	0.04
With a casual partner	8	6.8	4	4.0	17	14.2	13	11.2	11	9.1	0.03
With main partner alone	6	5.1	6	6.0	7	5.8	6	5.2	7	5.8	0.2

UAI unprotected anal intercourse
Source: Elford J, Bolding G, Sherr L 2002, 2003, 2004

12 months compared with 2% of HIV negative and 1% of never tested men. Corresponding figures for gonorrhea were 17%, 9%, 2% and for other STDs 25%, 15%, 5%, respectively (Bolding et al., 2002).

In addition to the men reporting non-concordant UAI, a further 15% reported seroconcordant UAI in 2002. That is to say, they reported unprotected anal intercourse but only with another HIV positive man (Bolding et al., 2002). While this does not present a risk of HIV transmission to an uninfected person, it may result in exposure to other STIs or drug-resistant strains of HIV for the positive men themselves. The percentage of HIV positive men reporting seroconcordant UAI has increased since 1998 (See Table 9.1). This increase was seen only with casual partners and not with a main partner. Among HIV positive men, those who looked for sex through the Internet were significantly more likely to report seroconcordant UAI with a casual partner than those who did not seek sex in this way (Elford et al., 2001b, Bolding et al 2002). This raises the possibility that HIV positive men use the Internet to meet other positive men for casual unprotected sex. In 2002 HIV positive men (65%) were significantly more likely to have used the Internet to look for sex than HIV negative (49%) or never-tested men (29%).

London Bars, Clubs, and Genitourinary Medicine Clinics

In a survey conducted among more than one thousand gay men attending bars, and clubs, as well as genitourinary clinics in London in 2002, HIV status was determined in two ways—by self report and by anonymous HIV antibody saliva testing. One hundred and twenty-seven men were HIV positive according to laboratory-confirmed saliva tests. Over a third of these HIV positive men (35%) reported non-concordant UAI in the previous year (Dodds and Mercey, 2003). There was no significant difference in the risk behavior of men who knew they were HIV positive and men who did not. However, HIV positive men were significantly more likely to report non-concordant UAI than HIV negative men (35% vs. 21%). They were also more likely to have had an STI in the last year (35% vs. 17%).

National Gay Men's Sex Survey

Of nearly 14000 gay men surveyed in England, Scotland and Wales in 2001 at Gay Pride events, through health promotion agencies and on the Internet, 735 (5%) said they were HIV positive. HIV positive men were more likely than other men to report high risk sexual behavior (Reid et al., 2002). For example, one third (33%) of HIV positive men said they had had insertive UAI in the last year with a non-concordant partner compared with one-in-five (20%) of the HIV negative or never-tested men. The corresponding figures for receptive UAI were 46% and 19%. Where condoms were used, HIV positive men were more likely to report condom failure than other men; 18% of HIV positive men reported condom failure compared with 13% of HIV negative men and 10% of those who had never been tested.

The authors noted that those who were diagnosed positive were more likely to report sexual behavior which could present a risk for HIV transmission. However, HIV positive men only accounted for five percent of the total sample. Consequently, in the sample as a whole the number of men reporting high risk behavior who were not HIV positive actually exceeded the number who were. This highlights the importance of not only considering relative risk, which compares men who are HIV positive with other men, but also attributable risk which takes into account the size of the HIV positive population.

HIV Treatment Clinics in London

In a survey of 420 HIV positive gay men attending a London outpatient clinic in 1999–2000 (median age 38 years), 39% reported UAI with one or more new partners in the past year and 13% reported UAI with a primary partner who was HIV negative or untested (Stephenson et al., 2003). Nearly one-third (31%) of the men also reported an STI in the last 12 months. The HIV positive men in the study were more likely to report a bacterial STI in the last 12 months than HIV negative men who took part in another study conducted in the same genitourinary clinic at about the same time (Imrie et al. 2001). Behavioral and clinical risk factors for HIV transmission were consistently lower in men taking HAART than men not on HAART. For example, 35% of men on HAART reported UAI with one or more new partners in the last year compared with 48% of men not on HAART. Men on HAART were also less likely to report an STI in the previous 12 months (27% vs. 40%). After adjusting for age, subjective wellbeing, CD4 count and time since HIV diagnosis, these differences were attenuated such that there were no significant differences between men who were on HAART and men who were not. There was no evidence that taking HAART was associated with elevated levels of high risk sexual behavior in this group of HIV positive men.

Just over 500 HIV positive gay men were surveyed in a north London outpatient HIV treatment clinic in 2002–2003 as part an MRC-funded study of the Internet, HIV and risk (Elford et al., in preparation). One third (34%) reported UAI in the previous 3 months; 11% reported UAI only with another HIV positive man while 22% reported UAI with a person of unknown or discordant HIV status. In multivariate analysis there was no association between high risk sexual behavior and either taking HAART or having an undetectable viral load.

Internet

In May–June 2002 gay and bisexual men using UK chatrooms or personal profiles on gaydar and gay.com were invited to complete an anonymous self-administered questionnaire online as part of the Internet and HIV study (Elford et al in preparation). Just over 1200 London gay men completed the online survey of which 12% were HIV positive (Elford et al., 2004a). Of the 142 HIV positive men, 47% reported non-concordant UAI in the previous 3 months. HIV positive men were significantly more likely to report high risk sexual behavior than HIV negative or never-tested men. In multivariate analysis, there was no association between high risk sexual behavior and either taking HAART or having an undetectable viral load (Graham Bolding, personal communication).

People from African Communities in the UK

It is only in the last few years that we have seen an increase in the number of people living with HIV among African communities in the UK. Consequently, investigators have only just begun to collect information on their sexual behavior. Research to date has focused primarily on heterosexual men and women in the UK African communities. However, there is an increasing awareness that HIV risk behavior among African MSM living in the UK also merits exploration.

Two surveys were conducted in London in 2002–2003 where respondents were asked to complete self-administered questionnaires concerning treatment and care, living with HIV, as well as sexual health and behavior. Both surveys reached the same conclusion: a substantial number of people from London's African communities who are living with HIV engage in sexual behavior that presents a risk to themselves and their sexual partners.

Padare

In 2002, 214 HIV positive black Africans living in London were recruited from community groups and outpatient clinics in Camden and Islington which covers central and northern parts of the capital (Chinouya and Davidson, 2003). Three-quarters of the respondents were female and most were aged 25–39 years. The majority were from Zimbabwe, Uganda, Zambia and the Congo; two-thirds had lived in the UK less than five years. Most of the respondents (80% of men, 93% of women) said their sexual partners were usually of the opposite sex. The remaining 20% of the men and 5% of women reported same sex partners while 2% of women reported both male and female partners.

Nearly two-thirds of the respondents (61%) reported having unprotected sexual intercourse with one or more partners in the previous year. Information was not available on the HIV status of their sexual partners so it was not possible to establish whether they were non-concordant. One third of the respondents said they had not used condoms with their most recent sexual partner. By way of comparison, in a survey of nearly 750 people from African communities recruited in central London social venues in 1999 of unknown HIV status, nearly 60% reported unprotected sexual intercourse with their most recent partner (Chinouya et al., 2000).

Forty percent of respondents in the Padare study said it was difficult to use condoms during sexual intercourse with a new partner. One of the problems the respondents faced was disclosure of HIV status. While two thirds said they had told their primary care physician or social worker about their positive diagnosis, only a third had told their partner. The authors wrote "Our data suggest that a significant number of people from London's African communities who are living with HIV engage in sexual behavior that is of significant risk to themselves and their sexual partners". They noted that the rates of unprotected sexual intercourse reported in the Padare study were similar to rates reported among HIV positive gay men, but lower than those seen in an African community sample.

Shibah

In 2002–2003, 124 Black Africans diagnosed with HIV, living in south London or using services there, completed a detailed questionnaire concerning treatment and care, living with HIV and sexual health (Chinouya et al., 2003). Two-thirds of the respondents were women. Respondents came from 19 countries, half from Zimbabwe or Uganda. Just over half had lived in the UK for less than 5 years. The sample was older than might have been expected with 44% being aged 40 years or more.

While just over half the respondents (56%) had consistently used condoms in the last 12 months, the remainder reported using them sometimes (34%) or not at all (10%). No information was available on the HIV status of their sexual partners so it was not possible to examine concordance and non-concordance. There appeared to be a low level of knowledge about sexual health. More than a third of respondents believed they could not pass on HIV if they had an undetectable viral load while nearly three quarters thought you could always tell if you had an STI. Seventy-four people had a regular sexual partner and 66 said they knew their partner's HIV status. Nearly two thirds were HIV positive. It seems that the choice of a positive partner was deliberate. Respondents said they often met HIV positive partners in support groups thus removing the need for disclosure.

African Women with HIV in London

Disclosure of HIV status was also explored in a qualitative study conducted in 2001 among 62 black African women with HIV living in London (Anderson and Doyal, 2004; Doyal and Anderson, 2003). Women were recruited from outpatient HIV treatment clinics. Disclosure of their HIV status was a major concern for all the women in the study. Six said they had made a conscious choice not to disclose their HIV status to former or current sexual partners. The main reason was the need to protect themselves from being abandoned or from physical or verbal abuse. Many reported that their male partners were unwilling to discuss HIV and related issues. These findings support those from the Padare and Shibah projects concerning the problems Africans with HIV living in London face disclosing their HIV status to partners.

SWITZERLAND: HEINER C. BUCHER, UNIVERSITY HOSPITAL BASEL, SWITZERLAND

Efforts in Switzerland to counteract HIV/AIDS have proved successful and gained worldwide recognition. From 1993 to 2001 HIV infections have decreased by more than 50% in Switzerland (Swiss Federal Office of Public Health, 1999). Access to potent antiretroviral therapies has been made possible in early 1996 to all HIV infected residents in Switzerland. Morbidity and mortality from HIV has substantially decreased in Switzerland (Egger et al., 1997; Ledergerber et al., 1999). As a consequence awareness of HIV in the public and in individuals living with HIV has changed and the former deadly infection is now being recognized as a chronic, treatable condition (Kelly et al., 1998; Kravcik et al., 1998). In 2002, for the first time a 25% increase in the incidence of HIV infections was recorded (789 new cases of HIV infection) and preliminary data from 2003 indicate that for the first time in years the country will additionally face an increase in new AIDS cases (BAG Bulletin, 2003). The federal government has recognized the latest developments of HIV infection and has approved the National AIDS Program. Considerable efforts will be taken to reverse these worrisome trends, including the start of a new national STOP AIDS campaign.

The Swiss HIV Cohort Study (SHCS)

The SHCS is a prospective cohort study of individuals with HIV infection aged 16 years or older (Sudre et al., 2000). Patients are followed every 6 months at outpatient clinics in 5 university hospitals, 2 tertiary care centers and private practices that serve large groups of HIV infected individuals. In a cross sectional study, the prevalence of unsafe sexual behavior and factors associated with unsafe sexual behavior was investigated with a newly introduced questionnaire (Wolf et al., 2003). The questionnaire included questions on protected or unprotected sexual intercourse, type of partnership (stable partnership or occasional partners) and known or unknown serostatus of a stable partner. Answers to these questions were voluntary and were recorded on an anonymous form.

The study included all participants in the SHCS who responded for the first time to the new outpatient questionnaire over a period of 12 months after its introduction. In this study reported 'unsafe sex' was defined if individuals indicated that they did not always use condoms when having sexual intercourse. 'Denied unsafe sex' was defined if individuals indicated that they either had no partner or they had no sexual intercourse with their partner or they always used condoms when having sexual intercourse. 'Possible unsafe sex' was defined if individuals neither reported nor denied unsafe sex. This definition was used to identify a possible reporting bias. Clinical and demographic information including gender, age, ethnicity, education, HIV transmission group, CDC stage, type of potent antiretroviral therapy and plasma HIV RNA (Morandi et al., 1998).

Trends in Sexual Behavior among HIV Positive Cohort Members

In April 2000, 4948 individuals were registered and not known to have left the SHCS. Of these, 4767 (96%) had at least one follow-up visit and 4723 (95%) responded to the sexual behavior questionnaire. The percentage of females, intravenous drug users, and individuals with only basic education was higher among those who did not respond than among those who did respond. Of those who responded, 55% had a stable partnership and 19% had occasional partners during the preceding 6 months, and 6% had both. Of those with stable partners, 82% reported sexual intercourse and of those reporting sexual intercourse, 76% said they always used condoms. Of those with occasional partners, 87% reported sexual intercourse and of those reporting sexual intercourse, 86% said they always used condoms. Overall 12% of the individuals reported unsafe sex, 81% denied unsafe sex, and the remaining 7% neither reported nor denied unsafe sex. Among those that responded 78% received antiretroviral therapy and 25% had optimal viral suppression with viral load measurements below 50 copies/mL during the preceding 12 months.

In multivariate analysis, reported unsafe sex was not associated with optimal viral suppression, antiretroviral therapy, diagnosis of an AIDS-defining disease or education. However reported unsafe sex was associated with gender, age, ethnicity, HIV transmission group, HIV status of the stable partner, having occasional partners, and living alone. After adjusting for all other covariates, the odds ratio for reported unsafe sex in individuals with optimal viral suppression was not significant. Men, individuals age over 40 years, and individuals living alone were less likely to report unsafe sex. Individuals from ethnic groups other than Caucasian, intravenous drug users, individuals with HIV infected partners, and those with occasional partners were more likely to report unsafe sex.

With unsafe sex not denied as the response, there was less evidence of associations with age and occasional partners and more evidence of associations with education and antiretroviral therapy. Most odds ratios suggest that the nature of any association was similar for both responses. For both reported and not denied unsafe sex, odds ratios were lower for individuals on antiretroviral therapy and for individuals with higher education. However odds ratios differed between the two responses for men having sex with men and for those with occasional partners. Compared to other HIV transmission groups, MSM were no more likely to report unsafe sex, but were more likely to not deny unsafe sex. Individuals with occasional partners were more likely to report unsafe sex, but were no more likely to not deny unsafe sex.

The interaction of gender and drug use was evaluated because female drug users may sell unsafe sex for drugs. As a replacement for gender in multivariate analysis, female drug users were more likely to report unsafe sex and not to deny unsafe sex. With this interaction included, gender was then not associated with either response.

Limitations and Summary

In this study of a large and well described HIV-infected population there was no evidence of an association between unsafe sexual behavior and optimal viral suppression. Intravenous drug users, women of other ethnic groups than Caucasian and those with occasional partners were amore likely to report unsafe sexual behavior. The study has limitations because information about sexual behavior was self-reported and patients were interviewed by their physician or study nurse. Individuals who responded to the questionnaire were different from those who did not respond, which suggests this study may underestimate the prevalence of unsafe sexual behavior. However, inferences from this study are strong due the large sample size and very high response rate. The study further allows us to explore to some extent the possibility of reporting bias. Similar odds ratios are seen for both responses, except for individuals with occasional partners and for MSM. The study underlines the importance of epidemiological data on sexual behavior in HIV-infected populations. In the SHCS four out of five HIV-infected individuals report safer sexual behavior with their partners. Sexual health programs targeting subgroups with increased risk behavior should complement programs aimed at the general population.

AUSTRALIA: PATRICK RAWSTORNE, ANDREA FOGARTY, PAUL VAN DE VEN, AND SUSAN KIPPAX, UNIVERSITY OF NEW SOUTH WALES, AUSTRALIA

By the end of March 2003, 22,775 people had been infected with HIV in Australia since the beginning of the epidemic (NCHECR, 2003a). Of these people, 9039 had developed AIDS, among whom 6,277 had died following AIDS (NCHECR, 2003a). There were approximately 16,498 people living with HIV in Australia in the first quarter of 2003.

The majority of people living with HIV/AIDS in Australia are men who acquired the virus through male-to-male sexual contact (NCHECR, 2003a) and who live in the three major cities along the east coast: Sydney, Melbourne and Brisbane. Of these cities, Sydney has the highest number of people with HIV. These cities also have the largest populations of gay community in Australia and are where the majority of HIV infections occur. Since the beginning of the epidemic, HIV transmission cases have occurred through male-to-male sexual contact (77.4%), heterosexual contact (11.0%), and through injecting drug use (8.5%), with other exposure risks less common (NCHECR, 2003a).

New HIV diagnoses have gradually risen in Australia over the last five years, after a long period of decline (see Figure 9.1, NCHECR, 2003b). In 1998, there were 650 people newly diagnosed with HIV compared with about 800 in 2002 (NCHECR, 2003b). The proportion of HIV transmission attributable to male homosexual contact may be rising: between the years 1998-2002, at least 85% of cases of HIV transmission occurred in this way (NCHECR, 2003b). As the majority of people living with HIV and HIV

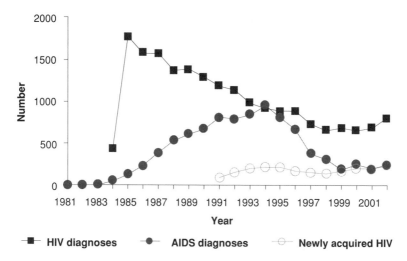

Figure 9.1. Number of diagnoses of HIV infection adjusted for multiple reporting and AIDS adjusted for reporting delay in Australia.

transmission cases are among MSM, the main focus of this section is with this group.

Australia's response to threat of HIV/AIDS is structured according to a tripartite relationship involving three separate partners: government, research centres, and community-based organizations. The relationship is reflexive (Kippax & Kinder, 2002). That is, research drives the health promotion work of community organizations which in turn informs research activities. Here we focus on the research in Australia based on risk practices among MSM.

A discussion based around risk behavior among people living with HIV/AIDS is very timely given the current increase in HIV infections in Australia. Unprotected anal intercourse (UAI) will be used here as a marker of risk, as it is the major route of HIV transmission between MSM. Within this discussion, UAI will be contextualized as much as possible by partner type (regular or casual), partner serostatus, and/or sexual positioning (insertive or receptive) and/or by the number of episodes or partners with whom one engaged in these practices. Some of the data presented in this section are shown for capital cities and other areas of Australia. Where it is not as important to provide an Australian overview, data are shown for one city only, usually Sydney.

As UAI between MSM is the major marker of HIV transmission risk in Australia, trends in UAI across Australia will be addressed first. There is evidence of a steady increase in UAI with casual partners (UAI-C) in most of the major cities in Australia up to the end of 2002 (see Table 9.2). The studies

Table 9.2. MSM engaging in unprotected anal intercourse with casual partners by serostatus Australia[1]

Source	1998 N	%	1999 N	%	2000 N	%	2001 N	%	2002 N	%
Australia										
Male Out										
Positive					69	62				
Negative					936	34				
HIV Futures			828	52	818	59				
Sydney										
HIM										
Negative							360	37	656	37
PH										
Positive							151	52	159	56
Periodic										
Positive	502	38	481	43	404	51	375	61	337	59
Negative	1526	19	1647	21	1519	27	1521	28	1521	29
Melbourne										
Periodic										
Positive	135	33			110	36	115	49	122	57
Negative	1019	15			864	22	909	23	972	24
Brisbane										
Periodic										
Positive	86	30	74	27	68	42	74	48	96	47
Negative	735	17	696	19	696	24	869	25	963	30
Perth										
Periodic										
Positive	33	33			42	26			18	33
Negative	440	16			530	27			381	28
Adelaide										
Periodic										
Positive	28	42	25	32			24	41		
Negative	260	20	216	18			293	23		
Canberra										
Periodic										
Positive					10	—[2]				
Negative					175	21				

[1] Excludes men whose serostatus was unknown, either because they reported that they had not been tested or because they did not provide information regarding serostatus. The difference between positive and negative men in the percentage who reported unprotected anal intercourse with casual partners is statistically significant throughout, except for the Perth 2000 *Periodic Survey* data.
[2] Number of men too small to give a reliable percentage. Source Van de Ven et al., 2003.

Table 9.3. Unprotected anal intercourse with regular male partners among men living with HIV/AIDS, by serostatus of partner Australia[1]

	1999		2001		2002	
Partner Type	N	%	N	%	N	%
HIV Futures (Nationwide)						
Regular male (HIV-positive)	123	83	122	91		
Regular male (HIV-negative)	125	34	121	41		
pH (NSW and Victoria)						
Regular male (HIV-positive)			52	71	65	73
Regular male (HIV-negative/unknown)			67	40	80	20

[1] Shows the number and the percentage of men living with HIV/AIDS who reported unprotected anal intercourse with regular partners in the six months prior to the survey. N is the number of people who answered the question (that is, who had a partner of the type shown).

reported in Table 9.2—an anonymous, cross-sectional survey of the sex practices of gay community attached men (Periodic survey), a cohort study of HIV-negative men in Sydney (HIM), a cohort study of HIV-positive men (pH) in NSW and Victoria, and a nationwide cross-sectional survey of MSM from urban, regional and remote areas of Australia (Male Out), and a national survey of people living with HIV (Futures)—indicate that a higher proportion of HIV-positive men than HIV-negative men report UAI-C (NCHSR, 2003).

Compared with rates of UAI-C, rates of UAI with regular partners (UAI-R) are generally higher (see Table 9.3), as men are more likely to be sure of their primary partner's serostatus. Drawing on data from Futures and pH studies, it can be seen that UAI-R with seroconcordant regular partners is more common than UAI-R with non-concordant or seronon-concordant regular partners. Although not reported in Table 9.3, data from the Periodic Survey across cities in Australia shows that there has been a significant increase in rates of UAI-R over the last 5 years (Van de Ven et al., 2002).

HIV Testing

Men's sexual practice is informed by knowledge of their own HIV status and that of their partners. There are a relatively high proportion of homosexually active men who have ever been tested for HIV, usually over 80% in major cities since 1996. In Sydney where seroprevalence is highest testing rates have been between 85% and 95%. The majority of younger men (less than 25 years) in each of the large cities have been tested for HIV. Most homosexually active men in Australia undertake regular HIV testing. A high proportion of HIV-negative men have an HIV antibody test in every 6 month period—in the order of 30%–50% depending on the city.

Factors Related to UAI among People Living with HIV in Australia

A number of factors help contextualize the practice of UAI. This section will discuss a number of strategies that HIV-positive men employ in their attempt to manage risk while engaging in UAI. These strategies might reduce harm, some more than others, but to an unknown extent.

Strategies Employed to Manage Risk of HIV Transmission when Engaging in UAI

HIV-positive men have adopted a range of strategies in an attempt to reduce the risk of HIV transmission when engaging in UAI. Some of these strategies carry a risk of HIV infection, yet some men may not be aware of the extent of the risk. Two of the three strategies discussed here require a sophisticated knowledge of medicine and its relationship to HIV transmission risk. Such knowledge is much greater among HIV-positive men than HIV-negative men (Rosengarten, et al., 2000). The strategies that will be discussed here include seroconcordant ('pos-pos') UAI, viral load as a gauge of HIV infectivity, and strategic positioning (receptive or insertive or both).

Seroconcordant (Pos-Pos) Sex

One of the reasons there are higher rates of UAI-C among HIV-positive men is that a sizeable proportion of UAI-C is with a seroconcordant partner—which poses no risk of HIV transmission to an uninfected partner. In contrast, the same act among men who believe they are HIV-negative carries considerable risk, as there is no assurance that a partner's most recent negative HIV test results reflect their current serostatus. To explore how much UAI-C is occurring with concordant partners, we need to look at data from the interview-based HIV-positive cohort study, pH.

Data from the pH cohort study shows that a large proportion of UAI-C acts occur with seroconcordant partners: of 338 HIV-positive men, 42% of these men reported 4,959 acts of UAI-C over a six-month period. Of these acts, 2111 (42.5%) were with other HIV-positive men, posing no risk of HIV transmission (Rawstorne, et al., 2004a). The remaining 2,848 acts of UAI-C were with HIV-unknown (2451 acts) and HIV-negative (397 acts) partners, posing a risk of HIV transmission (Rawstorne, et al., 2004a).

Locating other HIV-positive partners for the purpose of pos-pos sex is made easier in cities such as Sydney and Melbourne where there is a relatively large population of people with HIV/AIDS. Some of the sex-on-premises venues in these cities have a large number of HIV positive partners. It is common at these premises for assumptions to be made about a partner's serostatus and for men to engage in UAI in the absence of verbal disclosure. Sometimes the assumptions can be wrong. For example, results from a qualitative study suggest that the non-use of condoms for UAI may be read differently by HIV-positive and HIV-negative men. This is evidenced from the comments of an HIV-positive man in Sydney (Rosengarten, et al., 2000, p. 17):

> "...I assumed he was HIV-positive because he didn't want to use a condom. He assumed I was HIV-negative because I didn't want to use a condom."

Disclosure of HIV status to casual partners often occurs in the context of negotiating anal intercourse without condoms. HIV-positive men disclose more often than HIV-negative men (NCHSR, 2003) and this is consistent with the higher rates of UAI-C reported above. Disclosing one's HIV status can be extremely problematic for HIV-positive men, as reflected in the results of a nationwide cross-sectional survey of MSM, Male Out (Van de Ven, et al., 2001). In that study, participants were asked whether they avoid having sex with people they think have HIV. Among the HIV-negative or HIV serostatus unknown participants, over 80% answered 'yes'. Eighty percent of the same men answered 'yes' when asked whether they expected a man with HIV to tell them his status before having sex.

Viral Load as a Gauge of Risk

HIV-positive men are making assessments of HIV-transmission risk based on their knowledge of viral load. This knowledge informs their sex practice. Drawing on data from a qualitative study of men in Sydney and Brisbane, an HIV-positive man explains the absence of condoms with a non-concordant regular partner (Rosengarten, et al., 2000, p. 18):

> "I've been undetectable now for six months and I've been pretty happy about that...My partner understands the risks he's taking [by not wearing a condom],...he's being very careful and constantly gets tested."

Being asked to elaborate, he confirms that his partner's 'being careful' means being 'a top' or 'insertive'.

Data from quantitative studies suggests that there might only be a small proportion of HIV-positive men who rely on their own viral load to inform their sex practice with casual partners. For example, data from the pH cohort study shows that viral load is unrelated to engaging in UAI-C in the previous six months. Also, differences in viral load made no difference to the number of UAI-C acts men engaged in the previous 6 months. Although the use of viral load in guiding sex practice in casual contexts may be minimally used, it is likely that a minority of men rely on this strategy in non-concordant regular relationships.

Strategic Positioning

HIV-positive men are using their knowledge about HIV transmissibility to guide their sexual positioning. This is evidenced in a number of studies and is illustrated particularly well by an HIV-positive man from the same qualitative study mentioned above (Rosengarten, et al., 2000, p. 18):

> "Yeah, if um I'm being receptive, if I'm being the passive partner, um and it's a one nighter... I will leave it up to the other person who is being the active partner to put on a condom... if they don't [use a condom] I figure well obviously they know the risk... I also know the risk of them getting infected from me is very minimal. If on the other hand I'm being the active partner I'd always put a condom on...".

Strategic positioning is also evidenced in the quantitative survey data (Van de Ven, et al., 2002). In the context of UAI-R with a non-concordant regular partner, HIV-positive men are more likely to be receptive-only than either insertive-only or both insertive and receptive. Adding validity to these results, HIV-negative men show a complementary pattern: they are more likely to be insertive-only than either receptive-only or both receptive and insertive. These results cannot be explained on the basis of a positioning preference, as when these same men's sexual practices were analyzed with condoms, the most common mode was both receptive and insertive (Van de Ven, et al., 2002). Strategic positioning is also evident in the context of UAI-C and in combination with another strategy to reduce risk—withdrawal before ejaculation (NCHSR, 2003).

The Effects of HAART on Sex Practice

Data in Australia show a relationship between using HAART and sex practice. Consistent with results from a sample of HIV-positive homosexual men in London (Stephenson, et al., 2003), taking HAART is associated with lower HIV transmission risk among Sydney HIV-positive men (Rawstorne, et al., 2004b). Drawing on data from 621 HIV-positive men who participated in the Sydney Periodic Survey in 2003, men were classified into two groups based on whether they had engaged in UAI-C (48%) or not (51%) in the previous 6 months. Bivariate analyses showed that engaging in UAI-C was associated with: not taking HAART, having a greater number of sex partners, and poorer self-rated health. There were no associations with viral load, age, and having a regular partner. Logistic regression analysis found that UAI-C was significantly and independently associated with not taking HAART, and having a greater number of sex partners (Rawstorne, et al., 2004b).

INDIA: MARIA EKSTRAND, UNIVERSITY OF CALIFORNIA SAN FRANCISCO, SHALINI BHARAT, TATA INSTITUTE OF SOCIAL SCIENCES, MUMBAI, JAYASHREE RAMAKRISHNA, NATIONAL INSTITUTE OF MENTAL HEALTH AND NEUROSCIENCES IN BANGALORE

The number of HIV infections in India is difficult to ascertain and the subject of ongoing controversy. In 2001, India's National AIDS Control Organization (NACO) estimated that there were 3.9 million Indians infected with HIV. UNAIDS published this figure in its 2002 global update, but included an estimated range between 2.6 and 5.4 million (UNAIDS, 2002). Another 2002 report by the US National Intelligence Council estimated that the current number of infections is between 5 and 8 million and projected that this range will increase to 20 to 25 million by 2010 (US National Intelligence Council, 2002). In 2003, NACO revised its prevalence estimate to 4.5 million.

Because India has a population of over one billion, all the current HIV/AIDS figures cited above represent relatively low prevalence. According to UNAIDS, adult HIV prevalence was 0.8 percent at the end of 2001. However, low overall prevalence masks crucial differences among regions, states, and subpopulations. There are growing localized HIV epidemics in India (UNAIDS, Jan, 2002). Although HIV is currently concentrated among marginalized groups such as sex workers, MSM, Injection Drug Users, truck drivers and migrant workers, it is spreading rapidly to the general population (World Bank, 1999).

In 2003, NACO released a study of cumulative AIDS cases reported since 1986. It found that 85% of HIV infections were transmitted sexually. Perinatal transmission accounted for 2% of infections, IDU 2%, and unsafe blood and blood products 3%. Patterns of HIV differ by region. Among high-prevalence states such as Maharasthra, Tamil Nadu, Karnataka, and

Andhra Pradhesh, sexual transmission reportedly accounts for the majority of HIV infections, whereas injection drug use has been driving the epidemic in Manipur and Nagaland. Nevertheless, prevalence rates among IDUs are also high in the State of Tamil Nadu and in the city of Mumbai in Maharasthra (33% and 39%, respectively).

It is difficult to determine actual prevalence among MSM in India, given that NACO has only recently collected data on MSM and in only two surveillance sites. In 2001, MSM prevalence was 23% in Mumbai (Maharasthra) and 2% in Chennai (Tamil Nadu). Many public health professionals working in the area of male-to-male transmission have noted that the 3:1 proportion of male-to-female HIV cases does not fit with the reported prevalence of heterosexual transmission, given that male-to-female transmission is much more efficient than transmission from women to men. They therefore suggest that the prevalence figures reflect higher than reported levels of male-to-male transmission, a significant underreporting of infections among women, or unidentified co-factors.

Sexual Risk Behaviors in India

There are no behaviorally-based cohort studies of HIV infected individuals in India. We recently conducted a small study of the prevention needs of HIV-infected male STD patients in Mumbai, India in order to develop an effective and culturally-specific risk reduction intervention for this population (Ekstrand et al., 2004). One hundred and four HIV-infected men were interviewed at 3 and 6 months following receipt of their diagnosis. All participants received standard HIV pre- and post-test counseling following CDC guidelines and modified based on local conditions. Preliminary analyses of baseline data showed that sexual activity decreased following diagnosis, with 41 % of the men reporting no sex in the last 3 months, 58% reporting sex with women, and one person reporting sex only with a trans-gendered person. Condom use was inconsistent. Among those who were sexually active, 50% said that they always used condoms, 36% reported that this occurred "sometimes" and 22% said that they never used them. Unprotected sex was associated with lower self-efficacy, less condom comfort, and a greater likelihood of attributing one's health status to "chance". Men who reported a loss of interest in sex were also significantly less likely to report any sexual behaviors than men who reported no loss of interest (33% vs. 81%). However, loss of interest was not associated with condom use. The participants reported high levels of depression, with only 23% scoring in the normal range of the Beck Depression Inventory, 21% scoring "mildly" depressed, 38% "moderately" depressed, and 19%

"severely" depressed. Depression was not associated with sexual activity or with condom use.

Counselor notes indicate that the men expressed fears about AIDS-related stigma and discrimination and worried about their ability to get married, have children, and disclose their HIV status to prospective partners. Although both married and single men reported that marital and family issues were critically important, specific issues varied by marital status. Married men reported being unable to disclose their HIV status to their wives due to fears of rejection. The pressure of having children was reported to be an additional stressor for the married men who were unable to disclose. Unmarried men feared disclosing their status to family members and future partners and as a result, either chose to remain single or were pressured into marriage without disclosure. Among both groups, failure to disclose frequently resulted in an inability to introduce condom use.

Regardless of marital status, HIV-infected men were concerned about marital issues and needed help to overcome their fears of stigma and discrimination in order to comfortably disclose their status to wives, family and future partners. These results suggest that prevention interventions targeting HIV infected men in Mumbai need to use a comprehensive approach, addressing not only safer sex issues, but also psychological distress and the consequences of AIDS-related stigma and discrimination, such as legal issues and access to health care, in order to meet their needs.

A study of psychosocial and sexual adjustment among persons living with HIV was recently completed in Bangalore, India (Chandra, 2003). The sample included 27 women and 18 men, who were interviewed quarterly over a 12 month period regarding nature and frequency of sexual activity, sexual practices, sexual satisfaction and safer sex. The mean age of the sample was 28.6 years. The majority of the sample (55%) were of urban origin, 25% were from rural areas and 20% were from semi-urban areas. The study found that there were striking gender differences in the frequency of sexual intercourse, with men being more sexually active and women choosing to remain abstinent. Consistency of condom use depended largely on the HIV status of one's spouse. The eight non-concordant couples were found to be more motivated to use condoms regularly. In contrast, the seroconcordant couples reported both less of a need and less actual use of condoms. These couples reported that as both of them were already positive they would rather enjoy the rest of the life to the maximum possible extent. They considered condom use as a barrier to their enjoyment during sex.

There was an immediate increase in number of men who were abstinent during the first interview following receipt of diagnosis. This is consistent with the Mumbai STD study. Reasons given for this decrease included fear and shock. This reaction was shown to wear off gradually as time progressed and this change was accompanied by reports of increased sexual activity. A similar increase and subsequent gradual decrease was observed in condom use and masturbation among men.

Among women, both sexual activity and safer sex practices decreased over a period of one year following diagnosis. The former may be due to the worsening of health or death of their spouse, while the latter seemed to be associated with poor negotiation and communication with their spouses. Female sex workers who continued having unprotected sex typically stated that the decision to use condoms depended on their clients. However, the fear of losing business may contribute to an inability to convince clients to use condoms.

HIV Care and Treatment

A study by the S. Singh found that among 252 HIV-infected individuals, an HIV-positive spouse was the only risk factor for acquiring HIV in 82% of women, compared to only 2% of men. Among all women, 75% were "completely unaware" of the risk to themselves from their husband, only 19% had received primary education, 75% had never heard of HIV before being tested, 25% women were widows whose spouses had died because of AIDS.

Prior to HIV/AIDS, there were already strong gender biases in access to health care. Female children are the most disadvantaged. Girls are less likely to be brought into hospitals than boys and are almost always brought in at a later stage of illness. Given the intra-household nutritional biases, girls take longer to recover from diseases and have higher rates of mortality within hospitals, seriously affecting their education and employment. Moreover, women face serious occupational hazards, especially in rural areas, where they perform hard physical labor, both within and outside the house. Such labor has serious effects on adolescent girls with underdeveloped bone structures and high rates of malnutrition.

The International Alliance for HIV/AIDS (2002) has found that when both a husband and wife are infected with HIV/AIDS, men routinely receive care and treatment ahead of their wives. Lack of money and distance to treatment are also constraints (Alfred et al., 2002). The Lawyers Collective HIV/AIDS Unit, the leading organization analyzing HIV/AIDS and human rights in India, has reported on how HIV/AIDS is exacerbating gender inequalities and how Indian laws perpetuate gender inequality and are ill equipped to resolve the varied difficulties faced by women with HIV/AIDS. In a study of 70 cases involving women living with HIV/AIDS, it found that most women were between 18 and 30 years of age and that over 50 percent were widows, economically dependent and unemployed. Among the most critical issues was women's struggle to obtain maintenance from husbands or in-laws; other major issues included property rights, custody of children, discrimination in health care, consent and confidentiality, and harassment.

AIDS Stigma in India

AIDS stigma in India has been perpetrated by legal efforts and at the level of communities and individuals. One example of the former was the Indian Supreme Court's 1998 decision that a person with HIV/AIDS has no right to marry and start a family, life events of utmost importance in Indian culture. Another policy decision that may have far-ranging consequences for people with HIV were recent decisions to require pre-marital HIV testing. Indian media has also reported widespread AIDS stigma and discrimination in several Indian states. In one instance, an entire village became the target of stigma after one of its bus drivers tested positive for HIV, resulting in villagers being unable to find employment, being dismissed from nearby colleges, and having difficulty arranging marriages. Similar stories have been published of discrimination within villages. In Bihar, a family was boycotted when villagers blocked the road to a house, in which three people had died of AIDS, and decided not to have any contact with the family. The family members reported that their children were sick, yet they never received any help from anyone in the village. This discrimination appeared to be due to misconceptions regarding infection routes and one village member stated that "we are apprehensive about getting the disease ourselves" (Kumar, 2002).

However, fear of infection does not always seem to be the reason for AIDS-related discrimination. In 2002, three HIV positive children were refused admission by three different schools in Hyderabad, even though administrators acknowledged that "there may be no real risk" of HIV transmission to other children" (Sudhit, 2002). A similar incident happened in Assam, when one woman decided to speak out about her infection and work for AIDS awareness after losing her husband and daughter to AIDS. She was evicted from her home and unable to find another one. Her landlord said: "Media has made HIV look so frightening that we are scared. I understand that it's not contagious, but neighbors had put a lot of pressure. So I asked her to leave." (Bhattacharjee, 2002).

Several newspaper reports have described denial of health care services for people living with HIV/AIDS. The Health Institute for Mother and Child (MAMTA) in Delhi reported of a young woman, 8 months pregnant and living in Delhi, who was unable to find a private or government hospital that will agree to deliver her baby. Another one of MAMTA's clients was taken to the hospital with a severe breathing problem. While in the midst of emergency treatment, the doctors discovered that he was HIV positive. They screamed and jumped away from him, discontinuing treatment. The patient died within an hour. This kind of treatment appears to occur in other urban settings as well.

The largest study to date of AIDS stigma and health in India was conducted by Bharat (2001) among individuals who were infected, affected, and who were working with HIV/AIDS in Bangalore and Mumbai. This qualitative study identified many issues of vital importance for our understanding of the culturally specific nature and manifestations of AIDS stigma. In both sites, both overt and covert stigma and discrimination were identified in the health care setting. In an attempt to avoid having to provide care, health care staff sent patients from hospital to hospital. There was uncertainty among health care staff about basic HIV transmission information and about the need for, and purpose of, universal precautions. Staff typically overestimated the infectiousness of HIV, which profoundly affected their ability to provide good care. Treatments were thus selected, not based on what would be best for the patient, but what would guarantee complete elimination of any transmission risk, such as fumigation of operating and delivery rooms. In general, refusal of care for HIV positive individuals was common, especially for antenatal care and surgery, and confidentiality was frequently breached. Bharat's work also showed that stigma was greater in the case of sex workers, homosexuals, and "eunuchs" in both Mumbai and Bangalore, illustrating that AIDS stigma adds to and magnifies preexisting prejudices.

SOUTH AFRICA: LEICKNESS C. SIMBAYI, HUMAN SCIENCES RESEARCH COUNCIL, CAPE TOWN SOUTH AFRICA AND SETH C. KALICHMAN, UNIVERSITY OF CONNECTICUT

In the past decade, the numbers of HIV infections and deaths associated with AIDS have dramatically risen in South Africa. It is currently estimated that there are 1600 new HIV infections and 600 AIDS-related deaths in South Africa each day. The HIV epidemic in South Africa has recently been described by a nationally representative household HIV sero-prevalence study (Nelson Mandela/HSRC, Shisana and Simbayi, 2002). The South African national seroprevalence study, funded by both the Nelson Mandela Foundation and the Nelson Mandela Children's Fund, estimated that the overall HIV prevalence in the South African population is 11%, with the highest HIV prevalence (21%) occurring among people living in informal urban townships. HIV prevalence among those aged 15–49 is over 15%. HIV prevalence among women is 13% and prevalence for men is 9%. Among youth (aged 15–24), double the number of females (12%) are infected as males (6%). In terms of race, HIV prevalence among Black South Africans (Africans) is highest (13%) as compared to 6% among Whites as well as among Coloureds.

In South Africa research has repeatedly shown that only one in five South Africans are tested for HIV antibodies, and among those tested about one in five test HIV positive; 76% of South Africans who are HIV posi-tive are not aware of their HIV status (Shisana and Simbayi, 2002). Thus, a small minority of those infected with HIV are aware of their positive HIV status. In addition, it is most common for people who are HIV in-fected in South Africa to seek HIV testing only after they have become ill, late in the stage of their HIV infection. The low uptake of HIV testing in South Africa is probably accounted for by multiple factors including the historical unavailability of antiretroviral therapies, some misinformation and misperceptions about HIV/AIDS, and AIDS-related stigmas. In addi-tion, people may not get tested simply because they do not believe they are at risk for HIV. In the national HIV prevalence study, 63% of people who were found to be HIV positive did not even perceive themselves to be at risk (Shisana and Simbayi, 2002). It is worth noting that testing in the survey was done completely anonymously and results were not di-vulged to participants. HIV prevalence rates in some areas of South Africa are as high as 30% with HIV testing rates as low as 20%, indicating that HIV prevention will most likely reach HIV infected individuals when in-terventions are directed at all people, not just those who have tested HIV positive.

Nevertheless, there remains interest in developing HIV prevention interventions for South Africans who are aware that they are HIV positive. When people test HIV positive, their HIV prevention needs differ and there should be targeted interventions available to meet these needs. In addition, as antiretroviral medications become increasingly available there will be more people tested earlier in their HIV disease process. Clinics and hospitals where people with HIV receive care are viable points of contact for intervening with HIV infected populations.

HIV Infections in South Africa

Like many countries, South Africa has historically relied on surveillance of HIV infection rates among pregnant women attending antenatal
clinics to estimate and model their HIV epidemic. Although certainly a
useful data source, antenatal clinic data provides its best estimates for HIV
among demographic groups attending sentinel clinics and may be most
limited when estimating infection rates among men. HIV surveillance using population-based representative sampling provides an important additional data source for monitoring HIV infections. As was mentioned
earlier, the Nelson Mandela/HSRC Household HIV seroprevalence study
provides new information about the rates and distribution of HIV infections in South Africa. According to this study, the HIV prevalence in the
population of South Africa was 11.4% (Confidence Interval, 10.0%–12.7%),
indicating that 4.5 million people in South Africa are living with HIV infection. When restricted to individuals between the ages of 15 and 49,
representing 80% of people with HIV/AIDS, the HIV prevalence is 15%
(Confidence Interval, 13.9%–17.5%, Shisana and Simbayi, 2002). Among
this age group, HIV infections are highest in urban informal settlement
areas—communities that often surround Townships that are densely pop-
ulated and most impoverished—where HIV seroprevalence can reach 30%.
        HIV affects all South Africans, but not equally. The overwhelming ma-
jority (77%) of the South African population is indigenous in origin and
classified as African. This is the population segment clearly most affected
by HIV/AIDS, with 18% of all adult (15 to 49 years of age) Africans HIV
positive. Among the rest of the population there are people that descended
from Europe and are designated White (12% population) and those descended from the Indian sub-continent and are classified Indians (2%).
The national HIV prevalence study showed that 6% of Whites and nearly
2% of Indians were HIV positive. Another significant racial minority group
in South Africa is known as Coloureds and is mainly made of people who
are of mixed race or aboriginal in origin, a group with 7% HIV prevalence.
        Thus, racial classification continues to be used in South Africa due to
the existence of many disparities in all spheres of life including health status
and access to health services that reflect the legacy of the Apartheid era
when Whites enjoyed more privileges than their other counterparts from
the other races. The racial lines of South Africa are also demarcated by HIV.
However, there has been a false sense of distance from HIV/AIDS among
other races especially Whites and Coloureds. The finding that there also
exist some generalized HIV epidemics among both Whites and Coloureds
suggests that HIV could rapidly grow in these communities unless risks
are recognized and prevention steps are taken.

HIV Transmission Risks among People Who Know They Are HIV Positive

There are limited data available on HIV risks and risk behaviors among people living with HIV in South Africa. The Nelson Mandela/HSRC Household Survey once again provides some useful data in this regard. The sample was divided in two, those who tested HIV positive and those who tested HIV negative in the study. However, participants were not informed of their study test results. Comparisons could be made, however, on the proportion of persons who knew their HIV status within behavioral subgroups. For example, with respect to numbers of sexual partners, 20% of HIV positive individuals who were abstinent from sex were aware of their positive status compared to 6% of people who were HIV negative. When it came to numbers of partners, the rates of knowing one's HIV status were nearly mirror images: 25% of both HIV positive and HIV negative persons who had one sex partner were aware of their status and 16% of both HIV status groups who had multiple sex partners were aware of their HIV status. Among HIV positive individuals, 30% of those who had discussed HIV prevention with sex partners knew they were HIV positive, and among HIV negative persons 26% who had discussed HIV prevention with partners were aware of their status. In addition, among HIV infected persons who knew their partner's HIV status, 68% were aware that they were HIV positive compared to 66% of HIV negative persons who knew their partner's status. The study also found that 33% of people with HIV who had used a condom during their last sexual encounter were aware of their HIV status compared to 26% of people who did not have HIV and had used a condom. Thus, there was an apparent benefit of being aware of one's HIV status observed in these data, but the differences were only slight. However, participants in this study were not asked their HIV status. Therefore, these data might actually test the hypothesis that simply knowing one's HIV status irregardless of the actual diagnosis is enough to promote behavioral change among people that are tested in South Africa.

The national prevalence study also showed that 39% of people who had an STI in the previous 3 months were HIV positive. In addition, 40% of those with a genital ulcer and 25% of men with an abnormal penile discharge were HIV positive (Shisana and Simbayi, 2002). These data not only strongly support the link between HIV infection and other sexually transmitted infections in South Africa, they also provide a sense for the high rates of continued sexual risks among people who are HIV positive.

A study by Olley et al. (2003) reported data from an urban clinic that cares for people with HIV infection in South Africa. The study is unique in that it reports a health clinic sample of 148 patients that could be similar to populations that will be accessed by clinic-based interventions for people living with HIV/AIDS. Results indicated that 68% of people living with HIV/AIDS were sexually active during the previous six month period. Among those who were sexually active, more than half did not report using condoms during their last occasion of sexual intercourse. Thus, it can be inferred that about one in three people living with HIV reported engaging in unprotected intercourse during the past six months. In addition, Olley et al. found that 67% of individuals who did not use a condom at their last sexual encounter also did not know the HIV status of their sex partner. Engaging in unprotected intercourse was most closely associated with being HIV infected for a shorter duration of time and expressing a greater use of a denial style of coping.

People living with HIV/AIDS who contract new STI may represent the individuals at highest risk for HIV transmission. Data from a small convenience sample of 19 HIV positive men and 13 HIV positive women receiving STI diagnostic and treatment services in Cape Town provide some sense for this potentially important population. This sample was composed of Africans and only three men and one woman were married. With respect to sexual practices, 69% men and 23% women reported having two or more sex partners in the previous month. A total of 53% men and 77% women also reported engaging in unprotected vaginal intercourse during that time period. Ten men (53%) and one woman (8%) had used alcohol in a sexual context during the past month. It was also found that three men and four women had engaged in sexual intercourse during the past month when their genitals were bleeding, and 12 men reported that they had sexual intercourse during the past month with a woman whose genitals were bleeding. We do not, however, have data on the HIV status of their sex partners. It was not common for these individuals to be involved in trading sex for money or materials, with two women reporting that they had ever received money or materials in exchange for sex and three men reporting that they had given money or materials to obtain sex.

Taken together, findings from these studies show that there is very limited data on the rates and patterns of sexual risk practices among South Africans living with HIV/AIDS. From what information is available, the rates and patterns of sexual risk appear similar to other countries, with about one in three HIV infected adults reporting sexual behaviors that can potentially transmit HIV. An aspect of the HIV epidemic in South Africa that may be similar to some other countries, such as India, but quite different from countries in North America and Western Europe is the pervasiveness of stigmas against people living with HIV/AIDS. Stigmas create a context in which people with HIV are unlikely to get tested and those who do test HIV positive are unlikely to disclose their HIV status.

AIDS Stigmas in South Africa

HIV stigmas are pervasive in South African society. The Nelson Mandela/HSRC Household Survey found that 26% of respondents would not be willing to share a meal with a person living with AIDS, 18% were unwilling to sleep in the same room with someone with AIDS, and 6% would not talk to a person they knew to have AIDS (Shisana and Simbayi, 2002). In a study of 500 people living in a Cape Town township we found that individuals who had not been tested for HIV held significantly greater AIDS-related stigmas than individuals who had been tested (Kalichman and Simbayi, 2003). People who had not been tested were significantly more likely to agree that people with AIDS are dirty, should feel ashamed, and should feel guilty. Individuals who were not tested were also more likely to believe that people with AIDS must have done something wrong to have AIDS and were more likely to endorse that they would rather not be friends with someone who has AIDS. Finally, individuals who had not been tested were significantly more likely than those who had been tested to agree that people with AIDS should not be allowed to work with children. Thus, having been tested for HIV was related to less endorsement of stigmatizing beliefs against people living with HIV/AIDS, but those tested were not free of endorsing these stigmas.

Among people living with HIV themselves, we have found that some individuals endorse AIDS-related stigmas. In the STI clinic survey described above, we found that 48% of men and 39% of women stated that people living with HIV/AIDS should feel guilty about being HIV positive. Twenty-one percent of men also indicated that people living with HIV should feel ashamed of being HIV positive. In addition, 53% of men and 77% of women indicated that people who test HIV positive should expect to experience at least some restrictions on their lives. These high rates of endorsement of AIDS-related stigmas among people living with HIV/AIDS suggest that culturally held stigmas become internalized for some people living with HIV and that these internalized stigmas likely pose problems in the daily coping, disclosure, and perhaps practicing of safer sex (Lee et al., 2002; Parker and Aggleton, 2003).

CONCLUSIONS

The sample of countries represented in this chapter illustrate the cultural differences and similarities of AIDS. The available data indicates that roughly one in three people living with HIV/AIDS engage in unprotected intercourse. For developed countries, HIV prevention for people living with HIV occurs within a context of life improving antiretroviral medications. Studies in the UK, Switzerland and Australia were unable to detect any associations between taking antiretroviral medications and high risk sexual behavior. These findings are in contrast to research conducted with HIV positive MSM in the US, indicating potentially important cultural differences. For developing countries, AIDS-related stigmas are a recurring theme, clearly impeding HIV testing efforts and creating huge barriers to disclosing HIV status potential sex partners, as we saw among African communities living in the UK (see above). Additional research conducted within and across cultures is therefore needed to further identify the factors associated with HIV transmission risks among people living with HIV/AIDS.

REFERENCES

Alfred, D., Vijaya, S., and Alfred, R. (2002). "Women beyond the accessibility of treatment: the social, cultural and family barriers in accessing services in the rural parts of AP." Abstract no. WePeF6651. XIV International Conference on AIDS, Barcelona.

Anderson J, and Doyal L. (2004). Women from African living with HIV in London: a descriptive study. *AIDS Care*, 16:95–105

BAG Bulletin. 6-3-2003. Berne.

Bharat, R. (1998). AIDS: not a disease of morals. *Business Line* 11.

Bharat, S. (2001). *India: HIV and AIDS-related Discrimination, Stigma and Denial.* UNAIDS.

Bhattacharjee, K. Closed doors: HIV positive ostracized in Assam, (October 12, 2002); <http://www.ndtv.com/>

Bolding, G., Elford, J., and Sherr, L. (2002). *Gay men's survey in London gyms 2002.* London, City University London (http://www.city.ac.uk/barts/gymsurvey).

Chandra, P. (2003). Psychosocial and sexual adjustment among living with HIV: A Study Conducted at PRAYAS (an NGO) Pune, India. Report to NIMHANS Dept. of Health education Small Grants Programme for Research on Sexuality and Sexual Behavior. Coordinator Dr. Jayashree Ramakrishna, Funder; Ford Foundation.

Chinouya, M., and Davidson, O. (2003). *The Padare project: assessing health-related knowledge, attitudes and behaviors of HIV-positive Africans accessing services in north central London.* African HIV Policy Network, London.

Chinouya, M., Davidson, O., Fenton, K., and on behalf of the Mayisha team (2000). *The Mayisha Study: Sexual attitudes and lifestyles of migrant Africans in Inner London.* Horsham, Avert.

Chinouya, M., SSanyu-Sseruma, W., and Kwok, A. (2003). *The Shibah report: a study of sexual health issues affecting black Africans living with HIV in Lambeth, Southwark and Lewisham.* Health First, London.

Dodds, J., and Mercey, D. (2003). *Sexual health survey of gay men London 2002.* Royal Free and University College Medical School, London.

Doyal, L., and Anderson, J. (2003). *My heart is loaded: African women with HIV surviving in London.* Terrence Higgins Trust, London.

Egger, M., Hirschel, B., Francioli, P., Sudre, P., Wirz, M., Flepp, M., Rickenbach, M., Malinverni, R., Vernazza, P., and Battegay, M. (1997). Impact of new antiretroviral combination therapies in HIV infected patients in Switzerland: prospective multicentre study. Swiss HIV Cohort Study. *BMJ* 315:1194–1199.

Ekstrand, M., Gandhi, M., Setia, M., Rawade, S., Bob, J., Paul, S., Han, L., Lindan, C., and Jerajani, H. (under review) Examining the prevention needs of HIV-infected male STD patients in Mumbai, India.

Elford, J., Bolding, G., Davis, M., Sherr, L., and Hart, G. (manuscript in preparation). The Internet and HIV: design and methods.

Elford, J., Bolding, G., Maguire, M., and Sherr, L. (1999). Sexual risk behaviour among gay men in a relationship. *AIDS* 13:1407–1411.

Elford, J., Bolding, G., Maguire, M., and Sherr, L. (2001a). Gay men, risk and relationships. *AIDS* 15:1053–1055.

Elford, J., Bolding, G., and Sherr, L. (2001b). Seeking sex on the Internet and sexual risk behaviour among gay men using London gyms. *AIDS* 15:1409–1415.

Elford, J., Bolding, G., and Sherr, L. (2002). High risk sexual behaviour increases among London gay men: what is the role of HIV optimism? *AIDS* 16:1537–1544.

Elford, J., Bolding, G., and Sherr, L. (2003). Authors' response to letter from IG Stolte and NHTM Dukers concerning the paper "High risk sexual behaviour increases among London gay men between 1998-2001: what is the role of HIV optimism"? *AIDS* 17:2012–2013.

Elford, J., Bolding, G., Davis, M., Sherr, L., and Hart, G. (2004a). Trends in sexual behaviour among London gay men 1998–2003: implications for STI/HIV prevention and sexual health promotion. Sex Trans Infect, submitted for publication.

Elford, J., Bolding, G., Davis, M., Sherr, L., and Hart, G. (2004b). Web-based behavioural surveillance among men who have sex with men: a comparison of online and offline samples in London, UK. *JAIDS* 35:421–426.

Health Protection Agency (2003a). Epidemiology—HIV and AIDS. Health Protection Agency London. http://www.hpa.org.uk/infections/topics_az/hiv_and_sti/hiv/epidemiology/introduction.htm

Health Protection Agency (2003b). Survey of prevalent HIV infections diagnosed (SOPHID) data for 2002. HPA, London.

Health Protection Agency (2003c). AIDS/HIV quarterly surveillance tables, cumulative UK data to end September 2003 (Rep. No. 60: 03/3). HPA, London.

Imrie, J., Stephenson, J., Cowan, F., Wanigaratne, S., Billington, A.J., Copas, A.J., French, L., French, P.D., Johnson, A.M., and the Behavioural Intervention in Gay Men Project Study Group. (2001). A cognitive behavioural intervention to reduce sexually transmitted infections among gay men: randomised trial.*Brit Med J* 322:1451–1456.

International HIV/AIDS Alliance (2002). *Improving Access to HIV/AIDS-related Treatment: A Report Sharing Experiences and Lessons Learned on Improving Access to HIV/AIDS-related Treatment*. London.

International Collaboration on HIV Optimism (2003). HIV treatments optimism among gay men: an international perspective. *JAIDS* 32:545–550.

Kalichman, S., and Simbayi, L. (2003). HIV testing attitudes, AIDS stigmas, and voluntary HIV counseling and testing in the Western Cape, South Africa. *Sex Trans Inf* 79:442–447.

Kelly, J. A., Hoffman, R. G., Rompa, D., and Gray, M. (1998). Protease inhibitor combination therapies and perceptions of gay men regarding AIDS severity and the need to maintain safer sex. *AIDS* 12:F91–F95.

Kippax, S. & Kinder, P. (2002). Reflexive practice: The relationship between social research and health promotion in HIV prevention. Sex Education, 1, 91–109.

Kravcik, S., Victor, G., Houston, S., Sutherland, D., Garber, G. E., Hawley-Foss, N. Angel, J. B., and Cameron, D. W. (1998). Effect of antiretroviral therapy and viral load on the perceived risk of HIV transmission and the need for safer sexual practices. *J. Acquir. Immune. Defic. Syndr. Hum. Retrovirol.* 19:124–129.

Kumar M. (October 6, 2002) Bihar family boycotted after members die of AIDS <http://www.ndtv.com/>

Ledergerber, B., Egger, M., Opravil, M., Telenti, A., Hirschel, B., Battegay, M., Vernazza, P., Flepp, M., Furrer H., Francioli, P., and Weber, R. (1999). Clinical progression and virological failure on highly active antiretroviral therapy in HIV-1 patients: a prospective cohort study. Swiss HIV Cohort Study. *Lancet* 353:863–868.

Lee, R., Kochman, A., and Sikkema, K. (2002). Internalized Stigma Among People Living with HIV-AIDS. *AIDS Behav* 6: 309–319.

Morandi, P.A., Schockmel, G.A., Yerly, S., Burgisser, P., Erb, P., and Matter, L. (1998). Detection of human immunodeficiency virus type 1 (HIV-1) RNA in pools of sera negative for antibodies to HIV-1 and HIV-2. *J Clin Microbiol* 36:1534–1538.

Murphy, D. (2002). In a minority of gay men, sexual risk practice indicates strategic positioning for perceived risk reduction rather than unbridled sex. *AIDS Care* 14(4)471–480.

NCHECR: National Centre in HIV Epidemiology and Clinical Research (2003a). *Australian HIV Surveillance Report* July, 19(3).

NCHECR: National Centre in HIV Epidemiology and Clinical Research (2003b). HIV/AIDS, viral hepatitis and sexually transmissible infections in Australia Annual Surveillance Report 2003. Sydney: National Centre in HIV Epidemiology and Clinical Research, The University of New South Wales, Sydney, NSW.

Olley, B., Gxamza, F., Seedat, S, Theron, H., Taljaard, J., Reid, E., Reuter, H., and Stein, D. (2003). Psychopathology and coping in recently diagnosed HIV/AIDS patients—role of gender. *S Afr Med J* 93:928–931.

Parker, R. and Aggleton, P. (2003). HIV-AIDS-related stigma and discrimination: A conceptual framework and implications for action. *Soc Science Med* 57:13–24.

Rajendran, R., and Hariharan, S. (1995). Profile of intersex children in south India. *Indian Pediatr.* 32(6): 666–671.

Rawstorne, P., Fogarty, A., Crawford, J., Prestage, G., Grierson, J., and Kippax, S. (2004a). Esoteric sex practices and less education distinguish HIV-positive men who 'frequently' compared with 'occasionally' engage in risky UAIC acts. Abstract submitted to the XV International AIDS Conference in Bangkok.

Rawstorne, P., Hull, P., Van de Ven, P., Prestage, G., Crawford, J., and Kippax, S., (2004b). Taking HAART is associated with less sexual risk with casual partners. Abstract submitted to the XV International AIDS Conference in Bangkok.

Reid, D., Weatherburn, P., Hickson, F., and Stephens, M. (2002). *Know the score: findings from the national gay men's sex survey 2001 London.* Sigma Research, London.

Rosengarten, M., Race, K., and Kippax, S. (2000). Touch wood, everything will be okay: gay men's understanding of clinical markers in sexual practice. Monograph 7/2000, National Center in HIV Social Research. The University of New South Wales, Sydney, NSW.

Shisana, O. and Simbayi, L. (2002). *Nelson Mandela/HSRC Study of HIV/AIDS: South African National HIV Prevalence, Behavioral Risks and Mass Media, Household Survey 2002.* Human Sciences Research Council, Cape Town South Africa.

Stephenson, J. M., Imrie, J., Davis, M. M. D., Mercer, C., Black, S., Copas, A. J., Hart, G. J., Davidson, O. R., and Williams, I. G. (2003). Is use of antiretroviral therapy among homosexual men associated with increased risk of transmission of HIV infection? *Sex. Transm. Infect.* 79(1):7–10.

Sudhit, T. S. AP to make pre-marriage HIV tests mandatory, (October 3, 2002), http://www.ndtv.com/.

Sudre, P., Rickenbach, M., Taffe, P., Janin, P., Volkart, A. C., and Francioli, P. (2000). Clinical epidemiology and research on HIV infection in Switzerland: the Swiss HIV Cohort Study 1988–2000. *Schweiz.Med.Wochenschr*. 130:1493–1500.

Swiss Federal Office of Public Health. HIV and AIDS, National Program 1999–2003. Document 311.930.e. 1999. Berne, Switzerland.

UNAIDS, 2002a, <http://www.unaids.org/partnership/pdf/INDIAinserts.pdf>

UNAIDS, 2002b, Report on the Global HIV/AIDS Epidemic. Geneva: 2002 http://www.unaids.org/barcelona/presskit/barcelona%20report/table.html.

US National Intelligence Council, 2002, The Next Wave of HIV/AIDS: Nigeria, Ethiopia, Russia, India, and China. Report no. ICA 2002–04 D. Washington, DC, (September 2002); http://www.cia.gov/nic/pubs/other_products/ICA%20HIV-AIDS%20unclassified%20092302POSTGERBER.htm.

Van de Ven, P., Rawstorne, P., Crawford, J., and Kippax, S. (2001). Facts and Figures: 2000 Male Out Survey. Sydney: National Centre in HIV Social Research, NSW, The University of New South Wales, Sydney.

Van de Van, P., Rawstone, P., Treloar, C. and Pirchters, J. (2003). HIV/AIDS. Hepatitis C and related diseases in Australia: Annual Report of behavior. National Centre in HIV Social Research, The University of New South Wales, Sydney, NSW. Population Reference Bureau. 2002. World Population Data Sheet 2002. Washington, D.C. http://www.prb.org.

Wolf, K., Young, J., Rickenbach, M., Vernazza, P., Flepp, M., and Furrer, H. (2003). Prevalence of Unsafe Sexual Behavior among HIV-Infected Individuals: The Swiss HIV Cohort Study. *J Acquir Immune Defic Syndr* 33:494–499.

World Bank, India—Second National HIV/AIDS Control Project. Project Appraisal Document. Report no. 18918. Washington, D.C. (May 13, 1999); http://www-wds.worldbank.org/servlet/WDSServlet?pcont=detailsandeid=000094946_99060905302420.

Index

Advancing HIV Prevention initiative, 5, 60, 66, 193, 214
Adolescents, 8, 11, 72, 76–77, 80, 84–85, 92–93, 144, 163–167, 171, 173, 175, 177, 188, 197, 266
Africa, 40, 46, 50, 55, 58, 60, 137, 236–237, 245–246, 268–237
    Congo, 252
    South Africa, 236–237, 268–273
    Uganda, 252
    Zambia, 33, 50, 252
    Zimbabwe, 252
African Americans, 45, 65, 73, 78, 80–82, 84, 99, 117, 150, 163, 166, 196–199, 202, 212–214
AIDS Drug Assistance Program (ADAP), 205
AIDS Risk Reduction Model, 174, 188
Alcohol, 76, 87, 15, 124, 135, 148, 150, 152, 154, 174, 178–180, 219, 225, 229, 238, 273
Altruism, 147
Antiretroviral therapy, *see also* Highly active antiretroviral therapy, (HAART), 3–4, 10–11, 13, 20, 68, 87, 91, 101, 135, 137, 164, 167, 170, 197, 223, 227, 230, 236–237, 247, 253–255, 269, 274
    adherence, 3, 5, 12–13, 17, 20, 57, 135, 149, 152, 167, 169, 170, 174, 176–177, 197, 206, 225, 230–231
    drug resistance, 12, 20, 92, 100, 117
Asia, 137, 140, 245
    Burma, 146
    China, 140, 146
    India, 144, 146, 237, 263–268, 272, 274
    Thailand, 137, 140, 145–146
    Vietnam, 146
Australia, 74, 99, 245, 256–260, 262, 274

Bareback sex, 68, 102, 114–20, 127–128, 150
Bathhouses, 103, 105, 107, 109, 122, 127

Canada, 116
Case management, 10, 15–16, 183, 188, 194, 197, 199–201, 212, 230
Circuit parties, 119, 121, 123–125, 149, 154
Commercial sex, 102–108, 110–112, 119, 121–122, 127, 154
Community Promise Program, 212
Coping, 9, 15, 55, 76, 81, 113, 168, 170, 173, 179, 186, 196, 198, 208, 229, 230, 238, 272–273
Coping Effectiveness Training, 55
Couples, 32–33, 36–37, 43, 47–50, 56, 60, 66–67, 89–90, 104, 121, 265

Depression, 14, 154, 172–173, 184, 229, 234, 238, 264–265
Diffusion of innovations, 137, 147, 197, 211, 214
Disclosure of HIV, 14–17, 20, 34, 36, 55, 65–79, 80–82, 84–94, 101, 145, 153, 168, 170, 173, 186, 196, 200, 203–204, 209, 212, 223, 230, 252, 253, 261, 265, 273
    Disease Progression Theory, 70
    laws pertaining to disclosure, 67
    Self-Disclosure Theory, 69–70
Discrimination, 19–20, 67, 174, 204, 210, 265, 267–268
Drugs
    club drugs, 103, 110, 120–127, 136, 149–151, 154
    cocaine, 65, 121–123, 124–125, 135–136, 141–142, 149, 150
    ecstasy, (MDMA) 103, 111, 121–124, 127, 149
    GHB, 121, 123–125, 149
    heroin, 65, 139, 141
    ketamine, 121–125, 149
    marijuana, 110, 150, 174

Drugs (*cont.*)
  methamphetamine, 103, 111, 116, 121–128,
    136, 141, 149–150, 152, 176–177
  Viagra, 109, 111, 113, 124, 151

Europe, 46, 90, 99, 137, 139, 245, 270, 272
  Germany, 141
  Netherlands, 107, 112–113, 137, 139, 140,
    141
  Russia, 140
  Scotland, 145, 249
  Switzerland, 141, 253, 274
  Ukraine, 146
  United Kingdom, *see also Scotland*, 107,
    109–112, 246, 248

Family, 13, 18, 70, 145, 163–164, 167, 169, 173,
    181, 187, 205, 208, 265, 267
Female condom, 143

Gender power, 49, 66, 67, 71, 90, 224, 236

Harm reduction, 15, 100–101, 126, 128, 197,
    200, 203, 208
Health Belief Model, 173
Healthy Living Project, 51, 55, 60, 230
Healthy relationships, 14–15, 196–197, 202,
    212
Hemophilia, 16, 75–76, 167–168
Hepatitis, 100, 128, 136, 142, 148, 170
Highly active antiretroviral therapy
    (HAART), 4, 11, 13, 17, 19, 30–31, 50–51,
    59, 101, 139, 142, 143, 150–153, 164, 247,
    250–251, 259, 262–263
Hispanics, (see also Latinos) 72, 77, 136, 197,
    202
HIV testing, 30, 60, 260
  rapid test, 30, 107
  regular testing, 30, 58
Holistic Harm Reduction Program (HHRP),
    197, 203, 205, 208, 229, 232
Homelessness, 12–13, 165–166, 172, 176,
    210

Information-Motivation-Behavioral Skills
    Model, 174, 226–229, 232–234, 237,
    238
Injection drug users (IDU), 45–47, 136–139,
    141, 144–146, 148, 150–153, 165–166,
    232, 235, 263–264

Internet, 102, 104, 108–116, 119, 120, 127–128,
    154, 177, 183–184, 188, 246–247, 249–251
  chat rooms, 109–113, 119–120
Irrational beliefs, 117–118

Latinos, *see also* Hispanics, 34, 36, 38, 70, 82,
    99, 104–105, 109, 111, 120–121, 150, 163,
    166, 198, 212

MD 4 Life program, 231
Message framing, 91, 205, 222, 230–231
Meta-analysis, 29–30, 51, 146–147
Microbicides, 119, 120, 153
Motivational interviewing, 91, 119, 126, 128,
    154, 200, 231

Needle exchange, 87, 92, 118, 138, 140, 142,
    154, 194, 209, 232, 272
Negotiation, 67, 85, 89, 94, 108, 181, 229,
    232–233, 266
Networks, 138, 144–145, 175, 188, 201,
    211–212

Optimism, 101–102, 118, 150–151, 224–227
Options Project, 232–237
Outreach, 38, 94, 106–108, 113, 120, 138, 140,
    143–144, 153

Partner notification, 17, 67, 82, 113
Partnership for Health, 230–231
Peers, 13, 106, 119, 144–145, 148, 166–168,
    174–176, 195–196, 199, 205, 210, 224,
    230, 237
Prevention case management (PCM), 16,
    195, 199–201, 212
Protection Motivation Model, 59
Public sex environments, 87, 102, 104–108,
    110

Rational risk taking, 70, 117
Relapse, 114, 139, 172, 175–176, 178–180
Replicating effective programs, 194, 201,
    206, 210–211
Rural environments, 182, 203–207, 213–214,
    237, 265–266, 274

Self-efficacy, 13, 167–168, 174, 182, 187, 199,
    229, 231, 238, 264
Self-regulation, 179
Self-report, 57–58, 87

Sensation seeking, 123, 150, 154
Serosorting, 101, 105, 110–111, 115, 117, 125
Social Action Theory, 168–170
Social Cognitive Theory, 14, 56, 147, 173, 187
Social influence, 144–145
Social support, 13, 69, 71, 113, 147, 168, 170,
    173, 196, 230
South America
    Brazil, 144
Stages of Change (Transtheoretical Model),
    2, 59, 167–168, 174, 254, 266, 269
Stigma, 7–8, 10, 18–20, 57, 67–70, 88–89, 165,
    170–171, 173–174, 180, 182, 188,
    203–204, 206–207, 210, 224, 236, 265,
    267–269, 272–274
Strategic positioning, 91, 100, 117, 260, 262
Study to Reduce Intravenous Exposures
    (STRIVE), 148

Substance treatment, 8, 19–20, 125–126,
    138–143, 148, 153–154, 170, 177,
    180–181, 194, 197
    methadone, 15, 35, 42, 139–142, 148, 194,
    197, 231–232
    therapeutic workplace, 142
Support group, 4, 14, 195–196, 199, 253
Swiss Cohort Study, 254

Technology transfer, 204, 210–211
Teens Linked to Care, 164, 170–171, 177–178,
    182, 197–198
Theory of Reasoned Action, 70, 167–168,
    173
Theory of Planned Behavior, 173–174, 188

Uninformed protection, 68, 73, 74, 75, 84,
    93–94